Praise for *HEALTHCARE FOR CHILDRE*

MW01010579

"HEALTHCARE FOR CHILDREN ON THE AUTISM SPECTRUM could only have been written by physicians with extensive knowledge of current research and standards-of-care, who also possess a deep and compassionate understanding of the everyday experiences faced by families of their patients. In this wonderful book, Drs. Volkmar and Wiesner prove that they are all of this, and more. Their book will be essential reading for every parent and professional working in our field."

—Michael D. Powers, Psy.D.
Director, Center for Children with Special Needs
Tolland, Connecticut
Assistant Clinical Professor of Psychology
Yale Child Study Center

"Drs. Volkmar and Wiesner offer a superb contribution to the care of children with autism spectrum disorders (ASDs) and sound information for their families. From their extensive clinical and research experience they bring a balanced approach to assessment, routine healthcare, frequent health problems in daily living, and medical treatment of children with autism, Asperger's syndrome, and pervasive developmental disorder not otherwise specified (PDD-NOS). This is not a book about only infants and toddlers, but offers information addressing the future immediate healthcare needs of adolescents and adults with autism spectrum disorders. Their tips for treating children, such as how to approach a trip to the dentist or the hospital, and suggestions for where parents can go to learn more, are levelheaded and substantive. Theirs are not the reflections of distant observers, but borne of the authors' close-up experience caring for real children and families. This is a volume filled with sensible advice for parents who want to better understand their child with an ASD and to help their child attain optimal health."

—Kenneth E. Towbin, M.D.
Professor of Psychiatry and Behavioral Sciences and Pediatrics
The George Washington University School of Medicine

"The first of its kind, this comprehensive guide addresses the often-overlooked medical and healthcare needs of children on the autism spectrum.Clearly written in a user-friendly format, the wealth of invaluable information found between the covers of this book will assist parents in making well-informed decisions, thereby becoming better managers of their child's medical care. I am happy to recommend this book to both parents and professionals."

—Lori S. Shery, President and Co-founder, ASPEN® (Asperger Syndrome Education Network, Inc.)

Topics in Autism

Healthcare for Children on the Autism Spectrum

A Guide to Medical, Nutritional, and Behavioral Issues

Fred R. Volkmar, M.D. and
Lisa A. Wiesner, M.D.

Sandra L. Harris, Ph.D, *series editor*

Woodbine House ◆ 2004

All rights reserved under International and Pan-American copyright conventions. Published in the United States of America by Woodbine House, Inc., 6510 Bells Mill Road, Bethesda, MD 20817. 800-843-7323. www.woodbinehouse.com

Publisher's note: The information contained in this book is not intended as a substitute for consultation with your child's healthcare providers. Although the authors, editor, and publisher made every attempt to ensure that the information in this book was up-to-date and accurate at the time of publication, recommended treatments and drug therapies may change as new medical or scientific information becomes available. Additionally, the authors, editor, and publisher are not responsible for errors or omissions or for consequences from application of this book. Any practice described in this book should be applied by the reader in close consultation with a qualified physician.

Library of Congress Cataloging-in-Publication Data

Volkmar, Fred R.
    Healthcare for children on the autism spectrum : a guide to medical, nutritional, and behavioral issues / by Fred R. Volkmar and Lisa A. Wiesner ; foreword by Lorna Wing. –1st ed.
       p. cm. – (Topics in autism)
    Includes bibliographical references and index.
    ISBN 0-933149-97-2 (trade paperback)
    1. Autistic children—Medical care. 2. Autistic children—Health and hygiene. 3. Autistic children—Care. 4. Developmentally disabled children—Medical care. 5. Developmentally disabled children—Health and hygiene. 6. Developmentally disabled children—Care. 7. Child rearing. I. Wiesner, Lisa A. II. Title. III. Series.

RJ506.M4V656 2004
649'.154—dc22

                                                                                        2003022953

Manufactured in the United States of America

First Edition

10 9 8 7 6 5 4 3 2 1

To Lucy and Emily,
who have taught us about being parents,
and to the many children
who have taught us about being doctors

TABLE OF CONTENTS

In my dual role as a parent of a grown-up daughter with classic Kanner's autism and a professional in the field, it was a particular pleasure for me to read this book and write this foreword. When my daughter was a small child in the 1950s, there were no books on autism and certainly nothing written for parents. Now, many books on the subject written by and for parents have been published. However, Fred Volkmar and Lisa Wiesner's book is special because it focuses on the problems of healthcare in all its aspects—a subject little touched upon by other authors in the field. It tackles everyday health concerns well known to all parents bringing up children but which present particular difficulties for parents of children with autism spectrum disorders.

The authors give detailed explanations of the nature of autistic conditions and the complexities of diagnosis and classification. They provide clear descriptions of the medical conditions that parents of children with autism spectrum disorders may need to deal with. The discussions of relevant aspects of child development and the changes in adolescence provide an essential and interesting context in which to understand the healthcare and behavioral issues. The advice on managing the problems (and interacting with professional advisers) is eminently practical. The chapter on the pros and cons of psychotropic medications is particularly useful for those parents who are faced with their child's seemingly intractable challenging behaviour. Given the complexity of the subjects the authors are concerned with, it is remarkable that they do not talk down to parents and write with such clarity, avoiding jargon and explaining any technical terms they need to use.

The last chapter in the book discusses so-called complementary and alternative treatments. The authors do an excellent job of presenting the known facts in a calm, objective, and scientific way. They point out that many of these unorthodox therapies have never been independently evaluated and those that have been properly researched have failed to prove useful. At the same time, they show understanding and sympathy for parents' desperate desire to find a cure for their beloved child. Fred and Lisa tell the truth with compassion.

Fred has a long and distinguished career in research into autism. Lisa has many years clinical experience as a pediatrician and has a special interest in this field. Together they provide the unusual combination of detailed medical knowledge with in-depth experience of children with autism spectrum disorders. They are just as understanding of the problems and feelings of parents. They also have the essential quality of common sense.

It would have been invaluable to us as parents to have had this book when our daughter was a small child. I am happy now to be able to recommend it to other parents and caregivers. It should also be essential reading for medical and other professionals whose work brings them into contact with children and adults with autism spectrum disorders. Not only will it give professionals important information about healthcare in autism, it will also give them some insight into what it is like to bring up a child with this puzzling but fascinating developmental disorder.

PREFACE

Raising a child who is healthy is one of the most difficult—and rewarding—challenges any parent can tackle. For parents of children with autism and other pervasive developmental disorders (PDDs) the rewards are just as great as for any other parents. However, the challenges can be more daunting because parents have to take the child's difficulties into account in almost all decisions made about her health. For example, how will your child react to having her teeth cleaned and is it worth the trouble? Should your child receive regular immunizations? What about medications to deal with behavior problems? Given the expense and trouble, is it better to wait and see the doctor only when the child is ill?

Children normally experience a number of illnesses. The parents of typically developing children often are not informed of all the possible problems their child might have. However, if your child has autism or another pervasive developmental disorder, the doctor may be even more likely to tell you about conditions for which your child is at special risk. This is because the doctor wants you to collaborate with him or her in providing the best possible care for your child. Sometimes knowing ahead of time that their child is at risk for some conditions, such as seizures, makes parents more alert to warning signs or problems. Sometimes it's important to know that some medical problems can worsen your child's behavior or can further contribute to developmental delays. For example, recurrent ear infections and hearing loss may further contribute to difficulties in communication. In these cases, early detection and treatment is important. It is also important to be aware of some of the other risks that any child has in growing up, such as accidents and injuries. Children with developmental problems are at least as much at risk for accident and injury as are typically developing children—and probably even more so, since they may get themselves into more dangerous situations due to poor judgment or failure to appreciate consequences. Accordingly, it's important that parents be aware of their child's need for safety and a safe environment.

Parents are an integral part of healthcare for any child. This is especially true for children with special needs. As a parent, you have an important role in helping manage your child's medical care. This includes spotting problems early on as well as helping by asking the right questions and communicating with doctors and other healthcare providers so that you can make informed decisions about your child's medical care.

This book reviews some of the common medical problems you will encounter, as well as problem areas you should look out for. It includes advice about working with doctors and other healthcare professionals. In addition, it reviews some basic information about autism and related conditions and how these disorders are diagnosed. It also discusses medications that are sometimes used to treat the symptoms of autism and similar disorders. Some medical problems are actually more likely in autism or are especially important in terms of their implications for the child's development, and these are also discussed.

Keep in mind that in this book we are trying to provide you with some *general* information that will help you obtain quality medical care. This book can't (and won't) substitute for having a good working relationship with a healthcare professional who can advise you about what is best for your child in particular. The information provided in this book should supplement but does not replace the need for your child to have an ongoing relationship with a doctor, nurse practitioner, or other healthcare provider who knows her very well. Also bear in mind that although every effort has been made to ensure that the information provided here is accurate and up-to-date, knowledge changes over time. Some of the treatments that are of little or no interest now may be of more interest in the future. As time goes on, we should have increasingly good ways of detecting and treating autism and related conditions.

In the meantime, although we do not yet know the cause or causes of autism, there have been important advances in understanding the syndrome and in treating its symptoms. We know now that we can recognize some medical conditions early in life and reduce negative effects of these conditions on the child's development and behavior. In considering any medical treatment, it is always important to weigh the risk against the possible benefit of the medication. As the saying goes, "The perfect is sometimes the enemy of the good." That is, sometimes it is better not to strive for perfection but for reasonable care and quality of life. As discussed in this book, many new treatments for autism also periodically become available. Sometimes these are well evaluated scientifically. Unfortunately, much of the time they are not. In a later chapter in this book, we will review some of these treatments and discuss how parents can make informed decisions about using them.

In each chapter we include questions from parents and our answers. We hope that these are a helpful way for you to learn from the experience of others. Throughout the book, we also include some tables and boxes with additional information. The final sections of the book include a glossary, as well as a list of resources, websites, and other sources of good information. There is a list of readings for each of the chapters, as well as a more general reading list. In each case we comment, briefly, on what the reading has to offer. In some cases we have "flagged" reading that your doctor or healthcare provider may be interested in. In reading this, or any book, it is important to interpret the information with *your child* in mind. In this effort, your physician or other healthcare provider is an important ally.

We have written this book to provide parents with information that we hope will help them get the best possible care for their child. The two of us approach this from slightly different perspectives. One of us, Fred Volkmar, is a child psychiatrist whose main area of clinical work and research is in autism. The other, Lisa Wiesner, is a pediatrician who has seen children with autism and other disabilities in her pediatric practice. In addition to bringing our professional perspectives to the book, the two of us are married and parents of two children, and, as such, we've had our own experiences with obtaining quality medical care. We hope that this book will provide parents of children with autism practical and useful information as well as tips on how you can work with healthcare professionals to optimize your child's healthcare.

In doing a book of this kind, we were very sensitive to the problem of how best to refer to healthcare providers as well as children. By "healthcare provider," we mean a professional who can be in charge of your child's healthcare and work with you to ensure your child a healthy future. Healthcare providers are commonly physicians, with either medical degrees (MDs) or osteopathic degrees (DOs). They include individuals with special training in working with children (pediatricians) or in working with the health problems of families (family practitioners). In addition to physicians, there are a growing number of other health professionals who can provide day-to-day care for your child. These include nurse practitioners and physician's assistants, as well as many medical specialists. A variety of other individuals may be involved in providing some aspect of healthcare. When we refer to healthcare providers, we are referring to all these individuals.

You will see that within each chapter we consistently refer to the healthcare provider as either male or female, but we vary this across chapters. Similarly, and to prevent confusion, we refer to the child as either he or she—picking one or the other pronoun and sticking with it throughout the chapter. This is not ideal but, to our minds, is better than the unfortunate term "s/he" and also reflects the diversity of both healthcare and autism.

We are grateful to a number of our colleagues who have reviewed parts of this book in our efforts to make it helpful to parents. We have profited from their wisdom and comments. They include: Tom Anders, Darron Bacal, Phyllis Cohen, Ami Klin, Kathy Koenig, Amy Laurent, Susan Levy, Wendy Marans, Andres Martin, Laura Ment, Georgia Morgan, James Morgan, Nancy Moss, Douglas Muller, Rhea Paul, Michael Powers, Emily Rubin, Celine Saulnier, Larry Scahill, John Schowalter, Stephen Simonson, Lynn Simonson, Bill Tamborlane, Ken Towbin, and Joseph Zelson. We also are grateful to our editor, Susan Stokes, for her help in making this book as parent friendly as possible. Finally, we are grateful to our children—who have taught us much about child development—and, of course, to our patients and their families—who have taught us much about autism.

Fred Volkmar, MD
Lisa Wiesner, MD

1 | Autism and Related Conditions: An Overview

A lthough most educated people today have heard of autism, the recognition of autism as a disorder is actually a relatively recent one. The disorder was first described in 1943 but not "officially" recognized until 1980. Other conditions such as Asperger's disorder were "officially" recognized even more recently and grouped in the same category as autism. In this chapter we discuss these disorders and how our understanding of them has changed over the years. This background information is important for several reasons. One is that you may hear many different terms used to describe your child's difficulties. Secondly, because knowledge has changed over the years there are some misconceptions about autism that you may encounter (particularly among people who haven't kept up with the field). Also, these different conditions sometimes have different medical concerns associated with them, so understanding which disorder your child has will give you insight into which health-related concerns he may have.

Some Terms

The term *pervasive developmental disorder (PDD)* refers to the overarching group of conditions to which autism belongs. Thus, PDD is a term for the class of disorder. As the term implies, a pervasive developmental disorder is one that affects many areas of a child's development, especially social and communication skills. Within this class, several disorders are now officially recognized:

1. *autism*—also referred to as autistic disorder, infantile autism, or childhood autism,
2. *Rett's disorder*—also called Rett's syndrome,
3. *childhood disintegrative disorder (CDD)*—also sometimes referred to as Heller's syndrome or disintegrative "psychosis,"
4. *Asperger's disorder*—also called Asperger's syndrome and previously called autistic psychopathy or autistic personality disorder, and, finally,
5. *Pervasive Developmental Disorder Not Otherwise Specified (PDD-NOS)*— sometimes termed atypical PDD or atypical autism.

The terms PDD and PDD-NOS sometimes confuse parents. The term PDD technically refers to all these disorders—that is, to the entire group of conditions. The term PDD-NOS, on the other hand, is a specific diagnosis included within the PDD category. It refers to a condition where the child has some troubles suggestive of autism but these don't seem to fit the better defined diagnostic categories. In other words, PDD-NOS is essentially a term used for conditions that are suggestive of autism but "not quite" autism. See Figure 1-1 below for an illustration of how the different types of PDD are related.

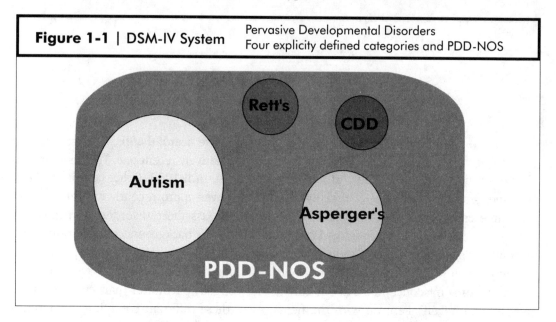

Figure 1-1 | DSM-IV System   Pervasive Developmental Disorders
Four explicitly defined categories and PDD-NOS

Although the term Autism Spectrum Disorder (ASD) is increasingly being used to mean the same thing as PDD, it is not an "official" term. That is, ASD means a disorder somewhere in the autism "ballpark." In this book, we use PDD and ASD interchangeably when we wish to refer to autistic disorders in general. We use the diagnostic categories listed above when we are discussing issues relevant to specific autistic disorders within the PDD category, such as autistic disorder or Asperger's disorder. The official guidelines for the diagnosis of each condition are included in Appendix A.

What is an "official" diagnosis? In the United States, it is most commonly one that is listed in the DSM – *The Diagnostic and Statistical Manual of Mental Disorders* of the American Psychiatric Association. It now exists in its fourth edition and is often called DSM-IV. The diagnoses in DSM-IV and the code numbers assigned to these diagnoses are used for many different purposes such as record keeping, public health information, and insurance reimbursement. As we'll discuss later in this book, these official systems are medical ones and sometimes schools and educators use different terms. Let us now review each of these diagnoses.

Autism

Leo Kanner and the First Description of Autism

The syndrome now known as autistic disorder, childhood autism, or infantile autism (all three names mean the same thing) was first described by Dr. Leo Kanner in 1943. Dr.

Kanner, the first child psychiatrist in the United States, reported on a group of eleven boys who appeared to exhibit what he called "an inborn disturbance of affective contact." By this he meant that, in contrast to typically developing babies, who find people to be the single most interesting things in the environment, these children came into the world without the usual interest in other people. He believed that the difficulty in dealing with the social world was congenital in nature. That is, the children were born with it.

Dr. Kanner gave a careful description of the unusual behaviors these boys exhibited. For example, he mentioned that these children exhibited "resistance to change" or "insistence on sameness." A child might require that his parents take the same route to school or church and become very upset if there was any deviation from this routine. He might panic if anything in his living room was out of place. He might be very rigid about what kinds of clothes he would wear or foods he would eat. The term "resistance to change" also came to include some other behaviors—for example, the purposeless motor behaviors (stereotypies) such as body rocking, toe walking, and hand flapping, often exhibited in autism.

Dr. Kanner mentioned that when language developed at all, the child's speech had unusual qualities. For example, the child with autism might fail to give the proper tone to his or her speech (that is, might speak like a robot) or might echo language (echolalia) or confuse personal pronouns (pronoun reversal). For example, when asked if he wanted a cookie, the child might respond, "Wanna cookie, wanna cookie, wanna cookie."

In his original report, Kanner thought there were two things essential for a diagnosis of autism: 1) the autism or social isolation, and 2) the unusual behaviors and insistence on sameness. As time went on, it has become clear that language-communication problems were also important. Including these problems along with the early onset of the condition that Kanner mentioned, we have what continue to be the four hallmarks of autism:

1. impaired social development of a type quite different from that in typically developing children (not just shyness or "nerdiness"),
2. impaired language and communication skills—again of a distinctive type (not just language delay, but very unusual communication development),
3. resistance to change or insistence on sameness, as reflected in inflexible adherence to routines, motor mannerisms, and stereotypies, and other behavioral oddities,
4. an onset in the first years of life before age three years.

Development and Behavior and Common Misconceptions

While Kanner's description remains a "classic," it was not, of course, the last word on the subject. Some aspects of his original report inadvertently served to mislead people for many years. For example, Kanner originally thought that children with autism probably had normal intelligence because they did rather well on some parts of intelligence (IQ) tests. On other parts, however, they did quite poorly or refused to cooperate at all. Kanner assumed that, if they did as well on all parts of the IQ test as they did on the one or two parts that they seemed to do well on, the child would not be mentally retarded.

Leo Kanner's First Description of Autism

The fundamental disorder is in the children's inability to relate themselves in the ordinary way to people and situations from the beginning of life. Their parents referred to them as having always been "self-sufficient"; "like in a shell"; "happiest when left alone"; "acting as if people weren't there"; "perfectly oblivious to everything about him"; "giving the impression of silent wisdom"; "failing to develop the usual amount of social awareness"; "acting almost as if hypnotized." This is not, as in schizophrenic children or adults, a departure from an initially present relationship; it is not a "withdrawal" from formerly existing participation. There is from the start an extreme autistic aloneness that, whenever possible, disregards, ignores, shuts out anything that comes into the child from outside.

The dread of change and incompleteness seems to be a major factor in the explanation of the monotonous repetitiousness and the resulting *limitation in the variety of spontaneous activity*. A situation, a performance, a sentence is not regarded as complete if it is not made up of exactly the same elements that were present at the time the child was first confronted with it. If the slightest ingredient is altered or removed the total situation is no longer the same and it is not accepted as such, or it is resented with impatience or even with a reaction of profound frustration.

From Leo Kanner (1943). "Autistic disturbances of affective contact." Nervous Child 2: 217-250.

Unfortunately, it turns out that cognitive or intellectual skills are often difficult to assess, in large part because they are very scattered. Put in another way, children with autism often do some things such as solving puzzles well but they may have tremendous difficulty with more language-related tasks. The degree of discrepancy or scatter between different skill areas is very uncommon in typically developing children, but very frequent in autism and related conditions. We now appreciate that many, perhaps as many as 70 percent or so, of children with autism function in the range of mental retardation when you combine all of their, sometimes quite different, scores.

On the other hand, the pattern of performance in autism is very unusual and quite different from what is usually seen in mental retardation without autism. Similarly, since the different abilities that go into estimating intelligence are often so different in autism, the use of a single score can be rather misleading. For example, sometimes a child with autism may have average or above average abilities when it comes to tasks that are not verbal, but very significant delays in verbal tasks. In such cases, which score is the right one? Both are, in some sense, but this means that you have to understand this and avoid using a single score to represent how the child functions. Sometimes schools or agencies will want to use a single overall score to describe the child's cognitive abilities, but in fact the single score may be very misleading.

Another source of confusion arose from Dr. Kanner's suggestion that autism was not associated with other medical conditions. We now know this is not true. For example, we

A Note about Terminology

In some countries, such as England, mental retardation is referred to as a learning disability. In the U.S., the term *learning disability* generally refers to a very specific problem in learning, such as in learning to spell or read. We use the term *mental retardation* in this book to refer to the combination of significantly subaverage intelligence (IQ) and impaired adaptive skills as defined in DSM-IV. We also occasionally use *intellectual disability* as a synonym for mental retardation, as this term is increasingly being used as an alternative to mental retardation in the U.S. We use the term *developmentally delayed* to refer to children, particularly young children, who seem to be at high risk for a later diagnosis of mental retardation.

now know that sometimes autism is seen with conditions such as fragile X syndrome or tuberous sclerosis (discussed in Chapter 3). In addition, children with autism frequently have seizures (see pages 13-14).

Dr. Kanner originally guessed that autism was a very distinctive condition and we now know that this is true. However, he chose to call the condition autism—a word which previously had been used to describe the unusual, self-centered, and self-contained thinking seen in major mental disorders such as schizophrenia. His use of the word autism suggested to many that perhaps autism was the earliest form of schizophrenia. It took many years for this to be clarified, but we now know that autism and schizophrenia are not related. Very occasionally, and no more than would be expected by chance, individuals with autism may, as adolescents or adults, develop an illness like schizophrenia. Autism differs from schizophrenia, however, in many different ways, including its clinical features, course, associated difficulties, and family history.

Finally, Kanner mentioned in his 1943 paper that in ten of the eleven families, the parent or parents were highly educated and successful. It also appeared that parents and children interacted somewhat unusually at times. This led to the idea, particularly in the 1950s, that some highly successful parents ignored or otherwise ill treated their children, causing autism. It is very clear that this is not true. Instead, it is clear that Kanner's original sample was a highly selected one. That is, in the 1940s, parents who were very educated and successful would be the most likely to find the one person in the country who was doing research on the kinds of problems their children had. It is also clear that unusual aspects of parent-child interaction are just as likely to come from the child as the parent. In addition, research has now begun to show that there is likely a genetic basis for autism.

Services for Children with Autism

Until the passage of the Education for All Handicapped Children Act in 1975, parents of children with autism often were at a loss as to how to educate them. Research began to suggest that structured educational programs were more effective than unstructured ones—that is, programs in which the adult had an agenda for teaching the child were better than if the child were left to his own devices to learn on his own. Before

1975, parents often were told by schools that there was no way their child could be educated. Often parents were advised to place their child in a residential or large state institution where the child got little in the way of intervention.

Now schools in the U.S. are mandated to provide a free and appropriate education for all individuals with disabilities. As programs have become increasingly sophisticated, schools have done an increasingly better job of providing education for children with autism. This means that schools often are now the major focus of intervention for children with autism.

Asperger's Disorder

In understanding Asperger's disorder, it is important to know where the concept came from in the first place, how it has been used over the years to refer to very different kinds of problems in children, and how it is used now. Hans Asperger was a medical student working at the University of Vienna during the Second World War. He had to write a paper on some aspect of research and he chose to write his paper on boys who had trouble forming groups. These boys had marked social problems, but their language and communication was, in some ways, very good. Asperger described them as being rather pedantic "little professors" who tended to intellectualize everything. Asperger also mentioned that they had unusual interests. For example, a child might know all the train or bus schedules into and out of Vienna.

These unusual and what are termed circumscribed (restricted) interests continue to be an important feature of the condition. They are unusual in that they are indeed highly circumscribed, but, more importantly, they interfere with other aspects of the child's life. In addition, Asperger mentioned that the boys were clumsy and awkward. He also mentioned that in several cases it appeared that other family members, particularly fathers, had similar kinds of problems. Asperger thought of the condition he described as something more like a personality trait, rather than a developmental disorder. He speculated that the condition was not usually recognized until after about age three.

Table 1-1 | Asperger's Disorder and Autism: Similarities and Differences

Symptom or Feature	Asperger's Disorder	Autism
Social Skills	Very impaired	Very impaired
Communication/language	A source of strength; talks early and often	A great weakness; speech delay
Motor abilities	Clumsy and poorly coordinated	Usually good early in life
Special interests	Very common; fact based	Not common; thing based
Recognition	Usually after age 3 years	Usually well before age 3

The name Asperger originally chose for the condition has been translated from the German either as "autistic psychopathy" or "autistic personality." That is, he used the word autistic in the same way that Leo Kanner, just a year before, had used the word autism. However, because of the war, neither Asperger nor Kanner knew of each other's work for some time. (Asperger used the word psychopathy because he also noted that these boys had difficulties being compliant and had some behavior problems.) In recent years, the practice has been to refer to this condition as Asperger's disorder or Asperger's syndrome (AS). Asperger, who lived for many years after describing this condition, saw many cases in his lifetime. And even until the end of his life, he felt that the condition was different from infantile autism.

Asperger's disorder received little recognition in English-speaking countries until the 1980s. Then Dr. Lorna Wing, a British psychiatrist and mother of a child with autism, wrote a paper on the disorder. She said that some aspects of Asperger's original report had to be modified. For example, she felt that AS could be seen in girls and in children with mild mental retardation. She also pointed out that the family histories could be more complicated than Asperger originally thought.

As time went on, several different views of Asperger's disorder came into being. Some people were confused about the relationship of Asperger's disorder and autism and wondered whether Asperger's disorder was just the same thing as "smarter" people with autism. Another set of investigators and clinicians equated the term with adults with autism. Yet another set of clinicians used the term Asperger's disorder interchangeably with the term Pervasive Developmental Disorder Not Otherwise Specified or atypical pervasive developmental disorder (this is a concept discussed subsequently in this chapter). Finally, some continued to use Asperger's disorder to refer to a specific set of symptoms which differed from autism in important ways. This is the only sense in which Asperger's disorder would merit a special category in a book such as DSM-IV.

Another set of problems came up because researchers outside the field of psychiatry also began to see very socially odd children who did not quite seem to have autism. A number of terms that had some degree of overlap with AS came into use. For example, some neurologists described something they called the right hemisphere learning disability syndrome; from within the speech/language literature came the concept of semantic-pragmatic processing disorder, and from the field of psychology came a profile of disabilities called the nonverbal learning disability syndrome. Within the field of psychiatry itself, there have been some attempts to describe children with problems similar to those described by Asperger, notably the notion of "schizoid personality," as described by Sula Wolf and her colleagues. It is perhaps not surprising, given all these factors, that there has been much controversy about Asperger's disorder.

As currently defined, Asperger's disorder shares some features with autism—most notably the social interaction problems—but early language and cognitive skills are relatively typical. In contrast to autism, the child's difficulties are not usually recognized for some years (often not until preschool) and usually the child has a very intense and all absorbing interest. In addition, children with AS often have a particular kind of learning disability—nonverbal learning disability—in which nonverbal skills can be quite impaired even when verbal skills are good. (See box on page 8.) Sometimes it is difficult to distinguish Asperger's disorder and high functioning autism. In both instances, however, an important point to highlight here is that the child's difficulties are not simply willful bad behavior but arise from a developmental problem. This is particularly important to recognize when a child has good verbal skills. Documenting the child's profile of strengths and weaknesses can be very helpful to schools.

One important treatment difference is that since children with Asperger's disorder have better verbal skills that children with more typical autism, we can sometimes use language-based treatments such as very structured and problem-oriented psychotherapy and counseling. If verbal skills are much better than nonverbal ones, we can also try to use this in teaching skills, such as social skills. In addition, if motor skills are not good, it is important to help the child learn to compensate for difficulties with fine motor demands (such as with handwriting).

Table 1-2 | Nonverbal Learning Disability (NLD)

A profile (pattern of strengths and weaknesses) on psychological testing. Both strengths AND weaknesses are present.

Strengths	Weaknesses
Auditory perception	Tactile perception
Rote verbal capacities (repeating things back)	Motor coordination
Verbal memory skills	Visual-spatial skills (e.g., solving geometric puzzles)
Verbal output	Nonverbal problem solving

- NLD impairs social skills.
- NLD is not an official diagnosis.
- NLD seems to be frequently associated with Asperger's disorder and PDD-NOS but *not* with autism, and is sometimes seen in other (non-PDD) conditions as well.
- There are important implications of the NLD profile for research.

Childhood Disintegrative Disorder

Childhood disintegrative disorder or CDD was first described almost one hundred years ago by a specialist in special education, Theodore Heller, who was working in Vienna. He noticed several children who had developed normally for some years and then had a marked and profound loss of skills. They seemed not to regain skills to previous levels. Originally, Heller termed this condition dementia infantilis. Subsequently, it was referred to as disintegrative psychosis or Heller's syndrome, but is now generally called childhood disintegrative disorder. (The term disintegrative psychosis captured the child's loss of skills, but the word psychosis implied some disconnect from reality which we no longer believe exists.)

This condition clearly is quite rare, although it's also probable that many children with the condition have not been adequately diagnosed or studied. Consistent with what Heller said in the first place, children with CDD develop normally for several years of life. Typically they talk and walk on time, acquire the capacity to speak in sentences, are normally socially related, and have achieved bladder and bowel control. Then, usually between the ages of three and four years, they experience a marked and enduring regression in skills. Many autistic-like behaviors develop, such as motor mannerisms (stereotypies) and a profound lack of interest in other people. We talk more about this condition in Chapter 15.

Table 1-3 | Childhood Disintegrative Disorder (CDD)

- First described by Theodore Heller in 1908
- Child has a period of normal development, usually three to four years, normal language, and self-care skills
- By definition the child has the capacity for speech
- Either rapid or more gradual regression occurs in multiple areas
- Child comes to exhibit many features of autism
- Sometimes a brain-based disorder is found which accounts for the regression
- Usually minimal recovery (outcome in general is worse than autism)
- Condition is rare but of much interest given potential for finding a specific cause

---

Rett's Disorder

In 1966, a Viennese physician, Andreas Rett, described a group of girls with an unusual history. They were apparently normal at birth and developed normally for the first months of life. However, usually within the first year or so, their head growth had begun to decrease in rate. In addition, they had started to lose developmental skills such as purposeful hand movements they had previously acquired. As the girls grew older, they lost more developmental skills and developed unusual hand-washing or hand-wringing stereotypies. In addition, the girls developed unusual respiratory symptoms such as breath-holding spells or air swallowing (aerophagia). Seizure disorders sometimes developed as well. Problems in walking and in posture were seen, and, over time, scoliosis (curvature of the spine) often developed. Often these children seemed to lose interest in other people—particularly in the preschool years—which is why there was the potential to misdiagnose the girls as having autism.

By adulthood, the girls had severe mental retardation. The degree of problems in breathing, in loss of hand movements and other motor difficulties, the problems of curvature of the spine, etc., suggested that this was a very distinct condition from autism. We discuss Rett's disorder in more detail in Chapter 15.

Table 1-4 | Rett's Disorder

- First described by Andreas Rett (1966)
- All cases were female in his original report (males have now been seen)
- Early development is normal
- Head growth slows (relative to rest of body)
- Purposeful hand movements are lost
- Some "autistic-like" features are present but tend to lessen over time
- Various associated problems are often present
    - Scoliosis (crooked spine) and movement problems
    - Unusual breathing patterns/breath-holding spells
- A gene has recently been identified that seems to be responsible for Rett's in at least some cases

Pervasive Developmental Disorder Not Otherwise Specified

Pervasive Developmental Disorder Not Otherwise Specified (PDD-NOS) is the so-called "subthreshold" pervasive developmental disorder. That is, this is the category that is used when a child, adolescent, or adult exhibits some features of a pervasive developmental disorder but does not meet all the guidelines for a diagnosis of one of the very specifically defined PDDs. This diagnosis is problematic because it is up to a clinician's judgment whether to use it or not. Probably not surprisingly, given the essentially "non-definition" definition, the term is used very inconsistently. Furthermore, the nature of this definition means that it's hard for researchers to get funding to study PDD-NOS. Somewhat paradoxically, this condition is almost certainly several times more common than autism, affecting perhaps one in several hundred children.

Although research on PDD-NOS is relatively sparse, some studies have appeared in recent years. Moreover, clinicians often have more experience treating and diagnosing PDD-NOS because it seems to be more common than strictly defined autism. Children with PDD-NOS have problems in social interaction but these are not as severe and pervasive as those in autism. For example, they may have problems in initiating conversation, in playing with other children, and in relating to parents or siblings. Unusual sensitivities are relatively common, although again usually not as severe as in autism. The term PDD-NOS is sometimes also used for children with very severe mental retardation, who often have some features of autism, particularly stereotyped motor movements. Except in these children with significant mental retardation, the outcome in PDD-NOS generally appears to be better than in most, if not all of, the other pervasive developmental disorders.

For a diagnosis of Pervasive Developmental Disorder Not Otherwise Specified to be made, the child should exhibit some problem in social interaction of the type usually seen in autism or other PDDs and at some problem either in language and communication skills *or* in unusual behavioral responses to the environment and restricted interests. A single symptom of autism is, by itself, not sufficient for a diagnosis of PDD-NOS; rather there have to be troubles both in the social area and either the language-communication or unusual behaviors category.

In practice, the diagnosis of PDD-NOS is used in several rather different situations:

1. It may be used for very young children who have some, but not all of, the features of autism. For example, at age thirty months a child may have marked social and communicative difficulties but not exhibit the unusual behaviors usually associated with autism. This child might be given a diagnosis of PDD-NOS. If he then went on to develop unusual mannerisms or movements or other unusual responses to the environment, the diagnosis of autistic disorder would be made.

2. Occasionally the term is used rather loosely. For example, someone may talk to you about "PDD" or "mild autism" when they mean PDD-NOS. In such situations, it is important to explicitly ask what is meant. Keep in mind that it is perfectly appropriate for a clinician to say that she doesn't know all the answers—what is important is that she realizes when she doesn't know!

Table 1-5 | PDD-NOS

- By definition the definition is a "negative" one (children who do not meet criteria for autism, Asperger's, etc.)
- The child must have problems in the social area of the type seen in autism and at least in one other area (communication, unusual behaviors)
- The relationship of PDD-NOS to autism remains unclear
- There may be several subtypes of PDD-NOS

How Common Are Autism and Related Conditions?

The first studies of the frequency or epidemiology of autism were conducted in the 1960s. Since that time, about thirty studies have been conducted—mostly in Great Britain and countries other than the United States. Given what we know about autism, there is no reason to suppose that the frequency of autism is vastly different here, although there has been concern, as we'll discuss in a moment, that the frequency of autism may be increasing in this country.

The various studies around the world have involved several million children. Estimates of the rate of autism vary somewhat from study to study because of the different methods used as well as the differences in diagnosis used over the years. If you lump all the studies together, a reasonable estimate of the rate is probably around 1 case of autism per 1,000 children.

Information on the frequency of other disorders on the autism spectrum is not nearly as good as that for autism. Both Rett's disorder and childhood disintegrative disorder are clearly much less common than autism. For Asperger's disorder, estimates have ranged from 1 in 500 children to 1 in 10,000. (The stricter the definition used for Asperger's disorder, the less common it appears to be.) PDD-NOS is almost certainly the most common form of pervasive developmental disorder. Some have estimated the frequency of PDD-NOS as high as one in several hundred, but again solid research data are lacking. Clearly at least one child in several hundred has some form of serious social disability consistent with autism or a related condition. This means that these conditions are a major public health problem.

Sex Differences in Autism and Related Disorders

It is clear that autism appears to be at least three to five times more frequent in boys than in girls. On the other hand, when girls have autism, they are more likely to also have mental retardation. We do not yet understand the basis for these differences. One theory is that perhaps on a genetic basis, girls are generally somewhat less vulnerable to autism (hence the greater frequency in boys), and that for girls to have autism, they must have greater genetic or central nervous system damage (hence the higher rate of mental retardation in girls). There is a male predominance in Asperger's disorder as well, but there does not appear to be such marked sex difference in PDD-NOS.

Is the Frequency of Autism Increasing?

The short answer is that we don't really know for sure. True, schools and departments of education have seen increased numbers of children qualifying for special services due to a diagnosis of autism. Centers that specialize in diagnosis and assessment of autism often now have long waiting lists. There is not much question that we are seeing more children who have been *diagnosed* with an autism spectrum disorder. It is not clear, though, whether these numbers represent an increase in the number of children who *have* autism.

Current approaches to diagnosis were specifically designed to diagnose children across the range of ages and developmental levels, whereas earlier systems tended to under-diagnose autism in more able children. Another issue is that public awareness of autism has vastly increased. (Twenty years ago when we talked to people about how we were interested in autism they might tell us how interesting it was to study *artistic* children! Now we get calls from day care providers worrying that a child might have autism.) A further complicating issue is that labels used for educational purposes may be more aimed at getting services than accurately pinpointing a child's diagnosis. Many educators understandably (from the point of view of giving services) lump autism and all related disorders together—this means that some of the "data" cited as indicating an increase in autism is really about the broader spectrum of autism and related conditions. Often when you hear about the "explosion of autism," you are really hearing about this.

Another problem is that methods of diagnosis have changed over time and there has been a real (and in many ways successful) effort to expand the awareness of teachers, healthcare professionals, day care providers, and others about autism. That is, part of the apparent increase may be due to the diagnosis of cases that were already there but had been overlooked. Finally, the lack of good epidemiological data on autism—particularly in the United States—makes it very difficult to answer the question in a way we could feel confident in. All this being said, it is concerning that estimates of autism around the world seem to have increased over time. It remains to be seen how much of this is a "real" increase, however.

What Causes Autism and Similar Disorders?

As we mentioned earlier, Kanner's first paper on autism was very influential—in both good and bad ways. The good ways had to do with the unusually clear way he described what he saw in autism (problems in social interaction and unusual responses to the environment). He also was clear in suggesting that autism was congenital—that is, that children were born with it.

On the other hand, the bad things about Kanner's description included some of his speculations or guesses. For example, he speculated that autism was not associated with mental retardation or other medical conditions. In addition, some aspects of his report misled other people—for instance, into thinking parents of children with autism might somehow cause the disorder. Kanner's early (and mistaken) notion that autism was more common in families where parents were more successful indirectly contributed to a very unfortunate development in the 1950s—that is, blaming the parent (usually the mother) for the child's troubles.

Beginning in the 1960s, and particularly in the 1970s, research began to show that autism was a brain-based disorder. Some clues that autism is brain based:

1. The prevalence of seizures: As children with autism were followed over time, it was clear that many of them went on to develop seizures.
2. The prevalence of neurological problems: Many children with autism exhibit unusual features on neurological examination such as persistent "primitive" reflexes (which are present at birth but typically disappear in children after a few months).
3. The high rate of prematurity or other birth problems: Some studies have reported that children with autism are more likely to have had complications during the pregnancy or birth.
4. The association of autism with a number of medical conditions that are known to affect brain development (see graph on page 14).
5. Increasing evidence that there is a genetic basis to autism: Studies have shown that if one identical twin has autism, the other is also likely to, and also that cognitive, language, and learning problems are common in siblings.

Seizure Disorders and EEG Abnormalities

Seizure disorders (also referred to as epilepsy or as convulsions) are a group of conditions which result from abnormal electrical activity in the brain. The symptoms of seizure disorders are quite varied. They can range from brief episodes in which the child seems to "tune out," to much more obvious convulsions in which the child falls to the ground, loses consciousness, and has alternating periods of muscle contraction and relaxation. There are many different kinds of epilepsy (see Chapter 9).

One of the ways doctors look for seizure activity is through the electroencephalogram (EEG), which measures electrical activity in the brain. Both early and more recent studies suggest that as many as 50 percent of individuals with autism have abnormalities in their EEG. There is no one EEG abnormality specific to autism, but the higher rates of abnormality suggest some basic problem with the way the brain is "wired." Even more dramatic are the rates of seizure disorder in autism, which some studies have put as high as 25 percent. In the "normal" population of children, rates of first seizure are highest around the time of birth and then greatly decrease over time. This is not the case in children with autism. Figure 1-2 presents information from two studies of children with autism or autism and PDD-NOS, as well as data from a large sample of typically developing British children. Compared to typically developing children, there are high rates for first seizures in children with autism at all ages, but especially between the ages of eleven and eighteen.

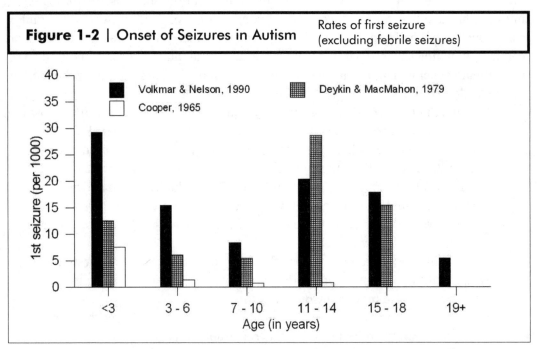

Figure 1-2 Rates of first seizure in two samples of individuals with autism (Volkmar & Nelson, Deykin & MacMahon) and a normal British sample (Cooper).

Other Neurological Problems

A number of other neurological problems are observed in autism. Again, these are of many different types. Not every child has every sign and some children will have none. Some children with autism have delays in the development of such skills as hand dominance (they may draw with either hand without having a preference for right or left). They can also have general decreases in muscle tone in the body and be somewhat "floppy" as babies (technically, this is called hypotonia).

Sometimes individuals with autism have unusual reflexes. Often these are reflexes that are usually seen only in very young babies but can persist into adulthood in individuals with autism. For example, if the doctor brings her reflex hammer towards a newborn's mouth, she may start to suck—as if anticipating the bottle or breast. This "visual rooting reflex" is sometimes seen even in adults with autism, whereas in most of us it disappears very early in childhood. Other neurologically based problems may be seen in the way that individuals with autism walk or with their posture.

Neuroanatomy and Brain Imaging Studies

Various methods can be used to study the brain. These range from actual studies of brain tissues obtained at the time of death (post mortem studies) to studies of the living and active brain through functional magnetic resonance imaging (fMRI). A number of findings support the idea that autism is a brain-based disorder.

Both autopsy and brain imaging studies have suggested that at least some individuals with autism have increased brain size. Several studies have suggested the possibility that there are some alterations in brain structure—particularly in those parts of the brain that process more emotional or social information (the limbic system) and possibly in the cerebellum. The cerebellum is the part of the brain that, among other things, helps coordinate and control movement. One investigator has, in particular, noted specific changes in the cerebellum in individuals with autism, but other investigators have generally not been able to find this.

In the last several years, several interesting findings have emerged from studies of MRI studies. A paper from our (Yale) group documented that children with autism and Asperger's disorder seemed to process the information in faces differently in the brain (Klin et al., 2002). Basically, they used the object-processing areas, whereas most of us use a very specialized face-processing center in the brain. Another possibly related finding is that higher functioning individuals with autism tend to look at mouths— rather than eyes and the upper parts of the face—when watching very intense social interactions. (Typically developing people focus on the eyes.) This may be because higher functioning people are using different brain mechanisms to process social information. (See Reading List.)

Neurochemistry

Nerve cells use different kinds of chemicals, or neurotransmitters, to communicate with each other. Some studies suggest that there may be alterations in these brain chemicals in individuals with autism. Probably the most work has centered on the chemical serotonin (also sometimes referred to as 5-HT or 5-Hydroxytryptamine). A number of studies have shown that levels of serotonin in the blood are often increased in individuals with autism. Unfortunately, the relationship between blood levels and brain levels of this chemical is not always clear. Other studies have focused on the chemical dopamine. This chemical is involved in parts of the brain that control movement and is part of a broader system which relates to levels of arousal. These differences in neurotransmitter levels may not be the *cause* of autism, but more likely may be the symptoms of some overall problem in the brain. Many of the drugs used to treat symptoms of autism affect these chemicals (see Chapter 13).

Table 1-6 | Neurochemistry of Autism

Neurotransmitter	Function Relevance to Autism
Serotonin	Regulates sleep, mood, body temperature High levels in blood of many individuals with autism Affected by some medications
Dopamine	Control of motor functions One class of medicines used in autism (neuroleptics) blocks dopamine function
Norepinephrine	Involved in arousal, stress response, memory, and anxiety, affected by some medications

---

Risks During Pregnancy and Childbirth

Could autism be caused by problems during pregnancy, labor, and delivery? A number of studies have looked at this question. Generally they have employed some rating scale that looks at the degree of risk during the pregnancy and/or during labor and delivery. Early studies seemed to show that there was an increased risk of autism based on the use of these rating scales. Factors that seemed to be associated with increased risk for autism included older age in the mother, prematurity, and some other problems during labor and delivery.

Several studies have also suggested that doctors or nurses may be more likely to notice something wrong—even if it is very minor—with newborns who eventually go on to be diagnosed with autism. This suggests an important point and a major problem in understanding whether problems during pregnancy or during labor and delivery might cause autism. This problem is that it would be just as reasonable to assume that if there were something wrong with the child from the moment of conception, it would be picked up at birth. Put in another way, we might be seeing problems at birth which may result from some vulnerability in the child. Thus, it would be just as reasonable to assume that problems in the child cause difficulties in the pregnancy as it would be to assume the reverse. The growing body of work on genetic factors in autism, which is discussed shortly, would be most consistent with this idea. At the same time, it is reasonably clear that horrendous difficulties during labor and delivery, particularly when associated with severe fetal distress, won't help any child—and have the potential to cause further trouble for a child who was going to have autism.

Medical Conditions and Autism

It took many years before people considered the possibility that autism could be associated with some medical conditions such as seizures. As knowledge about autism grew, it came to be associated with a number of other medical conditions and some people began to wonder whether perhaps some of these conditions caused autism. However, much of this work was based on what we call case reports—that is, from a doctor sending a letter or a short paper to a professional journal and reporting that he or she had observed that autism is associated with _____ syndrome (you can fill in the blank with essentially any known medical condition).

Case reports have some value, but also have many limitations since there is a bias for only positive reports to be published (this is really similar to the situation with the regular media!). The issue is not whether you ever see autism and condition X but whether in larger groups of individuals, the frequency of condition X is significantly greater in autism than you would expect, given how common condition X is in the general population. Another problem relates to the diagnosis of autism in the first place. Some researchers take a very broad view of autism; others a more narrow one. If you take a broad view, you will naturally tend to have higher estimates of the rate of autism. You also will tend to have an impression that rates of autism are more likely associated with other medical conditions. This comes about because when you use a broader definition of autism, you tend to make more diagnoses of autism in people with severe and profound mental retardation. In this group of people, about half the time you find an associated medical condition, and thus you are much more likely to conclude that various medical conditions are associated with autism.

If you look at the published research on medical conditions associated with autism, two rather different views emerge. If you take a very broad view of autism, perhaps one-third of people with autism might have some other condition in addition to autism, but if you take a narrow one, probably only 10 percent of people do.

Various conditions have been identified as possibly being associated with autism. These have included disorders such as phenylketonuria, congenital rubella, tuberous sclerosis, and fragile X syndrome. However, careful research has often caused us to rethink how strong these relationships are, and at present, the strongest associations are with fragile X and tuberous sclerosis.

Fragile X Syndrome

Fragile X is one of the more common causes of mental retardation, perhaps affecting 1 in 800 to 1,000 children. This condition particularly affects boys and has sometimes been associated with autism. Fragile X syndrome is called "fragile X" because the X chromosome in those who have it was noted to sometimes break or be "fragile" when examined under the microscope. The X chromosome is one of the so-called sex chromosomes that determines an individual's gender. Boys have an X chromosome (from their mothers) and a Y chromosome (from their fathers), while girls have two X chromosomes. Because boys have only one X chromosome, they are more likely to have the disorder (that is, there is no extra X to make up the difference). In girls (who have two X chromosomes), the disorder may be expressed in a somewhat milder form.

In fragile X syndrome, motor, attentional, and learning problems are very common and individuals may show varying degrees of social difficulty ranging from shyness to social withdrawal and avoidance and gaze aversion.

Early reports suggested a very strong association between autism and fragile X syndrome, with claims that as many as 60 percent of individuals with fragile X syndrome had autism. There was much optimism that a genetic cause of autism had been found. However, subsequent (and better) studies have suggested that the association between fragile X syndrome and autism is not nearly as strong as it first appeared. More recent work indicates that:

1. individuals with fragile X often have difficulties with social interaction,
2. perhaps 4 percent or so of individuals with autism have fragile X, and
3. about 1-2 percent of children with fragile X have strictly defined autism.

Thus, although it remains important to consider testing for fragile X, the rate of the condition in autism is relatively small and accounts for only a very small subgroup of children with autism.

At present, the main impact of diagnosing fragile X relates to the implications for genetic counseling of parents and sisters of affected individuals. That is, the treatment of children with autism who have fragile X is no different than for children with autism who do not have fragile X. However, for parents who know that they have a risk for subsequent children with fragile X, prenatal testing is available. In addition, it is important to remember that other children in the family may also have fragile X and that your daughters might be carriers, so that their children might be at potential risk.

In the past, the diagnosis of fragile X syndrome was made on the basis of an actual examination of the child's chromosomes—obtained through a blood sample and grown in a laboratory. This time-consuming and costly procedure has now been replaced in many centers by a more direct DNA test done on the blood, as the gene which causes fragile X has now been identified. A form of the test can also be used for prenatal diagnosis, early in the pregnancy.

Table 1-7 | Fragile X Syndrome

- Symptoms: social anxiety, "autistic like" symptoms, mental retardation or learning disabilities, and sometimes autism
- A small proportion (2-4%) of individuals with autism have fragile X
- A simple blood test can be used to determine whether fragile X is present
- The syndrome can be seen in boys and girls
- The genetic basis of this condition has been well described

Tuberous Sclerosis

This rather rare disease (1 in 10,000 people) has been noted to be significantly associated with autism. It is seen equally as frequently in boys and in girls. Symptoms of tuberous sclerosis include the growth of unusual tissue or benign tumors in the skin, eye, brain, and other organs. Over half of infants with the disorder will have white patches on their skin at birth. The tubers in the brain can be detected by computerized tomography (CT) or magnetic resonance imaging (MRI) scan. These growths are "benign" in the sense that unlike cancer they do not spread, but their effect on growth and development can be very serious.

The disorder is inherited as what is called an autosomal dominant trait. Autosomal means that it is on one of the "autosomes" (that is, on one of the twenty-two chromosomes other than the sex chromosomes), and dominant means that if you get one copy of this gene from either parent you are likely to have the disorder. Genes involved in causing the disorder have now been found.

The degree of severity in tuberous sclerosis is quite variable. Individuals with this condition often have developmental delay, speech delays, motor problems, and mental retardation (50 to 60 percent of the time), and seizures (about 80 percent of the time). Some individuals seem to be much less severely affected. It seems likely that this happens in some special circumstances—for example, as a result of spontaneous genetic change not inherited from the parents.

Interestingly, early reports on tuberous sclerosis which appeared in the 1930s described some problems suggestive of autism (which was not described until the 1940s!). These problems included stereotyped movement, abnormal speech, and social problems. Hyperactivity, aggression, and other behavior difficulties have also been reported.

Studies of individuals with autism show that a small number—probably under 1 percent—may also have tuberous sclerosis. This figure is higher if only individuals with autism and seizures are included. About 8 to 12 percent of these people may have tuberous sclerosis. If you look at the problem the other way around, roughly one-third of children with tuberous sclerosis have autism. The sex ratio of boys to girls in autism associated with tuberous sclerosis is about the same (boys and girls are equally likely); this is in contrast to autism in general, where the rate of autism is several times higher in boys than in girls. Studies of the small subgroup of children with tuberous sclerosis who do not have mental retardation suggest that they may not have an increased rate of autism or similar problems, but the final answers are not yet in. Promising work on the genetic causes of tuberous sclerosis is now underway.

Disorders of Metabolism: Phenylketonuria (PKU)

The relationship of autism to medical disorders of metabolism is somewhat complicated and controversial. One of the major problems in trying to sort out whether there truly is a relationship is that much research takes a very broad view of autism. Sometimes children who have severe mental retardation and some autistic-like behaviors are diagnosed with autism, when, according to a strict definition of autism, they really do not satisfy the diagnostic criteria. This is a particular problem because many of the disorders of metabolism, if untreated, result in very severe mental retardation where the diagnosis of autism can be complicated.

Some of these metabolic disorders are congenital and may be apparent at birth. In other cases, the condition may not be apparent for months or years. Of these disorders, PKU has probably received the most attention.

PKU (phenylketonuria) is caused by a problem in the body's use of the amino acid phenylalanine. As a result, levels of this amino acid build up in the body and eventually are excreted in the urine. This disorder is rather rare, affecting about 1 in 10,000 babies.

If it is not treated, PKU can cause severe mental retardation, growth problems, and seizures. Although the baby may otherwise appear normal at birth, symptoms gradually develop, including problems in feeding and development. Fortunately, the condition can be treated with a special diet which eliminates phenylalanine. This dietary treatment is one of a handful of dietary treatments medically proven to have a major role in preventing/treating developmental problems. PKU is now screened for at birth and two weeks of age in this country, since with prompt treatment children with PKU have normal and productive lives.

Early papers suggested that untreated PKU was a risk factor for autism. However, more recent research has questioned this view. Better controlled studies do not seem to suggest that there are higher than expected rates of PKU or other disorders of metabolism in autism. It seems likely that early reports of such associations probably equated "autistic features" (usually meaning stereotyped, self-stimulatory behaviors) with autism. It is still appropriate to consider screening children with severe developmental difficulties for inborn errors of metabolism, but there is not a clear relationship of these disorders to autism.

Congenital Infections

There have been some reports that autism is associated with infections either before or at the time of birth or shortly thereafter. These associations have been claimed for a wide variety of infections, including congenital rubella, cytomegalovirus, herpes simplex, and HIV (the AIDS virus). A few papers have also reported that there might be some association of autism with the time of year when children are born, suggesting that it might be caused by infections more common at certain times of year. However, other studies have not seen such associations. The infection that has probably drawn the most attention as a possible cause of autism is congenital rubella.

Congenital rubella occurs when a baby still in its mother's womb is infected with the rubella (German measles) virus. Woman who have not had rubella or who have not had the immunization for it are at very high risk for having a baby with congenital rubella if they are exposed to someone with the disease during pregnancy. The risk is greatest during the first eight weeks or so of the pregnancy (a time when women may not realize they are pregnant).

The virus often does severe damage to the developing baby. The baby may be born with problems in the heart, eyes, and ears. The head may be small and there may problems with other systems of the body. Deafness and blindness are relatively common, as are mental retardation and various behavior problems. While a few children do not have symptoms, most do.

Greater awareness of the seriousness of congenital rubella and the development of a vaccine have fortunately reduced the frequency of this condition. The vaccination of young children has been very helpful in this effort (one of the reasons why children are immunized against rubella).

Early reports on congenital rubella suggested that these children often seemed to have autism. However, as with other conditions, the presence of "autistic-like" features was taken as suggestive of autism. Remember, these children were often deaf or had impaired vision and severe learning difficulties. Follow-up studies have shown that, over time, the social and other problems of these children improve in ways that would not be typical of autism.

Does Genetics Play a Role in Autism?

In 1977, a study suggested that rates of autism in identical (or "monozygotic") twins were much higher than rates in same-sex fraternal (or "dizygotic") twins (Folstein and Rutter). (Same-sex fraternal twin pairs were studied, given the observation that autism is more likely in boys but more severe in girls when girls have it; identical twins are always of the same sex.) Since identical twins have exactly the same genes, while fraternal twins share some genes but no more than any siblings, the implication of this finding was that there was potentially a very strong genetic contribution in autism. A number of studies have now shown that this is the case.

As scientists began to look into the issue of genetics of autism, it became apparent that rates of autism were increased in the brothers and sisters of children with autism. Rates reported vary between a 1 in 10 and 1 in 50 chance that siblings of a child with autism will also have autism. This may not seem like a very high rate unless you compare it with the overall rate of autism, which is between 1 in 1000 and 1 in 2000. Although by no means common in siblings of children with autism, the rate is clearly increased— about 50- to 100-fold relative to the general population.

Even when siblings do not have autism, studies have found that there seems to be an increased risk for other problems—including language and learning difficulties. Recent research also suggests that there may be higher rates of mood and anxiety problems in family members, and, perhaps, more social difficulties. It was, and still is, not exactly clear what is inherited in autism. It is possible that what is inherited is a more general predisposition to difficulties rather than to autism as such.

Although research has increasingly highlighted the importance of genetic factors in autism, final answers are not yet in. The role of genetics in autism is not straightforward or simple, and it seems likely that multiple genes are involved. To make life complicated, all forms of autism may not have the same (or any) genetic basis but might come about through other ways. For example, there might be a specific problem at the moment of conception

---

Table 1-8 | Genetics of Autism

- Role for genetic factors suggested by:
  - higher rates in identical twins
  - increased risk for autism in siblings (between 2 and 10%)
- Genetic mechanism: Multiple genes seem to be involved
- Research has suggested promising leads for genes on several chromosomes
- It is likely that specific genes will be found in the next several years

when some genetic material might be lost or a genetic change (mutation) might occur. There is also a suggestion that some of a child's broad experiences (for example, early birth difficulties) might interact with genetic predisposition to cause autism.

Major efforts are now underway to identify potential genes in autism. It seems possible, and even likely, that some genetic cause (or causes) of autism will be identified over the next few years.

Environmental Causes of Autism

Can the environment cause autism? Currently, there is much interest in this idea, due to reports of "clusters" of cases and the possibility that immunizations or exposure to mercury in vaccines might "cause" autism. However, the evidence for environmental factors is very weak. We discuss the issue of vaccinations in Chapter 3 and review the evidence, which has not really shown a clear connection. This issue comes up particularly with regression in autism/ASD (see Chapter 15).

Reports of clusters of cases are very difficult to interpret since people (and the media) will pay a lot of attention to Town A, which may have an "outbreak" of autism, while Town B, the adjacent town, has no cases! Recent reports of an "upsurge" in autism are also difficult to understand. One possible explanation may be that we've done a good job of educating parents and professionals to look for autism and perhaps now we are just seeing "new" cases that were already there! Also, we now do a much better job of identifying individuals with autism or Asperger's disorder who are higher functioning, and it is likely that many of these diagnoses were missed in the past.

Understanding the Causes of PDDs Other than Autism

Our understanding of the causes of PDDs other than autism is not generally as far advanced as in autism—with the major exception of Rett's disorder (discussed in Chapter 15). We do, however, understand that all of the autism spectrum disorders have a basis in problems in the brain. This is suggested by such things as rates of seizure disorder, and, occasionally, other abnormalities as well.

Childhood Disintegrative Disorder

For many years, doctors presumed that some specific medical process could always be identified to explain why some children developed normally for several years and then had a major deterioration. It is clear now that this is the exception rather than the rule. Occasionally such a process is identified in an individual child, similar, in some ways, to the "dementias" of adults (like Alzheimer's disease, where there is progressive loss of functioning). However, in childhood disintegrative disorder, behavior and developmental skills usually deteriorate and then stay at the same, relatively low level. This kind of "plateau" is not usually observed when a progressive medical condition is present.

As in autism, the involvement of the brain is suggested by the high rates of EEG abnormality and seizure disorder. Information on brain structure and functioning is very limited, although research on this aspect of CDD is now underway.

Asperger's Disorder

There have been several reports of brain abnormalities associated with Asperger's disorder, but these are mostly based on reports of single cases rather than group studies. One interesting finding has been that Asperger's is frequently associated with nonverbal learning disability. This association with difficulties in nonverbal thought processes has been taken by some to suggest difficulties in the right part of the brain. (This is in contrast to autism, where the presence of language problems has often been taken to suggest problems in the left part of the brain.)

Although research on the issue of genetic contributions in Asperger's disorder is not as well advanced as in autism, there is already some evidence for a strong genetic component since there are high rates of social difficulty in members of the immediate family. Male relatives of individuals with Asperger's seem to be especially likely to have social difficulties. Female relatives are less likely to have these difficulties, but may be more likely to have problems with anxiety or depression.

PDD-NOS

Research on the causes of PDD-NOS is the least advanced of all the PDD conditions. There is, however, a strong suggestion of a possible genetic component, since many individuals with autism have relatives with language, learning, or social difficulties. It is possible that what we now see as PDD-NOS may someday be identified as a variant of autism—for example, one that comes about when some, but not all, the genes that cause autism are present. It is also likely that there really may be important distinctions within the broad group of PDD-NOS cases. For example, some cases may have more of a genetic basis and may be more closely related to autism, while others may have a different basis and might be closer to other conditions, such as language or attentional problems. It is also possible that some combination of factors might cause PDD-NOS.

Summary

This chapter has given some background information on autism and other PDDs. Relatively speaking, these are all fairly new diagnostic concepts, and, in some ways, it is surprising that we know as much as we already do about them. All these conditions share impairment in social interaction as a major feature, but also differ from each other in various ways. The best known of these disorders, autism, occurs in between 1 in 1000 and 1 in 2000 children. With the exception of PDD-NOS, the other conditions, such as Rett's disorder, CDD, and Asperger's disorder, are probably less common.

We know that autism is often, but not always, associated with mental retardation and is more common in boys than in girls. We also know that autism is frequently associated with evidence of brain impairment such as seizure disorders, and parents (and doctors) should be alert to the possibility of a child developing seizures. In addition, some children with autism have fragile X syndrome, so routine testing for this condition makes sense. It also makes sense to be particularly thorough when first evaluating a child for possible autism and in situations where the presentation is unusual and something "does not quite fit."

Although we are not yet sure exactly what causes autism, a number of promising leads are being investigated. We have now come to appreciate that genetic factors are very much involved in autism. There is evidence that the predisposition to develop autism can be inherited, and that a range of other problems—in language, learning, and social interaction—might also be inherited. Active research is being conducted around the world to look for the genes that cause autism. There is real hope that understanding what causes autism may some day lead to better treatments.

References

Cooper, J.E. (1965). "Epilepsy in a longitudinal survey of 5000 children." *British Medical Journal 1*: 1020-1022.

Deykin, E.Y. and B. MacMahon (1979). "The incidence of seizures among children with autistic symptoms." *American Journal of Psychiatry 136(10)*: 1310-1312.

Folstein, S. and M. Rutter (1977). "Infantile autism: a genetic study of 21 twin pairs." *Journal of Child Psychology & Psychiatry 18(4):* 297-321.

Kanner, L. (1943). "Autistic disturbances of affective contact." *Nervous Child 2:* 217-250.

Klin, A., W. Schultz, F.R. Volkmar, and D.J. Cohen (2002). "Visual fixation patterns during viewing of naturalistic social situations as predictors of social competence in individuals with autism." *Archives of General Psychiatry 59*: 809-816.

Volkmar, F.R. and D. Nelson (1990). "Seizure disorders in autism." *Journal of the American Academy of Child and Adolescent Psychiatry 29*: 127-129.

Questions

Q. Is there a "typical" child with autism?

On the one hand, we have information, particularly from epidemiological studies, which tells us about groups of children with autism. In this sense, we have information on the "average" child with autism. On the other hand, it is important to realize that this "average child" is not a real child, although it does give a sense of what is more frequently seen, and, importantly, a *range* of what is seen. It is the range of what we see in autism that is very unusual. As a diagnostic term, autism can be applied to the angelic-appearing, mute two-year-old who is sitting in a corner playing with a piece of string; it can also apply to a college graduate who does computer ordering for a small company.

If we had a large group of people with autism in a room together, we most likely would initially be struck by the differences, not the similarities. If, however, we spent more time, we would begin to notice the similarities. These would include major problems in:

1. negotiating through the social world,

2. communicating with others, and
3. responding to the nonsocial environment (that is, everything *but* people).

These three characteristics are what are seen in every person with autism.

Q. Did autism exist before Leo Kanner described it?

Undoubtedly there were cases of autism before Kanner first described the condition. For example, some people have argued that cases of so called "wild" or "feral" children like Victor the Wild Boy were really children with autism. It is possible that, before the improvements in childhood mortality in the twentieth century and before the increased concern with children, cases of autism had not been noticed. It was Kanner's genius to be a very careful observer and become aware of what we now know as autism.

Q. What will it mean if genes are found for autism?

A number of things will have to happen before the findings can translate into new treatments. These include discovering how the gene works and how it operates in development and in the brain, as well as the development of an animal model—that is, a mouse or other laboratory animal specially bred to have the genes for autism (which would enable us to operate on the animal and look at the effects on the developing brain). There *may* immediately be some important implications for screening. There also *may* be some possibility of understanding the broader spectrum of autism and related conditions.

Q. Someone told me that Asperger's disorder is the same as autism—Is this true?

There is much disagreement about the relationship of the two disorders, although both autism and Asperger's disorder clearly share severe social difficulties. Several different problems complicate this issue. One is that the term Asperger's disorder has come to be used for many different things; another is that various terms for disorders have come through other sources and overlap (at least in part) with Asperger's disorder. Our own view—and that of the DSM—is that these are separate disorders. Major differences have to do with the fact that language is so very good (in some ways) in Asperger's. Also in Asperger's, unusual preoccupations with fact-based knowledge about some topic is usually present. Finally, in contrast to autism, parents of children with Asperger's disorder tend not to be worried that something is "wrong" until the child enters preschool.

Q. I have one child with autism and am thinking about having a second child. What are the chances my second child could have autism?

In general, once you have had one child with autism, your risk of having another is increased—to an overall risk of probably between 2 percent and 10 percent each time you have a child (compared to the typical risk of about 0.1 percent). Put another way, your risk is between 20 to 100 in 1000 (2 to 10 in 100) compared to the typical risk of 1 in 1000. We have seen families with three and more children with autism, but we have also seen more families who have several children, only one of whom has autism. Keep in mind that this is a question we can only answer in general terms. For a specific answer relevant to you, speak with a genetic counselor who can take all the special factors in your situation such as family history into account.

Q: One of the teachers in my child's Sunday school made some comment to me about parents causing autism. Is there any truth to this?

No, there is no truth to it. In the 1950s, there was some thought that perhaps parental care might cause autism, but it became apparent that this was not true. Unfortunately, a whole generation of professionals (and parents) heard this erroneous theory and sometimes you will still find someone who was taught this. Give your friend a copy of this book or another recent one on autism!

Q: What is NLD and how is it related to Asperger's syndrome or Autism?

Nonverbal learning disability (NLD) is a *profile* of strengths and weaknesses on psychological testing. Areas of weakness include such things as coordination, understanding visual-spatial relationships, problem solving without words, and perceiving things through the fingers and hands. Areas of strength include aspects of hearing (auditory perception), the ability to memorize things heard, and to talk. Often individuals with NLD have difficulties with socialization, which is not surprising, since so much of social interaction is nonverbal. This profile often changes somewhat over time as the person learns to use his strengths to help cope with his areas of weakness.

Often, particularly in school-aged children, there may be a big gap (sometimes 30 or 40 points) between verbal abilities (or the verbal IQ) and nonverbal abilities (the performance IQ), favoring the verbal. This gap may narrow if the child learns to use verbal skills to compensate for difficulties with nonverbal skills. Ideally, teachers will be able to use the child's strengths in the verbal area for intervention, such as explicit teaching, use of rote (verbal) learning, and teaching specific problem solving strategies and well-rehearsed routines.

NLD is not an official diagnosis, although it may become one in the future. It has been described in relation to a number of conditions—notably Asperger's syndrome. Individuals with Asperger's syndrome (if this is strictly defined) seem to have a very high rate of NLD. Interestingly, children with autism, even high functioning children with autism, usually do not have this profile.

2 | Getting a Diagnosis

A diagnosis is a label that serves as a shorthand way for health professionals and others to communicate with each other very quickly. For example, if you have a cough and your doctor listens to your chest, he or she might be concerned that you have pneumonia and might ask you to have a chest X-ray. On the note for the X-ray, your doctor might write under reason for the X-ray "rule out pneumonia"; this would be a very fast way to explain to the technician who does the X-ray and the doctor who looks at the X-ray what the concern is. The "rule out pneumonia" note also has other uses—for example, it justifies to your insurance company why you should have a chest X-ray. If your X-ray reveals pneumonia, you then have an explanation for why you are not feeling well and your doctor has important information that will help guide treatment.

So far, diagnosis probably sounds pretty straightforward and uncomplicated. However, the diagnostic process is not always so cut and dried. In autism, unfortunately there is not (at least at the time this chapter is written) a simple blood or laboratory test that rules the condition in or out, although there are some tests for certain medical conditions, such as fragile X syndrome, which are associated with autism. As a result, we have to rely on the judgment of (hopefully) experienced clinicians who may do any of several things to help them arrive at a diagnosis.

Diagnosis of autism and related disorders has its uses as well as its limitations. It helps to "frame" the child's needs—for example, for educational and speech and language services. At the same time, there can sometimes be uncertainty about the diagnosis, particularly in very young children. Some clinicians, particularly less experienced ones, can make the diagnosis incorrectly (so can more experienced ones, although this is less frequent). It is important to realize that diagnosis only helps us to know the general kinds of problems or issues presented; it does not tell us a lot about the specifics.

As with many other aspects of life, life is lived in the details and it is the specifics about autism that are very important. For example, is the child verbal or nonverbal? Does she have any motor difficulties? How related is the child? And so on. These issues are particularly important for autism and related disorders, given the wide range of disabilities we see in children with these conditions. Since we don't yet know the exact cause of autism, we presently rely on observation and history to make the diagnosis. Various guidelines, rating scales, and checklists have been developed and they may help in making a diagnosis, but they never replace the importance of a skilled clinician.

This chapter covers aspects related to getting a diagnosis of autism and autism spectrum disorders. We discuss the uses and limitations of diagnosis, as well as what a good diagnostic evaluation consists of. We discuss some of the more common ways that parents and professionals become concerned about the child and the kinds of behaviors that very young children with autism exhibit. We also address some of the more frequent sources of disagreement on diagnosis, and, finally, what should happen after a diagnosis is made. As with other chapters in this book, it is important to realize that when we give examples, not every child will behave or develop in the same way and that the examples are just that. This chapter will be of greatest interest to parents of younger children, as well as to parents who are trying to understand what goes into an assessment of their child.

First Concerns

There are many ways that parents become aware that something is wrong with how their child is developing:

- Sometimes parents gradually become aware that there is something about their child that is different—maybe she seems less interested in her parents than they expect or has some unusual reaction to sounds.
- Other parents trace their concerns to a very specific event, such as seeing their child with other children of about the same age.
- Occasionally a grandparent or friend, or sometimes a daycare provider or the child's doctor, may mention that they are worried about how the child is doing.
- Sometimes parents will realize, upon reflection, that maybe there were some signs of trouble even earlier.
- Sometimes parents will say that their child was, as an infant, "too good," making few demands on them.
- At other times parents will tell us that the child had difficulties from shortly after birth—being difficult to console or being very demanding.
- Somewhat less commonly, parents will feel as if their child was doing reasonably well until, say, eighteen months of age, when either she lost ground or seemed to stop moving forward developmentally.
- Parents who have already had one child may make comparisons and realize that their new child is developing in a very different way.

Probably the most common cause of concern is speech delay. Concerns that the child may be deaf are also very frequent. Usually, however, children with autism seem to respond to some sounds, unlike deaf children. The child with autism may use pointing to get things or may pull a parent by the hand (often with no or limited eye contact) to get something, but does not seem interested in sharing attention. For example, she rarely points to show things to parents. Some parents, especially first-time parents, may not realize at first that there is anything unusual about this behavior and do not ask their doctor about it until eighteen or twenty months, when their child is still not speaking.

In other cases, parents may be worried about their child's development even earlier. When this happens, it is often the child's lack of social relatedness (or ability to "connect" with others) that causes concern. In our experience, parents are more likely to be concerned about this when they have had a fair amount of experience with children. Occasionally, parents will be worried because their child does not seem to enjoy contact with them, but she is instead interested in odd or unusual aspects of the environment, such as rocking by herself in a corner. Or parents may be concerned that their child has chosen an unusual transitional object to comfort herself. Rather than choosing something soft (and typical) such as a blanket or toy, she may choose something hard (and unusual). She may also be less interested in the actual object than in the "kind" of object (for instance, carrying a specific magazine around and taking it to bed with her but not caring which issue of the magazine it is). Sometimes the child will have dreadful and almost "catastrophic" responses to certain events in the environment. For example, when the vacuum cleaner is used, she runs upstairs crying and cannot be consoled for hours. Other children may have unusual aversions to food or certain smells. Some of the early warning signs for autism are listed in Figure 2-1 on the next page.

When parents of children with autism are asked when they were first worried about their child, it is clear that many are concerned by a year and most by sixteen to twenty months. By age two, about three-fourths of parents will be concerned and by age three, essentially all parents, even those of more able children with autism, will be worried.

For children with other ASDs such as Asperger's disorder, children are often even older before parents are first worried. In Asperger's disorder, parents seem to more usually become concerned when their child enters nursery school and is exposed to typically developing peers. Usually the child will have, if anything, seemed rather gifted and precocious (e.g., with an early interest in reading). However, the child's good verbal abilities may stand in contrast to difficulties with motor activities.

In PDD-NOS, the symptoms, at least early on, are usually not as dramatic as those of children with autism and, as a result, parents may wonder for some time about the child before expressing concern. The fact that the child often seems to do well in some situations may mislead healthcare and other professionals or make them fail to appreciate the child's difficulties. This may also reflect the fact that the child's problems may be most apparent at home rather than in the doctor's office or nursery school.

In the past, parents often had to fight to convince healthcare providers that something was wrong with their child. We've heard many stories of parents being told, "Oh, don't worry. She'll grow out of it." Fortunately, healthcare providers are usually now much more alert to developmental problems in general and autism spectrum disorders in particular, although occasionally a physician may still reassure worried parents that their child is "just language delayed." Children who have only language delay are, however, socially related and don't have the unusual behaviors we see in autism.

Making a Diagnosis

Although Dr. Leo Kanner first described several characteristics that were central for a diagnosis of autism in 1943, it was not until 1980 that enough work on autism had been done for autism to be included, for the first time, as an "official" psychiatric diagnosis in the United States. These diagnostic criteria were published in the third edition of

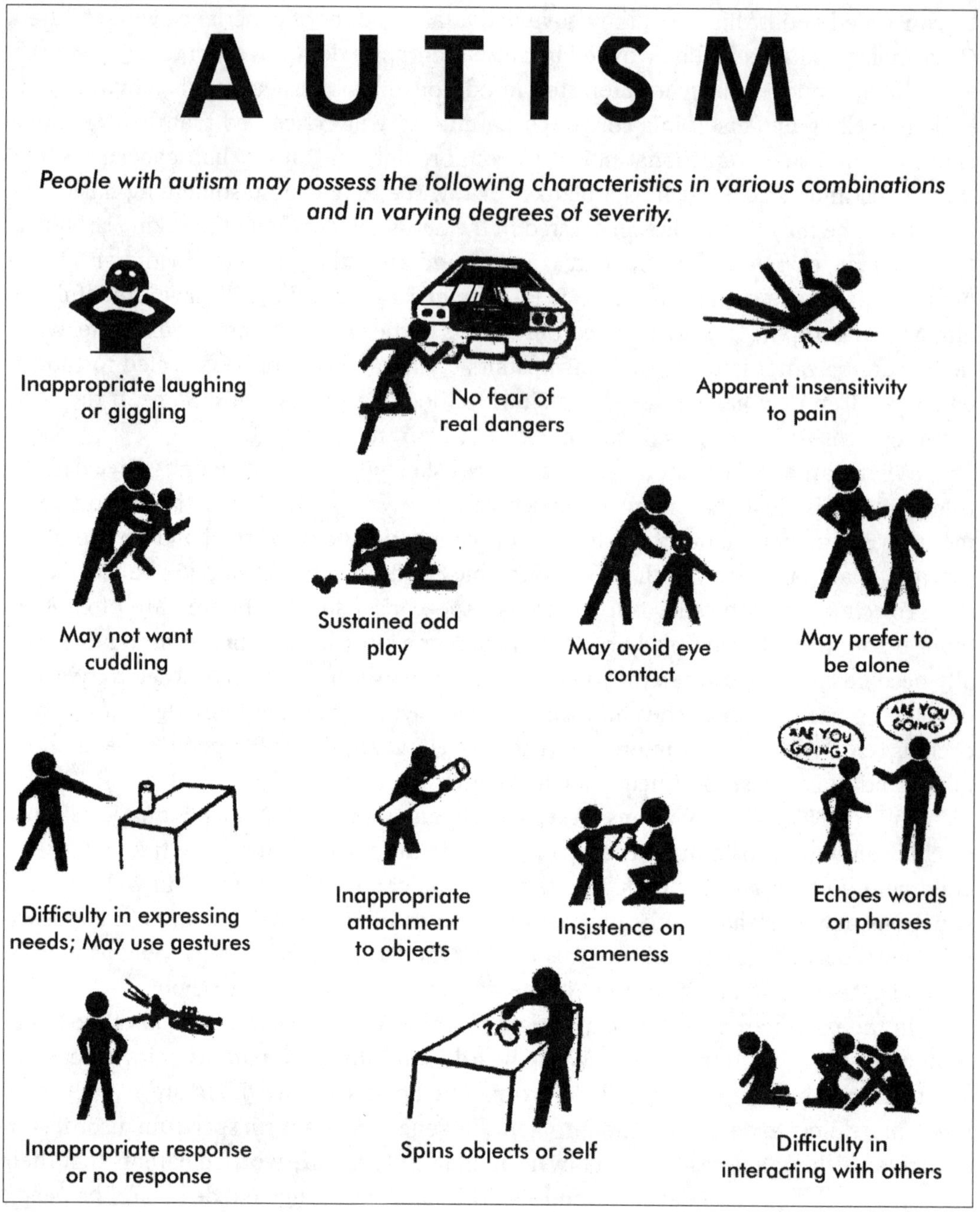

AUTISM

People with autism may possess the following characteristics in various combinations and in varying degrees of severity.

Inappropriate laughing or giggling

No fear of real dangers

Apparent insensitivity to pain

May not want cuddling

Sustained odd play

May avoid eye contact

May prefer to be alone

Difficulty in expressing needs; May use gestures

Inappropriate attachment to objects

Insistence on sameness

Echoes words or phrases

Inappropriate response or no response

Spins objects or self

Difficulty in interacting with others

Figure 2-1 Adapted from the original by Professor J. Rendle-Short, University of Queensland, Brisbane Children's Hospital, Australia. Reprinted with the permission of Autism Society of North Carolina (www.autismsociety-nc.org)

the *Diagnostic and Statistical Manual* of the American Psychiatric Association (also referred to as DSM-III). The current guidelines to the "official" diagnosis of autism in DSM-IV (see Appendix A) are intended to help doctors and educators by giving some *general* guidance about the features that ought to be observed. They do *not* replace the need for a careful examination. While a diagnosis of autism or other PDD may help parents and teachers think about general issues that may be relevant to the child, the diagnostic label is not a substitute for a careful and comprehensive evaluation which can serve as the basis for developing a detailed and individualized program of intervention.

Usually you should talk to your healthcare provider about obtaining an initial assessment. She will often know local resources and may be able to tell you how to be seen for an initial assessment through a state or local program fairly quickly—depending on your child's age, this may be through an early intervention program or through a public school. The purposes of this assessment usually include getting some basic information on your child's development and behavior and hopefully coming up with a provisional diagnosis or "working" diagnosis and establishing your child's eligibility for services. This initial assessment may be relatively brief; often parents will want to obtain an assessment at a more specialized center that has much experience in working with children with autism.

For Children Under Three

In the United States, there are specific agencies and often teams of people who can evaluate children suspected of having a disability. The names of these agencies vary from state to state; they may be called early intervention programs, or birth to three programs. In some states, these services are under the control of state departments of education; in other states, they are part of the departments of developmental disabilities or mental retardation or department of health. These organizations usually will provide a team of people to establish a need for intervention services for the child under three. Children over three are usually cared for within the public school system (see below).

Evaluation teams often vary considerably in terms of how much they know about autism. Typically, the team will establish your child's levels of functioning and potential needs by doing some initial assessment of your child, talking to you and getting a history, and, sometimes, completing special checklists or rating scales. Sometimes these teams feel confident about making a diagnosis; other teams may specifically wish to avoid giving a diagnostic label. They might do this for any of several reasons, such as to avoid the possible "bad" effects of labeling or because they might be worried about the difficulties of diagnosis in young children. However, for autism, in particular, it makes sense to start intervention as soon as possible, since it is clear that for many (although not all) children with autism, early intervention can make an important difference in the child's outcome. If your child will only receive appropriate services if she has a diagnosis of autism or pervasive developmental disorder (PDD) or autism spectrum disorder (ASD), it may be appropriate for you to make a fuss about the importance of an appropriate diagnosis in getting a good intervention program.

Sometimes the initial assessment team may suggest that you seek a more detailed and comprehensive diagnostic assessment at a specialized center. If so, see "Specialized Assessments for Autism," below.

Diagnosis and the School

Once your child reaches age three, responsibility for evaluating for disabilities falls upon the school system. Like early intervention programs, school systems employ teams of evaluators whose job is to determine which children require special educational and therapeutic services to learn. Parents can start the evaluation process by calling the special education department at their local public school and asking how to refer their child for an evaluation.

You should realize that school systems may use different labels that sometimes, but not always, correspond to the more typical medical ones. Increasingly, schools and state departments of education are recognizing autism (or sometimes PDD or ASD) as an acceptable label to get special services. Other states or school districts may not and may use other labels such as "other health impaired," "neurologically impaired," and so forth. Occasionally, particularly for higher functioning and somewhat older children, the school may want to use a label such as "social emotional maladjustment" (SEM). This can be very problematic, since it is a general term that refers to a range of children who have major problems in conduct. If this term is inappropriately applied to a child with an ASD, this can result in a very bad situation. For example, we've seen higher functioning children with autism and Asperger's disorder whose troubles at school were attributed by the school to emotional disturbance or "SEM" and who were then placed in classrooms with children with serious behavior problems—a perfectly impossible placement for a child with autism!

The diagnosis can be important for other reasons. Federal and state laws and regulations may require some services for children with autism or may specify specific kinds of treatment the child is entitled to. In other instances, insurance reimbursement issues come into play (see Appendix B).

Table 2-1 | Medical and Educational Labels

Medical Labels	Educational Labels
■ autistic disorder, autism, childhood autism	■ autism spectrum disorder
■ Rett's disorder	■ other health impaired
■ childhood disintegrative disorder	■ learning disabled
■ Asperger's disorder	■ social-emotional maladjustment
■ PDD-NOS	■ neurologically impaired
	■ multiply handicapped

Specialized Assessments for Autism

Various specialists and organizations around the country provide more comprehensive diagnostic assessments for children at risk of having autism. Sometimes these more detailed assessments are provided by specialists working as individuals, who may then suggest other assessments by members of other disciplines. It is increasingly common to find *groups* of specialists and interdisciplinary or transdisciplinary teams who work together to coordinate your child's assessment. (Interdisciplinary means individuals from different professions work together; transdisciplinary means that these individuals work very closely together, often watching each other work with the child.) There is tremendous variability in the country in terms of the level of expertise of such individuals and teams and the quality of the work they produce.

Good places to look for resources for assessment can include university-based medical schools or clinics or children's hospitals. Parent organizations (see Resources), including the Autism Society of America, often may be able to recommend people nearby. Working with an interdisciplinary team can be very helpful if you live in a rural or more isolated part of the country, since often you can coordinate with the team to do several things during your visit.

A comprehensive assessment will usually include a number of elements, varying a bit depending on your child's age and current levels of functioning:

1. **A history that you provide in response to the interviewers' questions:** This history is important for purposes of diagnosis and because it may suggest additional tests or evaluations that need to be done. It also provides information specific to your child and information relevant to your family and particular situation. This will include a history on the pregnancy, your child's early development and behaviors, medical history of your child, and history of other problems in family members.

2. **Psychological testing:** This includes testing of development and intelligence as well as other tests. This helps with the diagnosis as well as in planning treatment and intervention. This assessment will also look at adaptive functioning—that is, your child's ability to meet the demands of "real world" situations and take care of her basic day-to-day needs.

3. **A speech-language pathologist often will do an assessment of language and communication skills:** This may include tests of vocabulary and actual language ability. (Some children with autism may have a large vocabulary but don't always use their vocabulary on a regular basis.)

4. **Occupational and physical therapy assessments:** Evaluations of your child's fine motor skills (such as fastening zippers or buttons, handwriting, or using scissors) and of her gross motor skills (such as walking, running, using stairs) may be conducted as well, particularly if there are major difficulties in the motor area or many sensory issues/problems.

You may see any of a number of different professionals while your child is being assessed. These often include a psychologist, a speech-language pathologist, and a physician, but may include other individuals as well. Often a social worker or nurse may be involved in the assessment. The social worker may ask you for information on your family with a goal of helping you find the best resources and coordinate services; a nurse may be involved in taking the history and in working with the doctor in evaluating your child's physical health and developmental functioning. An audiologist may be involved in testing hearing, or an optometrist or ophthalmologist in testing vision. In the following discussion we will refer to these various people as "the professionals" since they may come from different disciplines and backgrounds. Some of these assessments are summarized in the box on the next page.

Table 2-2 | Evaluation Procedures: Autism and Pervasive Developmental Disorders

---

1. Historical Information
  a. Early development and characteristics of development
  b. Age and nature of onset
  c. Medical and family history

2. Psychological/Communicative Examination
  a. Estimate(s) of intellectual level (particularly nonverbal IQ)
  b. Communicative assessment (receptive and expressive language, use of nonverbal communication, pragmatic use of language)
  c. Adaptive behavior (how does the child cope with the real world)
  d. Evaluate social and communicative skills relative to nonverbal intellectual abilities

3. Psychiatric Examination
  a. Nature of social relatedness (eye contact, attachment behaviors)
  b. Behavioral features (stereotypy/self-stimulation, resistance to change, unusual sensitivities to the environment, etc.)
  c. Play skills (nonfunctional use of play materials, developmental level of play activities) and communication
  d. Various rating scales, checklists, and instruments specific to autism may be used

4. Medical Evaluation
  a. Search for any associated medical conditions (infectious, genetic, pre- and perinatal risk factors, etc.)
  b. Genetic screen (chromosome analysis and genetic consultation if indicated)—fragile X testing
  c. Hearing test (usually indicated)
  d. Other tests and consultation as indicated by history and current examination (e.g., EEG, CT/MRI scan)

5. Additional Consultations
  a. Occupational or physical therapy as needed
  b. Respiratory therapy and/or orthopedic specialists (Rett's disorder)

Adapted with permission from "Autism and Pervasive Developmental Disorders" by F. Volkmar, E. Cook, C. Lord in *Child and Adolescent Psychiatry: A Comprehensive Textbook*, M. Lewis, Ed. (Baltimore: Williams & Wilkins, 2002).

The History

The history will include a history of your child from birth to the present—including a history of the pregnancy, your child's development, and her medical and family history. Often the person talking with you will try to get a sense of what your child was like as a young baby. For example, was she "easy" and happy to be left alone? Did she smile responsively at you? Was she very demanding and difficult? When did you first become worried about your child and why were you worried? Don't be alarmed if people ask you about things you have never seen! Not all children with autism show every single features, and, to complicate life, some children who don't have autism may show a few signs that suggest autism!

Sometimes it may be difficult for you to remember specific developmental milestones or events. Feel free to bring a baby book or other information that would help you refresh your memory, or look at old videos of your child.

The medical history will include a review of any medical problems your child has had, such as frequent ear infections. The person talking with you will also be listening carefully for anything you mention that might suggest the need for special medical tests. She will also want to know about the kinds of programs your child has been involved in. If you have reports from schools or service providers, you should bring them to show the assessment team. The family history is important because we are now much more aware of the possible genetic aspects of autism. It is clear that a number of conditions, including problems in language, learning, and social interaction, seem to be more common in families of children with autism.

Issues in Assessment

Children with ASD typically exhibit some special challenges for assessment. Assessment of children with autism is both a science and an art. To do a good job, the people doing the assessment need to be able to do many things at the same time. They need to be able to see and interpret the results of their interactions with the child, keeping in mind both what is seen in typically developing children as well as in those with autism. Given the difficulties in social engagement and in learning, the examiners will have to use various methods to help ensure that the results are valid and reflect your child's "true" abilities at that specific point in time.

The science part of the assessment is that the examiner has to know exactly what the limits are that he has to work within (for example, the specific ways a test must be done). The art part of the assessment is that the examiner also has to be flexible in understanding how, within the constraints of what is "legal" on the test, he can help the child be interested and invested in doing well. Usually the goal for individually administered tests is that the examiner is trying to get the best possible performance out of the child while not violating the "rules" of the test. To this end, the examiner may use rewards or reinforcements (stickers, food, prizes, praise, opportunities to play). A very good examiner will quickly have a sense of how he must adapt himself to the child and will often quickly get into a rhythm where the work with child shifts easily from one task to another.

Parents often are concerned that their child's performance may not be typical or representative. We try to have parents observe the assessment either in the room with us, or, when possible, through a one-way mirror (you can see the child working but she can't see you). This gives parents a chance to observe what we do and tell us if they see things that are unusual. Occasionally parents realize that if they were to ask a question differently or with different materials, the child might be able to do better—again, something we want to know (although we also want to know what the child will do when we show her something in a very standard way). Sometimes parents are surprised both at what the child can, and sometimes can't, do.

If you are actually in the room with your child, please be sure *not* to interfere with the work of the people doing the assessment. Make notes to yourself about ways your child might have been able to answer a question if it had, for example, been asked differently. *Do not* answer for your child. Sometimes the wording of a question or the precise answer or response that is being looked for will seem to you perfectly arbitrary—sometimes because it really is. At other times, there will be several acceptable responses. If you can't observe in the room without interrupting, you should wait outside.

The importance of examiner experience in dealing with children who have autism spectrum disorders cannot be overemphasized. For example, some tests of intelligence are very verbal, and, given the problems with language, children with autism don't always do so well with these tests. On the other extreme, there are some tests that are done totally without language, and, while the results of these tests may be helpful, they don't tell us much about what the child can do with more language-based tests. Sometimes we'll see the results of an assessment where an examiner has used a test that is inappropriate to the child; in this case you'd get the same result (zeros) each time you used it and would have great reliability (you get the same results every time), but the results wouldn't tell you much about what the child actually could do!

As part of his work with your child, the examiner will try to get a sense not only of what your child is capable of, but also areas of strengths, weaknesses, or special interests that may affect programming. Also, the person doing the assessment will be alert to specific problem behaviors that are important either because they help with the issue of diagnosis or because they are important areas for intervention. For example, aggression, self injury, or stereotyped behaviors may be helped through behavioral (behavior modification) or pharmacological (drug) intervention.

Table 2-3 | Challenges for Assessment in Autism

- Tremendous range of variability in levels of function (within and between children)
- Great variability in functioning across settings
- Behavioral problems may complicate assessment
- Lack of social interest makes it hard to get the child's cooperation

---

Psychological Assessment

This part of the assessment is concerned with helping to establish your child's overall levels of cognitive ability (IQ), as well as describing her profiles of strengths and weaknesses. Any of a number of tests may be used (some of these are mentioned subsequently). Usually this testing will include—at a minimum—a test of cognitive ability or intelligence and some assessment of adaptive skills, as well as observation of the child and discussion with you.

Observation of the Child

Children with autism are quite variable in their behavior. As we mentioned previously, there are many issues in assessing a child with autism. New situations can be a problem, as can situations where the child is left to her own devices. Often the child's behavior is best in familiar settings and when her environment is very "structured" with clear expectations of what she is doing. The professionals evaluating your child should try to get a sense of the range of your child's behavior. You can also help them understand what is typical for your child.

Usually, for most of the assessment, the examiners will be working in a very structured way with your child in an effort to get her best possible performance within the limits of the test or assessment they are doing. We try to get the child's best performance by setting up a friendly but not overly stimulating environment and picking materials/tests that will be appropriate to the child's needs. As previously discussed, there is both a science and an art to doing assessment with children with autism! For some portions of the time with the child, the examiner must decide to "pull back" a bit to give the child more opportunities for less structured interaction. The examiner may also need to decide what the right pace of the assessment is—this again depends on the child; some children respond better to a rather rapid pace, while others like to take things slow and easy!

In our own assessment clinic for children with autism, we usually ask parents to observe all, or portions of, the assessment so they can tell us what is or is not so typical for their child. This has a number of advantages, including helping parents see what we and the child are doing. We do, however, have to remind parents of a couple of things. One is that, depending on the test or assessment we are using, we may have to ask a question in a very particular way. Sometimes parents will tell us afterward that the child could have answered the question if we'd asked it differently or used different materials. It is helpful for us to know this; at the same time we are interested in how the child responds to a very standardized question or item and so must work within the constraints of the specific test or assessment procedure we are using. At other times parents can be over eager to help their child—sometimes up to the point of answering the question for her! When this happens, we usually see if the parent can watch the examination through a one-way mirror in the next room and let us know afterwards what is typical or not.

Tests of Cognitive Ability

For younger children, developmental tests may be used; these tests provide information on the child's functioning in different areas relative to other children of the same age. For somewhat older children (those nearing five or six years of age and sometimes younger) more traditional intelligence tests may be used.

The distinction between developmental and intelligence tests is a somewhat arbitrary one and reflects, in part, the fact that results become more stable around the time most children traditionally enter schools. This is not a great surprise, since development of intellectual abilities stabilizes early in the elementary school years. Typically, psychologists administer more traditional tests of intelligence, while a range of professionals can administer developmental tests. Tests of intelligence usually provide an overall or "full scale" IQ score, as well as scores for verbal and nonverbal skills. Verbal skills often include such areas as the ability to define vocabulary words or explain similarities, whereas the nonverbal or performance skills can include areas such as the ability to recognize and reproduce patterns or assemble puzzles.

For typically developing children, the average (or mean) IQ is 100 with scores forming a "bell shaped curve" around this average. About 3 percent of the typical population of children will score above 130 and another 3 percent or so below 70. (The latter is usually taken as the cutoff for mental retardation, or intellectual disability, as it is sometimes called.)

In classical autism, particularly in younger children, nonverbal skills are usually much advanced over more verbal abilities. That is, it is common for children with autism to have a nonverbal IQ that is much higher than the verbal IQ. A child's nonverbal abilities might be, say, at a level corresponding to IQ 75 or 80 (standard score), while her verbal abilities might be at the IQ 40 level. For higher functioning children with autism, this gap is usually not as great, but may still, to some extent, be there. There is some indication that this situation is reversed in Asperger's disorder, where verbal skills are better than nonverbal skills.

Choices of IQ Tests

There are many different intelligence tests available. The specific test or tests chosen will depend on several factors. For example, how much language is required (either to understand or respond), how much does the test require transitions and shifting, what are the social demands of the test, and how important is speed of performance? Generally, children with autism do best on tests that require less language and social engagement and fewer shifts and transitions. Since IQ tests can vary widely in how much they emphasize these factors, it is possible that the same child could get very different results on different tests. Thus, it is important that the psychologist choose the tests carefully, keeping in mind the specific circumstances and needs of the child.

The choice of test (or tests) is up to the psychologist. He may try to start with something he thinks will be easier or more interesting to the child. Sometimes what seem to be minor differences in tests (more or less verbal tests) can actually be major changes for a child with autism; thus it is important that the psychologist have some experience in working with children with autism and be aware of the range of IQ tests available. Some of the more frequently used tests are listed in the box on the next page.

Adaptive Skills

In addition to tests of development and intelligence, often there will be some attempt to understand how your child does in more typical settings. This concern with *adaptive skills* is important because often children with autism can do something in a very structured way, but have more trouble generalizing the skills to real world settings. Tests of adaptive skills are usually done by interviewing parents. The results often add an important "real world" perspective and help identify areas the family and school can work on together.

Table 2-4 | Selected Tests of Intelligence/Development

Name	Comment
Wechsler Intelligence Scales	Excellent series of tests covering preschool (around age 4) to adulthood; provide separate verbal and performance IQ scores. Some tasks (both on the verbal and nonverbal sections) are timed—a challenge for many children with autism and related conditions. Typical profiles of ability are seen in autism and Asperger's disorder.
Stanford Binet Intelligence Scale	New version of a test that has been around for some time; can be used with somewhat younger children. Disadvantages include some timed tasks and emphasis on language, which limits its use with children with ASDs—particularly for children with more "classic" autism.
Kaufmann Assessment Battery	Excellent test, can be used from 2½ to 12 years of age. Some language is needed (but not much). Somewhat more flexible for children with autism (a small amount of teaching is allowed!). Limitations: some of the materials slightly dated; not quite as comprehensive as Wechsler scales.
Leiter International Performance Scale	A test originally developed for deaf children, recently redone. Provides assessment of nonverbal cognitive ability. (Can be used for children with no expressive speech.) Limitations: no verbal IQ and the revised materials are less interesting for children with autism.
Mullen Scales of Early Learning	Can be used with very young children. Provides scores in nonverbal problem solving, receptive and expressive language, and gross and fine motor skills. Scores from developmental tests like the Mullen are usually less predictive of later abilities.

Note: many other tests are available and tests are constantly being revised and reissued.

Adaptive functioning (adaptive skills) is a concept *distinct* from IQ. For example, we have an adolescent patient with Asperger's disorder who has a verbal IQ of 140 (genius level), one of whose major preoccupations is solving very complex mathematical equations. But this same young man cannot walk into McDonald's and get a cheeseburger and change! The latter skills—translating his mathematical ability into the real world—is what adaptive skills are all about. Assessment of adaptive skills is important both at the time of first diagnosis and also over time. Children with ASDs often have deficient adaptive skills and need specific and explicit teaching to make progress.

The most widespread test of adaptive behavior is the *Vineland Adaptive Behavior Scales,* which assess abilities in multiple areas including Communication (receptive, expressive, and written language), Daily Living Skills (personal, domestic, and community skills), Socialization (interpersonal relationships, play and leisure time, and coping skills), and, for children under six, Motor Skills (gross and fine). This test is done as an interview with a parent or caregiver; children only get full credit for things that they can do unprompted. Depending on how the assessment is set up, the psychologist may also engage your child in play or drawing or other activities. For some children, additional and even more specialized testing may be needed.

Speech-Language-Communication Assessments

Difficulties in communication are one of the central features of autism and a main focus of intervention. This is true even for higher functioning individuals with autism and Asperger's disorder, who have significant problems in the social use of language.

Typically developing children are quite communicative well before they begin to say words. In children with autism spectrum difficulties, these skills do not develop in the same way, so, for example, early (preverbal) methods of communicating such as reaching and pointing to show something to someone else may be quite deficient.

When children with autism do speak, their speech is remarkable in a number of ways. The prosody (musical aspects) of speech may be markedly off so that the child speaks in a somewhat robotic-like (what speech-language pathologists call monotonic) way. Use of pronouns (which are constantly shifting relative to who is speaking and being referred to) is an area of difficulty for many children with autism; often children with autism reverse pronouns, saying for example, you instead of I. Another very common characteristic is echolalia— repeating the same word/phrase over and over—such as saying "wanna cookie, wanna cookie, wanna cookie," having been asked, "Do you want a cookie?" Echolalia tends to persist over time, unlike in typically developing children where it gradually diminishes as the child becomes a more effective and sophisticated communicator. For the more able person with autism, difficulties in keeping up a conversation, in responding to more sophisticated language (e.g., humor, irony, sarcasm), may present significant obstacles. These are what speech-language pathologists refer to as *pragmatic* aspects (social aspects) of language.

It is important to realize that problems in communication do not exist in isolation. Rather, these difficulties have a major impact on the child's social and problem solving skills. For example, children who do communicate verbally may rely on very idiosyncratic communication, which further contributes to social difficulties. For example, the child may say "the mailman is coming" any time something unexpected happens because she remembers once when the mailman came unexpectedly early. Her parents may understand what this phrase means but most people would not!

Speech-communication assessments are important for all children with autism and related conditions, regardless of their level of functioning. For example, for children who are mute, an assessment of *comprehension* skills can be very appropriate. Speech-language pathologists (SLPs) are concerned with broader aspects of communication and not just speech, so might, for example, consider ways in which a child who is not yet speaking might be helped to communicate through some other means, such as picture exchange systems, sign language, communication boards, visual prompts, and so forth.

The communication assessment should include several components. As was true for psychological assessment, the choice of tests and assessment procedures must reflect an awareness of your child's unique circumstances. For example, the SLP may be interested in assessing your child's ability to produce sounds and words if it seems like this is an area of specific difficulty. Various standardized tests of vocabulary (both of receptive vocabulary—what your child understands, and expressive vocabulary—what she can say) are available, as are more sophisticated tests that look at exactly how language is used. For very young children, fewer assessment instruments are available. Instead, observation of social functioning (such as during play) may augment the results obtained with more standardized tests.

Table 2-5 | Commonly Used Tests of Speech-Language-Communication

Name	Comment
Peabody Picture Vocabulary Test, 3rd edition	Measures receptive vocabulary (what the child understands). Note: this score may overestimate child's actual language ability.
Expressive One Word Picture Test, revised	Measures expressive vocabulary (what the child can label). Again, may overestimate child's actual language ability.
Reynell Developmental Language Scales, U.S. edition	Useful from 12 months to age 6; provides measures of actual language use. Scores often lower than when single-word vocabulary is assessed.
Preschool Language Scale - 3	Used with parents (rather than child) to assess receptive and expressive language; frequently used in schools.
Clinical Evaluation of Language Fundamentals	Used for children from 3 to 21 (two versions). Assesses various language skills. Useful for older and higher functioning children.

Note: *many other tests are available.*

Depending on your child's age and ability to communicate, the speech-language pathologist will assess different, usually multiple, areas. These include measures of single-word vocabulary (receptive and expressive), as well as actual language use. There often is a significant gap between single-word vocabulary and the ability to use words regularly in conversation. As we mentioned before, sometimes the assessment will include evaluation of specific problems in language speech production (such as articulation) depending on the special needs of your child. Evaluation of your child's ability to use language socially should always be included.

The kinds of tests used are quite varied. Some of them rely on parental report of the child's skills, while others are based on assessment of the child by the SLP. (Some of the tests based on parent interview and report are listed in the table of Commonly Used Tests, above.) Various assessment measures have been developed specifically for children with autism and related disorders; often these employ a more play-based format, as is appropriate to younger children and those with more restricted communication skills.

For children who are not yet using words, the SLP is interested in the building blocks of language, including social interaction, play, and other behaviors with a strong communicative aspect. The goals include understanding what your child understands about communication with others (use of gestures and words), whether she displays communicative intent (the wish to communicate), and the kinds of ways your child communicates (behaviors, words, vocalization, gestures). The speech-language pathologist will also be interested in learning how effective and persistent your child is as a communicator. For instance, does she persist in trying when the other person does not understand, or does she use more or less conventional ways to communicate? In addition, the reasons why your child communicates will be noted. That is, does she communicate only to get things, to protest, or to engage other people? The social quality, as well as the rate of communications, is also important. For example, does your child pair her communication with eye contact or gestures?

When children are able to combine words, a different range of assessment tools becomes available. It becomes somewhat easier to assess the child's ability to understand receptive and expressive language and relationships between words. Specific tests are chosen based on both the child's age and her level of language. For this group of children, sometimes one needs to make compromises or accommodations to get information that is helpful for purposes of diagnosis and treatment planning. For example, if the child is older but has limited language, the SLP may choose to use a test originally developed for younger children. Or, if the child has specific issues that complicate giving the test the usual way, some accommodation may be made. These changes might include repeating instructions, using reinforcement, or giving additional cues to the child. When these strategies are used, it does complicate scoring and interpretation of the test but may give valuable information for treatment.

In addition to doing formal testing, the SLP will also usually include a period of play so that he or she can record a language sample. The latter, usually audio- or videotaped, can be used after the assessment to analyze the level and sophistication of the child's spontaneous language.

For older children and those with better language (including children with Asperger's disorder) the usual tests of vocabulary levels and language abilities may tend to overestimate or inflate the child's language skills and thus mislead school staff. For such children, the assessment should focus on more complicated aspects of language, including social uses of language, such as understanding humor and non-literal language (for example, "His eyes were bigger than his stomach"). For these children, often the results of the Vineland (see above) are more informative than many of the more usual language measures. For individuals who do speak, the SLP will often pay special attention to the child's ability to modulate or moderate her tone of voice and volume as relevant to the specific topic or place.

Medical Assessments

Depending on the specific situation, your child may be seen for a medical assessment as part of the comprehensive assessment or you may be referred for specific medical tests on the basis of the history and assessment of your child. Doctors may find correctable or treatable medical conditions (e.g., hearing loss or seizures) or other conditions (e.g., mental retardation, language disorders) that may produce symptoms suggestive of autism or autism spectrum disorders. Depending on the findings of the assessment, there may also be a search for genetic conditions such as fragile X syndrome or tuberous sclerosis. Testing hearing or vision (see Chapter 11) are also important. More specialized testing for seizures may include a brain wave test (EEG) or sometimes neuroimaging (MRI or CT scan). These tests are probably not routinely needed, however. Clearly, symptoms that suggest a possible seizure do suggest that more extensive assessment is needed.

There is no specific laboratory test for autism at the present time. However, the blood test for fragile X syndrome is almost always done. For children who have had a period of developmental regression, more extensive medical investigations are usually undertaken (see Chapter 15).

Occupational and Physical Therapy Assessments

Occupational and physical therapists may be involved either as members of the assessment team or in the school-based intervention program. Physical therapists are concerned with your child's ability to engage in gross motor (large muscle) movements, and occupational therapists are concerned with fine motor (hand) movements. They also may be needed to help assess your child if she has major sensory challenges. These specialists can provide input to classroom teachers as well as to parents on ways to help cope with, and understand, challenging behaviors, as well as motor difficulties such as with writing, and unusual sensitivities.

Rating Scales and Checklists for Autism and Related Disorders

A number of different rating scales, checklists, and other assessment instruments have been developed to help clinicians diagnose autism. Some of these scales are listed in the table on the next page. Some of them are really checklists for *screening* for autism. That is, they were developed for healthcare providers or others to use to determine which children who show some signs of autism should have a comprehensive evaluation. Others are more specifically concerned with *diagnosing* autism. These may take the form of either parent-completed rating scales or interviews, or they may be based on actual work with the child. That is, there are some checklists that are completed by professionals based on observation of and/or work with the child.

Many different issues are involved in the use of these instruments (again, a little knowledge can be a dangerous thing) and sometimes people will use them in ways that were not intended. For example, we've encountered a well-meaning teacher who got access to a rating scale, and, with no training in how to use it and very little experience with autism, decided a child "couldn't have autism" based on her (incorrect) completion of the rating scale. Some of the scales require specific training to complete. None of these scales are a substitute for a careful, thoughtful assessment by an experienced clinician. Be particularly wary if you hear that someone who "just got trained" on some instrument is going to diagnose your child. Often a little knowledge is a dangerous thing! We've seen well-meaning people who tried, often in the space of just a few minutes of reading, to prepare themselves to use a diagnostic instrument—sometimes with disastrous results.

The two instruments that are probably most commonly used at present are the *Autism Diagnostic Interview – Revised (ADI-R)* and the *Autism Diagnostic Observation Schedule (ADOS)*. The ADI is an interview done with parents that focuses on the child's social and communication skills, as well as other behaviors. This test, which can take a while to complete, was originally designed for research (to be sure that researchers in different parts of the world were diagnosing autism in the same way). It has the considerable advantage of being explicitly "keyed" or linked to the diagnostic criteria for autism in DSM-IV. The ADOS is a companion instrument to the ADI; it focuses on assessment of the child using various activities.

Other instruments commonly used at present include the *Childhood Autism Rating Scale (CARS)*, along with several others. These scales measure severity of autism either on the basis of parent or teacher report or observation of the child.

Table 2-6 | Frequently Used Instruments for Diagnosis of Autism

Name	Format and Comments
Autism Behavior Checklist	Teacher- or parent-completed checklist; useful for screening.
ADI-R (Autism Diagnostic Interview—Revised)	Interview with parents to verify diagnosis of autism based on history of child (requires substantial training). Very well done.
ADOS (Autism Diagnostic Observation Schedule)	Assessment of the child, covering wide span in ability levels; assesses behaviors and features relevant to diagnosis of autism. Companion instrument to ADI-R, also very well done. Requires significant training.
Childhood Autism Rating Scale (CARS)	Assesses severity of autistic behaviors; useful for screening. Requires some (minimal) training.
CHAT (Checklist for Autism in Toddlers)	Screening instrument. Tends to over-identify possible autism.

Understanding Test Results

When your child's evaluation is complete, a variety of numbers will be available to describe her performance. This is especially true if the tests used were based or standardized on the "normal population." The professional(s) who work with your child will be able to interpret these for you. Keep in mind that for scores to be valid the person doing the assessment has a number of rules he or she must follow in the assessment. Validity means that the test must actually measure what it is designed to measure. In addition, instructions which govern giving the test must be followed. If you gave the child the answer in advance, of course she'd do well, but the results would not be *valid*. Sometimes deviations from these rules are needed and can sensibly be made, but when this is done, it will tend to invalidate the results obtained.

Usually different kinds of numbers or scores will be produced. The most common scores you will hear about are age equivalents and standard scores. Age equivalent scores tell you that your child's work would be typical of a certain age child in the general or typically developing population. If your child has an age equivalent score of 4 years 2 months, it means that her performance on the given measure would be more typical, overall, of a child of that age in the general population. The beauty of this type of score is that it is pretty straightforward and understandable. The limitations are a bit less clear but very important. Namely, age equivalent scores do not take into account the actual or chronological age of your child. A score of 4 years 2 months would be a great score for a three-year-old and not so good for a seven-year-old.

To deal with this problem, the standard score is often used. It takes age into account, and, as a result, enables you to readily compare the results across children. Originally, standard scores such as the IQ (intelligence quotient) were computed by taking the child's age equivalent score (mental age) and dividing it by the child's actual chronological age and then multiplying the result by 100. Thus, a child with a mental age of 3 years and an actual age of 5 years would have been said to have an IQ of 60 ($\frac{3}{5}$ x 100). Nowadays tests are developed and "standardized" in more sophisticated ways, but the general idea is the same.

The distribution of standard scores falls on the famous (or infamous) bell-shaped curve. The average score will be in the middle, with other scores around it. (See Figure 2-2 below). For many IQ tests, the average or mean score in the general population is 100. That is, about 50 percent of people would score above 100 and 50 percent would

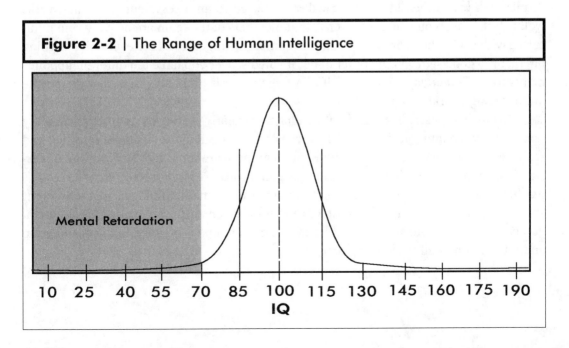

Figure 2-2 | The Range of Human Intelligence

Mental Retardation

10   25   40   55   70   85   100   115   130   145   160   175   190

IQ

score below it. These tests usually have what is called a standard deviation (measure of how the scores scatter around the average) of about 15. This means that most people (about two-thirds) taking the test will score within 15 points above to 15 points above the mean, or between 85 and 115. Only about 3 percent of people will score more than 30 points (two standard deviations) above or below the mean. That is, only about 3 percent of people would have scores of 70 or below. Some tests will have different means and standard deviations. You need to look both at the age equivalent and standard scores in interpreting the results of a test.

Integration of Findings

Due to health insurance issues, geographical location, and other factors, parents unfortunately do not always have that much choice when selecting a team to assess their child. If you can, try to connect with people who have worked together previously and who have considerable experience in diagnosing autism and related conditions. Other parents and often school staff will be able to give you good information about qualified professionals. Often, your primary healthcare provider is the person who provides an initial referral to a team and then helps you obtain local services and resources. He then works with the assessment team or private providers assessing your child, both by providing an initial referral and by helping you obtain local services and resources. He may or may not be able to direct you to a good team that has worked together previously and that is experienced in diagnosing autism and related conditions.

You should know that one danger of some diagnostic "teams" is that they really don't work so well together—rather than getting a single view of your child, the "team" members work as individuals who write up their own reports and do not discuss the results with each other. Ideally, you will be referred to an assessment team that works well together and you will have a sense that members of the team are actively communicating with each other. For example, if the team meets together as the evaluation is going on, that is a good sign. On the other hand, if you discover you have ten different appointments (on different days) with ten different doctors, it is probably a sign that the people are not really working together!

As much as possible, assessment results, particularly if done by an interdisciplinary team, should be integrated and used to translate the results into a single, sensible, and realistic view of the child. As a consumer and parent, you should feel as if you can understand the reports and that the results have implications for how you or your child's teacher and others can work with her. Sometimes one can't help but see many different specialists; in this case the lack of integration is often a major problem. In this situation, you can ask one of the specialists if he or she can assume a major role in coordination and integration of all the various reports.

Diagnostic Certainty and Uncertainty

To make life complicated, many conditions may be apparent in the first years of life and may be confused with autism. For example, significant mental retardation may result in language delay and lead parents and healthcare providers to suspect autism. Usually, however, these children have social abilities and language-communication skills that are pretty much on target for their overall intelligence or cognitive ability. At times, however, distinguishing between autism and mental retardation can be difficult. One reason is that we know that many children with strictly diagnosed autism also go on to exhibit mental retardation. Another reason is that sometimes children with mental retardation exhibit some of the same kinds of unusual self-stimulating behaviors (e.g., hand flapping) seen in children with autism. Yet another reason is that we know that the results of developmental and other tests only become stable as the child gets older.

Somewhat less commonly, language difficulties may be confused with autism. We often see children with very serious language problems who have been diagnosed with autism, but who are in fact very socially related and sometimes very "communicative" even when they do not have any words. Occasionally, such children may seem to develop their own sign language system. They usually are very much interested in communication even when their actual language is limited.

Although we continue to see that many children with autism have isolated areas of ability, professionals have become aware that when one looks at the *entire* intelligence test, often many—indeed, probably most—children with strictly defined autism do have some degree of associated mental retardation overall. This is important for several reasons. First, it disproves the notion that arose in the 1950s and 1960s that, rather than having some degree of developmental delay, children with autism were "choosing" not to respond (negativism). It also contradicts the related idea that they could not be tested. While there can indeed be many difficulties in assessing children with autism, these days when we hear that a child is "untestable," this often says more about the examiner than the child! It is now clear that assessment can be done if the person doing the testing is flexible and is prepared to test developmental skills using techniques adapted for children with autism.

Consistent with Kanner's original report, we often see children with autism who have some good skills, particularly in nonverbal problem solving. The observation of areas of "splinter skills" has been made repeatedly. The term splinter means just that—skills that are striking because they are so much better than other areas of the child's development. For some children with autism, these unusual abilities (e.g., in drawing, music, or calendar calculation) rise to the level of savant skills. Such skills tend to be very narrow and often involve visual-spatial skills (e.g., jigsaw puzzles) or memory for concrete events or trivial information (e.g., numbers, calendars). Many younger children with autism have an unusual interest in letters and numbers, with some children teaching themselves to "decode" words, although they are usually much less advanced at understanding what they read. Unfortunately, splinter skills often don't contribute much to the child's ability to meet the demands of daily life.

Table 2-7 | Conditions That May Be Confused with Autism

Condition	Features That Help Differentiate It from Autism
Mental Retardation (Intellectual Disability)	Generally even pattern of cognitive and language delay. Social skills not much different from cognitive level. (Note: mental retardation may co-exist with autism and related disorders, except for Asperger's disorder.) Problems arise in distinguishing autism from MR in individuals with very low IQ, who often exhibit self-stimulatory behaviors.
Language Disorders	Nonverbal and social skills often preserved; the child can be very communicative even when a severe language disorder is present. Differentiation from autism can be complicated in very young children.
Deafness	In contrast to more typical situation in autism, hearing difficulties are not very selective. (Hearing is affected in all/ most situations, not just in certain situations, as in autism.) Hearing testing is critical; occasionally children with autism are deaf or have other sensory impairment (see Chapter 11.) Some deaf children exhibit self-stimulatory movements.
Schizophrenia	In children, schizophrenia is very uncommon. Hallucinations (hearing voices) and delusions (bizarre beliefs) are present. Major deterioration in function may suggest childhood disintegrative disorder, but marked social problems and other unusual behaviors more typical of autism are not seen in schizophrenia.
Obsessive Compulsive Disorder (OCD)	Usually the child voices active dislike of the symptoms, in contrast to autism and Asperger's disorder, where repetitive behaviors or restricted interests seem to be preferred activities. Social skills are usually preserved in OCD.
Reactive Attachment Disorder (RAD)	Lack of social interest is common in children reared in very neglectful settings (e.g., some orphanages) and the child may exhibit some unusual behaviors, but usually development dramatically improves when a more appropriate environment is provided.
Selective Mutism	Child talks only in some situations. While some social difficulties are present, these are not as severe as in autism and the child can communicate in some settings.

For many parents, a diagnosis of mental retardation seems, if anything, even worse than a diagnosis of autism. Given the difficulties in assessment and the limitations of testing for young (preschool) children, often the term developmentally delayed may be used at first. The question of whether mental retardation is present is often settled only when the child is at or near traditional school age. Keep in mind that children with autism who also have some degree of associated mental retardation will continue to grow and develop. Less commonly, some children will make major gains over time—

particularly in the preschool years, and, to a lesser extent, in adolescence. Also keep in mind that although it is possible to drop a diagnosis of mental retardation if this is appropriate as a child grows older, it is rather harder to acquire a diagnosis of mental retardation as the child gets older and may otherwise be eligible for special services through state departments of developmental disability or mental retardation.

Special Issues

Autism in Very Young Children

A relatively common problem in diagnosing children under age three is that these younger children may exhibit *some* but not all of the features of autism. We usually encounter this problem when a child exhibits the required social and communication problems but does not yet have the unusual motor mannerisms and interests typical of autism. Often these children go on to develop more typical autism after age three, but sometimes they do not. More rarely, we see a child at two or even near three who appears to have autism, but as time goes on, the child seems to have some other problem, or, more rarely, appears perfectly normal.

The difficulties in early diagnosis partly reflect our real difficulties in assessment of younger children and partly reflect the fact that different kinds of problems can mimic autism early in life. Consequently, the assessment team may discuss with you a provisional or working diagnosis and make it clear that the issue of final diagnosis will be made with certainty only over time.

Table 2-8	Difficulties in Early Diagnosis

- Limitations of developmental tests and difficulties of assessment
- Some children with autism don't display all the features needed for diagnosis until after age 3
- Less commonly, a child seems to exhibit many autistic-like features but loses these after age 3

Asperger's Disorder

Of all the syndromes on the autism spectrum, probably the greatest diagnostic controversy has surrounded Asperger's disorder. Children with Asperger's usually do not have delayed language—instead, their language skills are often a source of strength. Probably, in part, as a result of their much better language, parents don't seem to be worried as early as parents of children with autism. It is more typical for parents to become concerned only when the child enters preschool, nursery school, or kindergarten and the combination of the child's major social difficulties and her unusual interests makes her stand out from her peers.

In Asperger's disorder, there may be an early fascination with letters and numbers. As time goes on, the child develops one or more highly specialized interests, such as in clocks, time, rocks, dinosaurs, snakes, or sometimes in much more esoteric areas, such as deep fat fryers or telegraph line pole insulators. The family will discover that its life revolves around the child's special interests and that these special interests dominate the child's life and interfere with learning.

Unfortunately, as discussed in Chapter 1, this diagnosis has been used in various and varied ways. For example, sometimes it is used to mean adults with autism or higher functioning people with autism. Although there are some data suggesting differences, the final work on the relationship between autism and Asperger's disorder is not yet in. Chapter 1 explains how Asperger's disorder is defined in DSM-IV. The DSM-IV definition undoubtedly will be improved as time goes on; it has been criticized as being overly restrictive. Diagnostic evaluations of children with Asperger's disorder are very similar to those of children with autism. One exception is that since the children are more verbal, often a wider choice of tests and other assessments are available.

Childhood Disintegrative Disorder (CDD)

In CDD, the child develops perfectly normally for at least two years and then experiences a marked loss of skills in multiple areas. The child develops many of the behavioral features seen in autism—and in some ways comes to look more classically "autistic" than most autistic children. The onset of this rather rare condition is usually between ages three and four. However, it is possible that current guidelines for the diagnosis are overly strict and that some children with "regressive autism" which develops before two years may, in some ways, be more similar to children with CDD. (This is an area where research is going on now.)

The onset of CDD is either gradual (weeks or months) or fairly quick (days to weeks). Parents will sometimes say that the child had a time when she seemed more anxious or agitated before the skill loss occurred. Information from the parents and documentation of early normal development are important in making a diagnosis of CDD; videotapes can be very helpful for this. We discuss this condition in more detail in Chapter 15.

Rett's Disorder

In Rett's disorder, there is a fairly brief period of normal development. The child (usually a girl) then experiences a loss of purposeful hand movements, her head growth slows, and development becomes very delayed. The main reason that this condition is included in the PDD group in DSM-IV is that there is a fairly short period of time during the preschool years when Rett's disorder may be mistaken for autism. During this time it may seem that the children are less related and thus possibly autistic. However, over time, the very characteristic course of the disorder clarifies the diagnosis. The recent discovery of a gene involved in Rett's disorder points out the importance of our trying to make distinctions among various conditions like autism, Rett's disorder, and CDD. Like CDD, the diagnosis of Rett's disorder is made on the basis of history and clinical examination. We discuss Rett's disorder in greater detail in Chapter 15.

PDD-NOS

Pervasive developmental disorder—not otherwise specified (PDD-NOS) (also sometimes called atypical PDD, or atypical autism)—is both an easy and a rather complicated diagnosis to make. It is easy in the sense that this category is reserved for children whose problems don't exactly correspond to the guidelines for autism or one of the other explicitly defined pervasive developmental disorders, but who have *some* problems in social interaction and either communication problems or stereotyped behavior patterns and interests. As a result, this is a category that really is very much based on the judgment and experience of the clinician.

One complication in making this diagnosis is that even though it is the most common of all the PDDs, it is also the least studied (mostly because it has been hard to define). The relationship of this category to more strictly defined autism and other disorders is now an area of much interest. Hopefully, research on it will increase in the next years. Another complication is that for those of us who deal with children with PDD-NOS, it is clear that there probably are many subtypes. For example, one possible subtype is a group of children with PDD-NOS who also have major problems with attention.

As a result of these issues, your child might get a diagnosis of PDD-NOS under several conditions:

- if she is younger,
- if she is evaluated by someone with less experience diagnosing children with autism spectrum disorders,
- if some aspects of the picture don't quite "fit" with the more usual presentation of autism or another autism spectrum condition.

The various rating scales and tests used for other disorders can still be used and may provide important information for program planning.

What Happens after the Assessment?

It is critical that you, as parents, feel involved in the assessment in a central way and that you meet with the individual or team doing the assessment to go over the results. The conference with you may occur right after the assessment, or the team or doctor doing the assessment may give you a brief feedback and then ask you to return later for a more detailed review of the report of the assessment.

It is important that you have adequate time to talk about the findings and your concerns for your child. The findings of the evaluation should be easily understood, detailed, and concrete, and realistic recommendations should be provided. If there is too much jargon or if you have questions, you should speak up. Also be sure to ask questions if you do not understand how the diagnostic assessment clarifies the interventions that may help your child. The results of the evaluation should provide you with a coherent picture of your child and her strengths and difficulties. Having many different individual reports may be less helpful than having a longer but more integrated single report. Whenever possible, you should ask if your child's teacher, speech-language pathologist, or some other member of the school or early intervention treatment team can come either to watch part of the assessment or come to the parent conference where the results are being discussed. This has several advantages. First, it may help the assessment team, since the teacher or person working with your child may be able to give new information. Second, it gives the teacher an opportunity to ask questions and understand the results.

Usually at the parent conference you will *not* want to have your child present so that you can really focus on talking about the assessment. (There are some exceptions to this, of course.) If you have had a positive experience, you may also want to discuss with the team how they can be involved over time. For example, can they consult to the school, if that is appropriate? When do they want your child to come back for another assessment? If your child's assessment was done by the school, you'll have the opportunity to review the results at the conference where you develop your child's Individualized Education Program (IEP). You are also within your rights to ask that you see the results before the IEP meeting.

Implementing the results of the assessment can be a very complex task. Many books have been written on this process and the efforts of consultants, other parents, and advocates may be helpful as you work with the school or intervention program. References to these are provided in the Reading List.

Summary

We have discussed both the uses and limitations of diagnosis and have reviewed some aspects of what a good assessment should include. Keep in mind that there will be considerable variability in diagnostic procedures and materials used, depending on your child and her specific needs, strengths, and weaknesses. As with other chapters in this book, it is important to realize that when we give examples, not every child will behave or develop in the same way and that the examples are just that.

Keep in mind as well that there are many good professionals to work with, but there are also many professionals with a lot to learn. You should pay attention to your experience of the assessment. If you do not feel that your child has been accurately seen or that your own views haven't been heard, think about going elsewhere. Unfortunately, the number of truly outstanding diagnostic centers around the country is relatively limited, but, as time goes on, more and more professionals are learning more about assessment of autism.

Questions

Q. Does the diagnosis really matter?

This is a good question. The answer is yes and a qualified no. The complication is that diagnosis is used for many different things—for research, for teaching people about commonalities in illnesses and disorders, for communicating rapidly, and for getting educational services. All of these are legitimate goals and the needs for diagnosis will vary somewhat depending on what the goal is. Essentially, the diagnosis grounds us in the general territory we are dealing with, but, of course, to come up with a program or treatment, we need to take the needs of the individual child into account. Some people advocate against giving a diagnosis to avoid giving premature or stigmatizing labels. On the other hand, it is just these labels that sometimes help a child get services. For purposes of research, rather strict diagnostic labels are often needed—that is to avoid what would be confounding or complicating issues in interpreting the results of a research study.

Q. Can autism be diagnosed from an EEG?

No, autism is diagnosed based on history and clinical examination. The EEG is useful in the diagnosis of seizure disorders—which are sometimes associated with autism. Seizure disorders are diagnosed on the basis of the EEG.

Q. Is a brain scan and EEG always indicated in evaluating a child with autism?

In general, the answer is no. Without a specific clinical reason to do the tests, the likelihood of finding something is small. If there are specific clinical reasons to do these tests—for example, if you suspect seizures or if the child's history and behavior are highly unusual—then they should be done.

Q. Are there any lab tests that diagnose autism?

At present, the answer is no. When genes for autism are found, there may, in the future, be some such tests. At the moment, the only lab test that makes sense is the test for fragile X syndrome (a blood test). Other tests may be needed, given the child's history and examination.

Q. What is the difference between DSM and ICD?

The DSM system is the American system of diagnosis (published by the American Psychiatry Association). DSM stands for *Diagnostic and Statistical Manual of Mental Disorders*. The DSM is now in its fourth edition. This book is used for both clinical work and research; it includes guidelines (or *criteria*) for diagnosis. The ICD published by the World Health Organization (based in Geneva, Switzerland) is the *International Classification of Diseases,* now in its tenth edition. Unlike DSM, there are two versions: one for clinical work and another for research. For autism and related disorders, there are no major differences between the two systems.

Q. My child has been diagnosed with PDD-NOS but the school has given her the label of autism. Is this OK?

Labels used by schools often differ somewhat from those used by medical professionals. These labels also vary considerably from state to state and sometimes within states! Often for purposes of getting appropriate services, the label of autism is used very broadly, so in this case it may be perfectly fine for your child. Keep in mind that you need to evaluate labeling issues in the context of your child's particular needs and that you can always ask to discuss the label and change or drop it.

Q. My daughter had a diagnosis of PDD-NOS when she was younger. Now she is ten years old and has been included in a regular class for two years. She has not needed special services. Can we now drop the label which used to get her special services that she no longer needs?

Yes, you can indeed drop the label. If it turns out, for whatever reason, that she needs some special services in the future, you can revisit this issue with the school.

Q. On the intelligence test, my son's verbal skills fell into the mentally retarded range, but his nonverbal skills were above the mentally retarded range. Does this mean he is mentally retarded?

It is very common for children, particularly with autism, to have greater delays in verbal than in nonverbal abilities. As time goes on, you will get a better sense of how stable this pattern will be (for some children the gap widens, for others it grows smaller). Often the overall abilities (full scale IQ) of children with autism go down over time. That is, the IQ score decreases because, although the child makes gains, the *rate* of gain is not as great as expected in typically developing children. Roughly 70 percent of children with "classical" autism also have mental retardation.

The diagnosis of mental retardation is made on the basis of the full scale (or global) IQ—usually a combination of the verbal and nonverbal parts of the test. This can be a misleading number in terms of program but is the number people use for diagnosis of mental retardation. In addition to having a full scale IQ (the combination of both verbal and nonverbal scores) of less than 70, the child also has to have deficits in adaptive (self-care, real world) skills. Often the diagnosis of MR is: a) less important than the profile of test results during the school years (as is the case for your child, where we'd want to use strengths in the nonverbal area to try to address weaknesses in the verbal area), and b) more important when thinking about longer term provision of services. That is, in many states adults who qualify for MR services often have the broadest range of services to choose from.

Q. My school wants to treat my child as if her primary disability is mental retardation, not autism. Is that OK?

In the best of all possible worlds (of which this is *not* one) we should be providing educational programming to children and not to labels. That being said, the problem in the real world is that a label of mental retardation (and not of autism) tends to imply the need for a general kind of intervention—for example, with many opportunities for learning, stimulating environments, and so forth. For a child with autism who also has mental retardation, it is generally better to go with the autism label since this label implies the need for special services. One of the problems with general stimulation programs and classrooms designed for children with MR is that they may be overstimulating for the child with autism and also often lack the intensive focus on behavior and communication that is needed. On the other hand, for some children with autism, particularly in adolescence, the differences can be less important. For example, in both conditions a lot of work has to be done on "real world" or adaptive skills. Talk with a parent advocate or an outside consultant about how best to work with your school on this issue with regard to your child's specific needs.

Q. My child wouldn't cooperate enough during intelligence testing for the school to obtain a score, but they decided she has mental retardation anyway. Is this OK?

The short answer is no. Sometimes children with autism spectrum disorders *are* difficult to test. However, psychologists who have had a great deal of experience are often able to test the child when less experienced psychologists are not able to.

3 | Raising a Healthy Child with an Autism Spectrum Disorder

Before your child was born, you may have expressed the hope that he would be "healthy." Fortunately, having an autism spectrum disorder and being healthy are not usually mutually exclusive. Although there are a few medical problems that are more common in ASDs, most children with autism are born with the same potential to live healthy lives as anyone else. However, the communication and behavior challenges that go along with autism can make it harder to detect, treat, and manage problems that might affect your child's health.

In this chapter, we discuss some of the issues involved in raising a healthy child with autism. First we discuss some of the challenges that autism often poses for children in terms of getting healthcare. We discuss your role as an advocate for your child and as a careful observer who can participate as a valuable part of the healthcare team. We also talk about routine preventive care, immunizations, and the help you can get from the pharmacist and the school nurse. Finally, we discuss a few of the medical conditions that are more common in autism.

Challenges in Providing Healthcare for Children with Autism

Not surprisingly, two of the major problems in autism—difficulties with communication and social skills—can pose major challenges in raising a healthy child. Particularly if a child with autism or similar disability is nonverbal, it may be difficult for him to communicate when he's feeling ill. An acute disease may actually present itself as irritability, refusal to walk, decreased appetite or refusal to eat, acute weight loss, behavioral deterioration such as head banging or self-injury, and so forth. Sometimes it seems like the opposite occurs and you may even be able to tell that your child is getting sick because he seems to be doing better! (See Chapter 4 for more information about behavior as communication.)

Social and communication problems can also cause other challenges. For example, your child may not understand what a doctor is asking him to do. Cooperation can be a major challenge—even getting your child undressed in a strange place can be a burden. The unusual sensitivities and difficulties with change are yet another problem. The child who avoids being touched by other people is not going to be too willing to have a doctor poke and prod him, much less let the doctor look in his ears! In addition, behavioral issues such as impulsivity, aggression, or self-injurious behaviors can make it more likely that the child will hurt himself (see Chapters 7 and 12).

Children with autism spectrum disorders may have other problems—such as in eating or sleeping—that may make more frequent doctor's visits necessary. Similarly, the need to monitor medications sometimes used for behavioral and psychiatric difficulties may mean more doctor visits. Having to take your child to a place that overwhelms him or that he dislikes can be very stressful to you *and* your child, but is necessary, of course. Accordingly, the information below is meant to help you and your child make your way through the health care system as smoothly as possibly.

Dealing with the Healthcare System

Although autism is still not as well understood as it should be in the medical community, more and more doctors know at least something about it. It is now very possible for parents of children with autism and other pervasive developmental disorders to find a doctor or other medical professional who is willing and able to work with them as part of a team. As a parent, you are ultimately responsible for your child's well-being. This is a responsibility you can share with competent, caring professionals, who should be selected carefully. You then have to work with them to obtain the best possible medical care and the healthiest, happiest future for your child.

Dealing with Medical Professionals

Dealing with medical professionals can be complicated for any parent—even when the parent is a doctor. It is even more complicated for parents of a child with significant developmental problems. While most parents occasionally have trouble getting their younger children to cooperate with routine medical procedures, even the most minor procedures pose potentially major problems for the parents of a child with autism or other PDD. Just sitting in the waiting room for a long period of time can be stressful for both child and parents. Because children with autism often need extra time getting used to the doctor and the setting, the usual rapid pace of medical care—which only seems to increase over time—may make examination more difficult.

It is important that you find healthcare professionals who understand you and your child's special needs, as well as your anxiety in taking your child to a doctor's office. A good relationship with a pediatrician or other primary care provider is important. You can work together to anticipate problems and keep them to a minimum. As we'll discuss shortly, working with the doctor during well or preventive visits also gives your child a chance to learn more about the doctor's office and the healthcare system. You can also work on this knowledge at home and at school. The long-term goal is to help your child participate as much as possible in the process of getting good healthcare and learning to be as informed as he can be about this process.

Probably the most important thing to look for in your child's primary care doctor (as well as any specialists your child might need to see) is her interest in your child and in making the relationship with you and your child a success over the long haul. Her willingness to make an effort to make the visits easy is a key. If your child had significant communication problems, the doctor often will need to spend more time than usual asking about your child's history and symptoms. The doctor should have a gentle and careful approach to interacting with your child, trying to reduce his anxiety whenever possible. Typically, the doctor should start with the less stressful procedures and move on to the more difficult or challenging ones as she gains your child's confidence.

Even the best doctor will occasionally have to treat or examine your child without his cooperation—for example, if an emergency arises and your child is too upset to cooperate. In an emergency, the doctor or other health professionals must do whatever needs to be done to assure the safely and health of your child. Even in these situations, you can provide some information that may be helpful—for example, about ways to approach your child. For non-emergency situations, you have the luxury of being able to plan ahead.

Selecting a Pediatrician or Primary Care Provider

By the time your child is diagnosed with autism, you will probably already have a pediatrician, family doctor, or other primary care provider. If you are quite satisfied with the care your child has been receiving from her, there is generally no reason to switch to another physician. Even if the doctor has never had another patient with autism, this shouldn't be an impediment to good care, as long as the doctor is willing to accommodate your child's special needs and to learn about autism. Flexibility, interest in your child, and a willingness of the doctor to learn are all positive signs. Other considerations (distance to the office, office staff, and other factors) may also be important.

If you are dissatisfied with your current pediatrician or need to find a new provider for another reason, you should spend some time looking. You probably cannot (and should not) pick a pediatrician right out of the phonebook. Find out which doctors in your area have experience in treating children with developmental problems. Ask for recommendations from other parents of children with developmental problems, teachers and members of the school staff, as well as members of an interdisciplinary evaluation team, local parent support groups, or Autism Society of America chapters. It is important to find a doctor who either has some experience with autism or is willing to learn about it. Sometimes doctors have major misconceptions about autism and related disorders. If they can "relearn" to correct these misconceptions it is fine; otherwise, find another doctor.

Once you have the names of several potential doctors, your first step is to call and ask for a visit. You may or may not wish to take your child to the first visit; you can discuss this with doctor and staff while setting up an appointment. Whether you go by yourself or take your child, the objective is to find out how much the physician knows about autism, to get a sense of how comfortable you are with the doctor and her office, and to review your child's medical history.

You should not feel shy or uncomfortable asking the doctor about her experience with autism. Explain what you are doing, then ask if she has cared for other children with autism or pervasive developmental disorders and what she knows about autism. If she has no first-hand experience with children with autism and PDD, try to get a sense of whether she's interested in learning more about it. You can also bring up special issues such as the use of medicine for dealing with behavior problems to see how the doctor's position compares with yours. Usually doctors are very willing to discuss their views with you. Pediatricians in particular often have experience in dealing with children with developmental issues. Signs that you should probably look elsewhere for a doctor might include:

- Communication problems (e.g., the doctor doesn't seem to listen to you)
- Lack of up-to-date information (e.g., a doctor who tells you that parents cause autism!)
- Distant or inconvenient location
- Office staff who are not "user friendly"
- Problems with coverage (e.g., you may find that you might be dealing with many different doctors on nights or weekends)

Just as important as the doctor's knowledge of autism is the way that you and your child are treated during your first visit. If the doctor is rushed, your child is more likely to be frightened or anxious. If the doctor and her staff are prepared to take an appropriate amount of time, particularly at the start of your relationship with them, future visits will be less traumatic. You may want to look for a smaller practice where your child can know the doctors and nurses individually, and they can know him. The sensitivity and tact of the doctor during a first visit provide important clues about her suitability as your child's physician.

Routine Office Visits for Preventive Care

All children should see their healthcare provider on a regular basis for preventive care. This is true for kids with autism spectrum disorders, as well as for all others. The pediatrician will monitor your child's growth and development and provide all the necessary immunizations. She can help you understand your child's behavior at different ages and help foresee his safety needs at different developmental stages.

Some medical problems have no early symptoms, so routine screening by physical exam and laboratory testing are important to detect the problems early—when treatments can be helpful and prevent more severe or permanent conditions. This is especially true for children with autism and other PDDs. In order to optimize their ability to learn and progress, we want to be sure that any treatable impairment is corrected. For example, hearing difficulties or eye problems such as strabismus (weak eye muscles that can lead to permanent visual impairment) can, if untreated, make learning more difficult. Poor growth, dental problems, crooked spine (scoliosis), and high blood pressure are a few of the other disorders that might be found at a routine preventive care exam. Also, because children with autism and related conditions often receive medications, we want to minimize possible side effects that might result from any underlying problems. For example, if a child has a low blood count (anemia) or has abnormal liver function, a medication might either worsen the condition, be ineffective, or cause side effects because of the underlying problems.

Your healthcare provider can also discuss with you the many options for childcare, at home or in various types of daycare. She may help you with school choices, transportation options for getting to and from school, after school programs, and summer programs and respite care. Partly because she sees many children, she will often know about these different programs in your area from other parents.

Finally, as we've mentioned, it is important that you and your child feel comfortable in your doctor's office and that the office staff feel comfortable with you and your child. Again, one reason routine office visits are important is that they give everyone a chance to see each other without the additional stress of an illness. Keep in mind that it will be easier to cope during a routine visit than during a visit when your child is not feeling well. For both kinds of visit, some advance preparation can be helpful.

Preparing Your Child for a Visit

If your child is new to the office, try to get some pictures of the staff ahead of time and even drive by the office to show your child where it is if that helps. (Some parents tell us it is better not to give too much advance notice if the child will start to obsess about the visit.) Also look in the library (or bookstores) for books about going to the doctor. There are some excellent books developed specifically for people with learning difficulties and developmental problems. (See the Reading List.)

For children with marked communication problems, using a visual storyboard or pictures of the doctor and the office may be helpful each time you visit. The storyboard might show pictures of things that will happen immediately before the visit and during the visit, as well as a rewarding thing that will happen right after.

Familiarity is a big key for children with autism/PDD. In addition to reading a picture book or storyboard, you may also want to prepare by getting in some practice at home with medical equipment. If you can get them cheaply, equipment like a stethoscope, blood pressure cuff, tongue depressor, and even an otoscope (the instrument doctors use to look in the ear) can help your child feel less anxious about what's in store for him. (Be careful, however, *not* to have your child put things in his ears). Show these instruments to your child and encourage him to touch and explore them so they don't feel so new or unfamiliar. If he is hesitant, use them on a stuffed animal or sibling.

If possible, schedule your child's visit for a time when your wait is likely to be minimal, such as the first appointment of the day. Once at the doctor's office, you may want to ask if there is a spare examination room that your child can become familiar with. Or, if there is more than one waiting area, ask for the smaller and quieter one.

Bring a couple of things your child will be interested in doing, even if he is a teenager. Even with the best of intentions, doctors often run late and they do not always stock their waiting rooms with activities that children with autism enjoy. You might bring a favorite toy, book, or activity. You might even try to find some special things that are only brought out for doctor's visits. For younger children, a treasured, favorite object may do the trick. Some parents find that planning something special after the appointment can be a good way of helping the child get through.

If your child is very anxious or has trouble with office visits, think about ways to help him relax. This can include the visual book but can also include social stories, relaxation training, and so forth. Don't dwell on any painful or uncomfortable procedures that he might be having in the office, but don't lie to him about what's going to happen either.

Sometimes parents are so worried about something like a blood test that they go to great lengths to "protect" their child and end up making things worse!

If you think you may need help keeping your child calm, bring another adult with you. This might be your spouse, a familiar staff member, or teacher if possible. A second supporter for your child can be reassuring for all concerned.

Physical Examination

Giving a child with an autism spectrum disorder a physical exam requires some flexibility on the doctor's part. The exam actually starts as the doctor enters the room and sees your child. The doctor observes how he moves, how he relates and communicates, and what he is doing in the room. Often staff will have already tried to weigh and measure your child and will have made observations about how cooperative he is. It is important that the doctor not unduly alarm your child. Because many children with autism and related disorders are very sensitive to touch, it usually is helpful if the doctor takes her time and approaches your child slowly, often with open hands, rather than with diagnostic instruments such as the stethoscope. When possible, it's best if your child can undress himself in the doctor's presence. This way, she can observe your child's motor skills and physical movements while he is undressing.

As with other children, explanations of what is going to happen are helpful. Giving your child a chance to become familiar with some of the instruments is a good idea. You might want to ask the doctor to demonstrate their use on you first. Work with your child in advance to teach important communication skills, such as words/signs/pictures for "stop" to give your child a way to let the doctor know to "back off" at least briefly. As a rule, it is best for doctors to examine the more sensitive areas, such as the ears or the mouth, at the very end of the examination.

Even with the best of intentions and procedures, children sometimes are intimidated and upset. They may attempt to grab the doctor, pull instruments away, push hands away, or throw things. Whenever possible, a parent or other caregiver who knows your child should be present and available to help calm him and make him feel comfortable. This will help the doctor in the long run. You can also help by letting the doctor know about your child's communication abilities or by serving as a translator between doctor and child.

Sometimes if your child is not cooperative, the doctor must modify the usual examination procedure. For example, a younger child may be more comfortable having his ears examined if he sits on your lap. If your child is going to have an injection or blood test, use of an anesthetic cream to numb the area may help. You always need to weigh the costs and benefits of persisting with a medical procedure that is traumatic for your child. For example, if you have to have four people hold your child down to look in his ears, is it worth it? (It may well be, if your child is having an ear infection and banging his head as a result; it may not be if there is no suspicion of ear infections.) Also keep in mind the best timing of procedures—saving the more complicated or uncomfortable things for last can be a help.

Laboratory Studies, X-rays, Scans

As part of regular physical checkups, periodic lab studies of blood and urine are usually needed. Sometimes these tests can be done in your pediatrician's office; other times you may be sent to an outside lab. As much as possible, you should request that these tests be done in the familiar setting of your doctor's office, even if that just means that the blood is drawn there and then sent to the outside lab to run the tests.

These tests become especially important if your child is receiving medication. Because children with autism and pervasive developmental disorders may sometimes eat non-food substances, a blood test called a lead screening should be part of the initial evaluation and then repeated periodically. This is particularly true for patients who are already known to eat non-food substances such as paint or dirt (a behavior called pica).

To minimize the pain from blood draws or shots, you can apply an anesthetic cream ahead of time. You no longer need a prescription for the cream. Ask the pharmacist if you have trouble finding it. You can also ask your doctor about using it.

Your healthcare provider or specialist may also recommend other tests such as X-rays, an EEG, CT, or MRI scans to follow ongoing problems or to understand new problems. These tests can be difficult for children with autism because they involve new and sometimes slightly intimidating equipment. As with other new experiences, familiarizing your child ahead of time with the equipment and procedures can help. Some places even have mock scanners to show children. It may be possible for your child to have a visit ahead of time. If your child needs an MRI scan, he may do better with an MRI machine that is open (the child doesn't have to be confined to a small space). For some children, sedation or even anesthesia may be needed before such procedures.

Immunizations

In the past, there were many childhood illnesses that almost all children had to suffer through in order to become immune to them. Many children in years gone by died from these illnesses and others suffered permanent brain damage. For example, Helen Keller became both blind and deaf as a result of a childhood infection that could, today, have been prevented. Now many infectious diseases can be prevented by vaccination. Some illnesses such as smallpox have been eliminated, which is why there is no longer a routine immunization requirement. Other illnesses, such as polio and measles, will hopefully be eliminated in the not-too-distant future. Sometimes the reason to immunize children is also to protect unborn children—for instance, so that pregnant women don't contract rubella and give it to their unborn child. Until these illnesses are eradicated, vaccinations are crucial: Around the world, about one million children will die this year from measles.

In the United States, there are currently eleven infectious diseases that children are routinely protected against by being immunized. In most states, ten of these immunizations are required before entry into daycare or school. There are a range of ages at which each vaccine can be given. The exact schedule will be influenced by several things:

- what your state or town requires,
- which combination the vaccines are given in,
- your pediatrician's preference as to how many shots to give at once, and, sometimes
- the availability of the vaccine to your doctor.

There have been shortages of several vaccines in recent years and the American Academy of Pediatrics and others have made changes in the recommended vaccine schedule to deal with these shortages. Some of these vaccines have been combined for some years now. Others have or will be combined in new ways—with the goal of giving fewer injections per child. The combinations of vaccines may also have different names in the future. Each company that produces vaccines has its own trade name for the individual vaccines. The names of the vaccines and the diseases they protect against are listed below with the approximate ages at which they are given. The following are the January 2003 recommendations of the Advisory Committee on Immunization Practices (www.cdc.gov/nip/acip), the American Academy of Pediatrics (www.aap.org), and the American Academy of Family Physicians (www.aafp.org).

- **DTaP – Diphtheria, Tetanus (lock jaw), Acellular Pertussis (whooping cough)**—Five shots in total are given at approximately 2, 4, 6, and 18 months and between 4-6 years; booster shots of tetanus and diphtheria are given every ten years to keep up your child's immunity. There is a new combination shot called Pediarix that includes five vaccines combined into one shot that has recently been licensed for use in the United States, and some doctors may be using it. It provides immunity against diphtheria, tetanus, pertussis, polio, and hepatitis B. There are many other combination vaccines being developed. If your child is hurt and the wound is felt to be dirty and at risk for tetanus, he will receive a booster shot if there have been 5 years since the last tetanus shot.

- **Polio (IPV – Inactivated Polio Virus)**—Four shots in total are given at approximately 2, 4, and 18 months and between 4-6 years.

- **Hepatitis B**—The series includes three shots in total. The first dose is always given at birth if a mother has hepatitis B, or sometime before two months if a mother does not have hepatitis B. Two more doses are given before eighteen months. It may also be given in combination with the Hib vaccine. If your child did not receive the Hepatitis B series starting earlier in life, he will be required by his school to get it in adolescence.

- **Hib (Haemophilus Influenza Type B)**—Before immunization began for Hib, it was the most common cause of childhood meningitis. The total is either three or four shots depending on whether it is given alone or in combination with the Hepatitis B vaccine. It is given at 2, 4, 6, and between 12-18 months, if given alone, or 2, 4, and between 15-18 months, if given in the current combination with Hepatitis B.

- **Pneumococcal Disease**—Bacterial pneumococcal disease can cause meningitis, serious blood infections, and pneumonia. It also causes some of the most difficult-to-treat-ear infections. This vaccine is the newest one and it is not currently required. It is recommended for all children less than 24 months and for those aged 24-59 months who are at increased risk for pneumococcal disease because of other medical conditions. The number of doses varies with the age of the child when it is started.

- **Varicella (chickenpox)**—One dose is all that is currently recommended unless the person receiving it is thirteen years or older, in which case he needs two doses four to eight weeks apart. Children are now receiving it between 12 and 18 months or later if they did not receive it at that age initially (a booster may be required in the future).

- **MMR – Measles, Mumps, Rubella (German Measles)**—Two doses are required, first between 12 and 15 months and second either before kindergarten or before junior high or middle school, depending on your state or local requirements.

- **Influenza**—This vaccine was recently suggested, although not formally recommended, for all children between the ages of six months and two years. It is not currently required to enter daycare or school. It may become available as a nasal spray, and when that happens and it is approved for younger children, it may be recommended and used more widely. It has long been advised for children with heart disease, diabetes, asthma requiring steroids, and disorders requiring aspirin therapy. This vaccine has to be given yearly in the fall before the flu season.

- **Hepatitis A**—This vaccine is recommended in some parts of the country and in certain situations.

As with blood draws for lab tests, you can use an anesthetic cream to numb your child's arm or leg before he is given shots. It will not prevent pain from shots as well as it does from drawing blood and placing an intravenous line, but it may help somewhat.

Your doctor will discuss the possible side effects of the vaccines with you before they are given. Many shots may cause some mild reactions such as redness or tenderness at the injection site. They may also cause fever and irritability, or at times, lethargy. If your child has a seizure disorder, your doctor may suggest that you give acetaminophen or ibuprofen before the shots to try to reduce the chance of a fever. This is because many children with seizure disorders are more likely to have a seizure when they have a fever. These medications also help reduce pain that may result from the shots. These reactions shouldn't be severe or last much longer than a day. If there are reactions that you are worried about, you should contact your doctor.

How Often to See the Doctor

Your doctor will tell you how often your child should come for preventive care visits. The frequency will depend on your child's age, whether or not he is your first

Do Vaccines Cause Autism?

At present, there is much concern that autism might sometimes be caused, or made worse, by measles immunization with the MMR shot. This was suggested in a study in which it was thought that persistent measles virus could be found in the gastrointestinal (GI) tract of a small number of children with autism. The fear that measles immunization (particularly the MMR combination) could cause autism led many parents, starting in Great Britain, to refuse the shot for their child.

It is true that some children with autism seem to be doing fine until some specific event—such as an immunization—after which they seem to regress. However, there are several things that make this whole business difficult to sort out. In the first place, it is possible that the apparent association between an immunization such as measles and the onset of regression is just that—only an *apparent* association. This possibility is even more likely since the vaccine is usually given at a time when parents start to notice possible developmental problems anyway. Secondly, the formulation of various vaccines has changed over the years and one would expect that changes in how the vaccine is made might be related to variations in rates of autism. Again, this is something that has not been demonstrated convincingly. In addition, in the original paper that suggested a possible association, the time between the measles shot and development of autism was as long as several months. A recent report from the National Academy of Sciences also did not find convincing evidence for the association of measles immunization with autism. A number of well-done scientific studies have now been done and do not support the idea that immunizations cause autism.

Some parents who are concerned about the MMR immunization arrange with their pediatrician to do the three immunizations separately—that is, as a measles shot at one time, a mumps shot at some other time, and a rubella shot at yet another time. The disadvantage with this is that it entails multiple shots instead of just one (and there is no specific information on exactly how far apart the shots should be given). It also has become harder to obtain the vaccines individually, and may become impossible in the future if the vaccines makers stop producing them individually. If your child has had an unusual reaction to immunizations or if you are concerned about the MMR immunization, you should discuss this with your child's doctor.

Yet another concern with immunizations relates to the use of small doses of mercury in a preservative called Thimerisol that was used in some vaccines. Again, this issue has been looked into and a number of studies are now available that do not support the idea that Thimerisol can cause autism. A committee for the National Academy of Sciences could find no evidence that Thimerisol was dangerous, but did suggest the elimination of mercury in vaccines just to be safe. (This has now been done, except in some flu vaccines.)

child, and whether there are concerns or problems that she is following. Typically your insurance company will only pay for a certain number of "well-child" visits per year—that is, visits when your child is coming in for preventive care and checkups rather than sickness. Usually the number the insurance covers will depend on your child's age.

A common schedule would be for your child to be seen daily in the hospital after his birth, then at two weeks, and then at two months, four months, six months, nine months, and a year. The second year, a child is usually seen at fifteen months and at eighteen months. Some pediatricians will also see children at twenty-one months. The next visits will be at two years and two-and-a-half years. Often it is between the ages of twelve and twenty-four months that parents, healthcare providers, or both first suspect autism. It is during this time that your healthcare provider is often most involved in helping you access specialists, assessment services, and early intervention.

Starting at age three, your child will often come only once a year for routine preventive care. Some insurance companies will only pay for a visit every two years starting at six years of age. This is actually rather unfortunate, since every visit helps your child get more familiar with the office.

Once your child reaches adolescence, some of the insurance companies will go back to covering annual check-ups. For children with autism, it is best if the child can be seen once a year for routine care. You may want to check with your insurance company to find out exactly how many preventive care visits they allow and at what ages they allow them. See Appendix B for information about health insurance.

Referrals to Specialists

Occasionally, your child's pediatrician may suggest laboratory tests or consultations with medical or nonmedical professionals (hearing tests, psychological tests, or tests of communication skills or of nutrition). Always feel free to ask why a doctor recommends a specific test or procedure. As a matter of course, your doctor should discuss with you if she feels another doctor should be involved. For example, your child's pediatrician might wish to have the opinion of a psychiatrist or a child psychiatrist if behavior modifying prescription medication is being considered. If your child has seizures, your pediatrician might suggest a consultation with a neurologist, who would then work with the pediatrician in the management of the seizures. Generally, your pediatrician or primary care provider will supply you with the names of specialists she feels would be appropriate; you may also get names from friends or other parents, but check with your pediatrician to be safe.

Sometimes specialists are located in your area. Other times they are some distance away. Usually the first time you meet a specialist, your pediatrician sends copies of any past records or a letter indicating why your child is being referred. You should take records of any past evaluations. As with your pediatrician, you should feel free to ask questions, particularly if medication is prescribed. Your pediatrician or primary care provider should be given the report of the specialist's recommendations and informed about new medications prescribed, since it is the primary doctor who will be most involved in your child's care. The pediatrician or primary doctor should serve as the manager for your child's health care; that is, she will gather information from all members of your child's healthcare team and coordinate treatment with educational and other professionals.

How to Get the Best Possible Care

The quality of your child's medical care depends a lot on you. You can often control not only who cares for you and for your child, but also how, when, and where that care is given. Always keep in mind that you know your child best, and you are responsible for making sure he receives good medical care. There are several steps you can take to make sure this happens.

1. **Always be a careful observer.** Often, indeed, usually, you're the primary source of information about your child. Particularly if your child has limited expressive language skills, the doctor, nurses, and other professionals have to rely on you for information. Not uncommonly, a change in your child's behavior may be the clue that an illness is beginning. As a careful observer, you can provide the doctor with important information.

2. **Discuss and try to anticipate your child's special needs.** Never hesitate to discuss any special needs or problems of your child. Try to anticipate what you and the doctor and her staff can do to make your child as comfortable as possible.

3. **Don't pass up the routine checkups.** It's particularly important for your child to see the doctor for routine checkups under circumstances that are less stressful. Routine (well child) visits also give you a chance to talk with the doctor in a situation that is less pressured than during a sick or emergency visit. In addition, these visits give your doctor a chance to observe your child when he is not ill.

4. **Ask questions and get information.** The doctor can provide you with valuable information, as much as you can provide the doctor. Most physicians are very sympathetic to your need and your right to know. They should explain medical terms, procedures, and issues in plain language. If you don't understand something, you should always ask. Unless you understand your child's needs and problems, you can't be sure he is getting the most appropriate care.

5. **Keep a record.** You may want to keep a notebook with reports of previous evaluations and past specialists; the information can be helpful to physicians who do not know your child.

   Especially during the first visit, the doctor may ask you to provide more extensive history about your child and family. You can feel comfortable talking about the results of past evaluations even if you don't agree with all parts of them. By showing the doctor that you can discuss differences of opinion reasonably, you encourage her to communicate just as openly with you. If the doctor resists open discussions with you, consider finding another physician.

   Often a careful history can be more helpful to the doctor than the physical examination when you have made an appointment to discuss a specific problem. Keep in mind that as time goes on, many parents accumulate a large notebook full of all kinds of information. Not all of this will be immediately relevant and might easily be overwhelming to the doctor. Try to give her the right amount of information; for example, if your child has been sick, she will want to know for how long, what the symptoms have been, what your child's current medicines are, etc. When you go to a specialist who hasn't seen your child before, be sure to bring along your notebook, so the specialist can, with your permission, copy whatever she wants to.

It is very helpful to put together a short (one-page) summary of important medical information, such as the one on the next page, that travels with your child and is readily available. This can come in handy if your child becomes ill or has an accident at school, at camp, or at a summer day program. This document should include a very short summary of your child's history and diagnosis, alerting the doctor to the nature of your child's disability and what special issues he has. This one-page summary should also list any chronic medical problems your child has, as well as past medical problems such as unusual responses to infection, neurological problems, seizures, past illnesses, hospitalizations, and surgeries. Be sure to list any allergies, particularly drug allergies. Also include a current list of any medications your child is on. The summary should also, of course, have your name and various phone numbers, as well as those of your child's primary doctor and other family members or friends who should be called if you are not available.

6. **Teach healthcare.** Teach your child about going to the doctor through books, pictures, play, videos, and other sources. Work with school staff to teach some basic aspects of personal self-care, including personal hygiene. Also work with the school staff on helping your child acquire important basic functional words and concepts—understanding body parts, the idea that something hurts, and so forth. (See Chapter 4 for ideas for teaching your child to communicate about pain.)

The Pharmacist's Role

An understanding and helpful pharmacist can make an enormous difference to your life. One who can compound (make up) medications can be especially important with children who are hard to get medication into. You are more likely to find such a pharmacist at a small, independently owned pharmacy, but occasionally you may be lucky enough to find one working for a large pharmacy chain.

Does your child give you a hard time about taking his medications? Do you dread the fight involved in getting medications or supplements into him? Does your child react to the coloring or additives in drugs? A compounding pharmacist may be able to help with those problems. He or she may be able to change the flavor of a medication or suggest tasty treats that a medication can be mixed in without compromising its effectiveness. Certain additives may be avoided if the pharmacist knows that it is important

Summary of Medical History Information

Child's name: _____ Date of birth: _____

Parents' names: _____

Address: _____

Home phone: _____ Work phone: _____

Healthcare provider name: _____ Phone: _____

Other person to contact in emergency: _____

School: _____

PDD Diagnosis: _____

Level of communication and behavioral issues: _____

_____

Medical problems (e.g., seizures, asthma): _____

_____

Medications patient is taking (name and dose): _____

_____

Allergies to medications: _____

_____

Other allergies: _____

_____

Unusual reactions to medications: _____

_____

Hospitalizations: _____

_____

Surgeries: _____

_____

for your child. You may need to ask around among other parents or your child's doctor to find a good pharmacist. The search will pay off in the end.

Using the same pharmacy for all prescription medications is important. Be sure to tell your pharmacist if your child has any medication allergies. That way the pharmacy computer will have all of your child's medications listed and indicate a problem immediately if a new medication should be avoided because of earlier allergy experiences or incompatibility with other medication that your child is taking. This is especially important if you have prescriptions from several different doctors. A psychiatrist may prescribe one medication to help with your child's behavior and a neurologist may prescribe something else for his seizures. At times these physicians may be unaware of the other medications that your child is on and prescribe something that cannot be mixed with the other medications. You should also mention to the pharmacist if your child is on any nonprescription medications that might interact with the prescription medicines. Many pharmacy computers will supply you with a list of all the possible side effects to look for with a new medication.

Whenever a doctor is prescribing a new medication for your child, be sure she knows of any medications that your child has had trouble with in the past. Some medications can cause side effects that are not allergies but that you would not want to have occur again.

As we have mentioned before, you are your child's best advocate and you can always provide the most accurate and up-to-date medical history on your own child. A good pharmacist can be an enormous help, however.

The School Nurse's Role

The school nurse can play a very important role in your child's life. She will often be the person at school who is most knowledgeable about your child's medical problems. She may be involved daily with your child if he needs to take medication while at school. She may be a great comfort to him because she knows him so well.

Most states require the school nurse to have a signed permission slip from a doctor before she can give medication to any child, even something used so often as acetaminophen (Tylenol®). Before school starts for a new year, you will need to have your doctor fill out a permission slip for each medication that your child will take at school on a daily basis or even just occasionally.

Alert the school nurse when your child changes medications (or when the dose is changed) so she can be on the lookout for side effects. You should also make sure that the nurse has information from your child's pediatrician about any possible emergency situations that may arise, such as serious food allergies or seizures. It is best if the nurse plus the teachers have a plan in place before school starts to deal with any of these possible emergencies. The nurse should know how to reach you in the case of an emergency and whether or not your child should be given any medication such as diphenhydramine (Benedryl®) or an EpiPen® to deal with the problem immediately. She should also know whether to call 911, and if so, exactly when she should do that. If your child does have known life-threatening allergies, treatment should be started and emergency medical services called to transport him to the hospital if he eats a food he is allergic to.

If your child has seizures, the nurse should know what to expect. Does he lose consciousness with the seizures or does he just "space out" briefly and then recover on his own? Does he usually need further medication to stop the seizures? See Chapter 9 for more information about seizures and autism.

Making a point of getting to know the school nurse usually helps parents feel more comfortable about leaving their child at a new school. If the school nurse is not at school full time, find out what the arrangements are for coverage. Sometimes nurses will cover several schools; in other school districts there will be a nurse at each school.

Medical Conditions More Common in Autism and Related Disorders

Fragile X Syndrome

Fragile X syndrome is a common syndrome associated with mental retardation, and, sometimes, with autism. It is probably second only to Down syndrome as the most identified genetic source of mental retardation. The condition is X-linked. That is, it is passed on in the mother's X chromosome to the child, and, like most X-linked disorders, it occurs more frequently in boys. The cause of the condition has been identified in a particular abnormality in a specific gene on the X chromosome.

Associated problems in fragile X syndrome include mild mental retardation (although sometimes IQ is in the normal range). Boys with the disorder may have some unusual body features such as large ears and genitals; the face may be long and narrow; and the palate (the roof of the mouth) may be unusually high and arched. Some individuals with this condition have seizures.

In addition to mental retardation, behavioral problems can include hyperactivity, difficulties with attention, anxiety, repetitive motor mannerisms (stereotypies), aggression, impaired speech and language skills, difficulty making eye contact, and extreme shyness. Children with Fragile X syndrome seem particularly likely to have greater degrees of attentional difficulty than other children with mental retardation. Medical treatments for many of these behavioral difficulties are discussed in Chapter 13.

Tuberous Sclerosis

Tuberous sclerosis is a disease that affects about 1 in 10,000 people, and, although rare, has been noted to be significantly associated with autism. As Chapter 1 explained, symptoms of tuberous sclerosis include the growth of unusual tissue (tubers) or benign tumors in the skin, eye, brain, and other organs, as well as white patches on the skin at birth. The tumors associated with this disorder are often seen in the preschool years and may increase in frequency during puberty. These growths are "benign" in the sense that, unlike cancer, they do not spread. Their effect on growth and development can be very serious, however.

Although the effects of the disorder can be severe, the degree of severity in individual children is quite variable. Sometimes the first symptoms are seen in infancy or early childhood—often with the onset of seizures. Between 50 to 60 percent of affected individuals show mental retardation and about 80 percent have seizures. Sometimes the findings include a specific abnormality in brainwave (EEG) testing. The seizures may include a specific kind of muscle spasm known as myoclonic jerks. See Chapter 9 for information about medical treatment of seizures.

Children with tuberous sclerosis may have speech delays and learning problems, even if they do not have mental retardation. They often have motor problems as well. All children with developmental delays and seizures should be carefully examined for the physical signs of tuberous sclerosis. See the Resource Guide for sources of additional information about tuberous sclerosis.

Seizure Disorders

Epilepsy (recurrent seizures) is the medical condition most commonly seen in autism and related disorders. Because as many as 25 percent of strictly diagnosed children with autism may develop epilepsy, we devote an entire chapter to seizure disorders and their treatment later in this book. Even if your child does not have seizures now, it is important to know something about them since they can develop as he gets older. Sometimes seizures are pretty difficult to miss; at other times it may be quite easy to miss them.

Optimal seizure management is important for healthcare in several respects. Their treatment is obviously important since having seizures can interfere with learning. On the other hand, there also are risks associated with treating seizures. The medicines used to treat seizures have side effects and the blood level of medications often must be monitored (and used to adjust the dose). Other blood work may be needed to rule out possible side effects. In addition, children with seizures, particularly seizures that are not well controlled, may be at increased risk for accident and injury.

Summary

In this chapter, we've reviewed some aspects of healthcare in autism. We have emphasized that finding a good healthcare provider is really important and worth spending extra time on. We also discussed the importance of helping your child become familiar with the doctor's office and office staff and of paying attention to routine care and immunizations. We advocated for keeping a short medical summary with your child—particularly if he has any important medical conditions. Even if he doesn't, it will be good to have a summary that can be used in case of emergency. We finished with a discussion of some of the most common medical problems you may encounter, as well as other disorders that have been associated with autism. The next two chapters continue the discussion of medical care for children with autism by delving into issues related to caring for your child when he is sick or injured.

Questions

Q. My daughter is really phobic about going to the doctor. She freaks out when she sees the stethoscope—not to mention the thing the doctor looks in her ears with. We get so anxious taking her to doctors. What can we do to prevent all this?

There are a couple of things you can do. You can attempt to gradually familiarize your child with medical "stuff." See if you can get her a doctor's kit to play with. Sometimes doctors' offices will have old stethoscopes children can see. One of the functions for typically developing children of "playing doctor" is to deal with their anxieties about going to the doctor. In that respect, your daughter's response may be pretty normal. She may, however, lack some of the abilities to put this into words. See if looking at some books about going to the doctor helps. You could also try taking pictures and/or developing a story about going to the doctor. If the problem persists, talk with the school psychologist or someone with experience in managing behavior problems to try to come up with a way to make the experience more positive for her.

Q. My husband's employment recently changed and we have a new insurance company. It seems like we'll have to change our son's pediatrician since he doesn't participate. Is this a good idea?

If you have had a good experience so far with your current pediatrician, it is *not* a good idea. Try to find out why your pediatrician doesn't participate or whether you might have a choice of insurance plans and still be able to have the same doctor. Although switching pediatricians is more and more common (for the reasons you mention), it is not a good idea for someone with chronic medical problems and with difficulties adjusting to new people and places.

Q. My child hates going to the doctor's office, so I usually go only when I have to. Is this a mistake?

Yes, it is a mistake. The more familiar you and your child are with the office, the less traumatic it will be to go—particularly when your child is not feeling well anyway. Talk to your child's doctor and maybe the office staff to see what they can do to help you (for example, giving you the first appointment of the day or giving your child a room of his own to wait in). Try to go just to get acquainted and have a special treat for your child waiting at the office. If need be, get the help of a behavioral psychologist so that you can work out a plan to help your child feel more comfortable. It will pay off in the long run!

4 | Coping with Common Medical Problems

In Chapter 3, we discussed some of the ways that routine medical care for children with autism spectrum disorders can be more challenging. In this chapter, we talk about common childhood illnesses and injuries and aspects of dealing with these problems in children with ASDs. Our emphasis is on the challenge of diagnosing these problems in children with autism spectrum disorders. We will mention some issues relevant to treatment, but remember, your child's healthcare provider is the most important source of information on treatment for your child.

Dealing with a Sick Child

Generally speaking, children with autism are no more nor less susceptible to the usual range of childhood illnesses. However, when children with autism *are* ill, the child's difficulties communicating what is wrong, dealing with the doctor and other medical professionals, and following through with treatment can complicate diagnosis and treatment.

This section reviews some of the medical problems most common in autism and other pervasive developmental disorders. Because we devote Chapter 9 to seizures, we don't cover that topic here. We also won't cover safety and accidents, since these are covered in Chapter 7. Although we talk about some of the more common problems, please bear in mind that your child will not necessarily have any of them. On the other hand, it is possible that your child will have some less common medical condition we do not cover here. It goes without saying—even though we are now saying it—that the information provided here is *general* information and your child's healthcare professional is the best source of information *specific* to your child. Also keep in mind that, as parents, you are an important part of the medical treatment team. You can provide information on history as well as your child's responses to previous treatments—which is an invaluable part of the healthcare process.

How Do You Know When Your Child Is Sick?

There are many different ways that parents can tell when their child is sick. The child can have a fever, a rash, a cough or runny nose, upset stomach with vomiting and diarrhea, or one of many other symptoms. Sometimes a change in behavior is the only sign of an illness. It can, at times, be a real detective project to find the cause of the changes that you notice. Many children who have an ASD are on medications to help with behaviors or to treat a seizure disorder. At times these medications can cause adverse reactions and sometimes this can complicate the task of figuring out what is really going on when your child is ill.

Children who are not yet talking present special problems for medical professionals. Of course, in some ways, these problems are similar to those faced by pediatricians every day as they deal with infants. For example, when the patient can't communicate very well, the doctor has to rely a lot on the history or information you provide about the illness. The doctor also can rely on what he sees while watching the child, as well as on what he finds on the physical examination, and, sometimes, on laboratory tests, X-rays, or other special procedures. There are some major differences, however, between dealing with a nonverbal eight-month-old and a nonverbal eight-year-old. Some of these are discussed below.

How to Know When Your Child Is in Pain

There are several reasons that it can be difficult to recognize that a child with an ASD is in pain. First, children with autism may not experience pain in the same way that other children do. And second, they can have a great deal of difficulty communicating about their pain.

Some children with autism don't seem to mind pain very much. We've known children with appendicitis who didn't complain at all. Sometimes the doctor may be surprised the child was not "acting sicker." (Some children seem to have a high tolerance for pain.) Other children may be bothered quite a bit even by a small amount of discomfort. For these children, difficulties with change and inability to deal with even minor annoyances can create major behavior problems. As your child gets older, you'll have an increasingly better sense of how she deals with pain.

Children who are not yet using words to communicate present the greatest challenges when they are ill. As the individual who knows your child best, be alert for any changes in your child's behavior or appearance. Behaviors that suggest pain in children with autism include:

- **Moaning, whimpering, unusual crying:** These vocalizations may or may not be associated with changes in facial expression suggesting pain.
- **Changes in eating or sleeping habits:** For example, your child may refuse favorite foods or seem to be sleeping more. Sometimes your child may seem sleepy much more of the time than usual.
- **Changes in activity or behavior:** This can include either unusual lack of activity or over activity. Some children may start to become self-abusive if they are in pain—for example, hitting their head on the floor or with their hand if they have earaches, dental pain, or sinus infections. Pain in an arm or leg might result in changes in your child's movement. Occasionally, parents tell us that their child's behavior actually improves when the child is sick. For example, the child may be more talkative (this is probably related to the stress of being ill).

■ **Changes in appearance:** Although it can sometimes be hard for you to put into words, you'll sometimes notice that your child just looks ill. As the person who knows your child the best, you may be the first one to realize this.

Sometimes, particularly when pain or discomfort is chronic, you and the doctor have to work together to try to track down the source of the behavior change. It can be helpful to take a broad view of your child. For example, for an adolescent girl who has behavior difficulties on a monthly basis, you might wonder about whether your daughter is having discomfort in relation to getting her period or to that time in the menstrual cycle when ovulation (passage of the egg from the ovaries) occurs. Similarly, changes in behavior in association with the seasons might suggest seasonal allergies. As we mentioned, the sudden onset of self-injurious behavior can also be the first sign of illness due to pain from an ear infection or new teeth (this can include the eruption of the "wisdom teeth" or third molars in adolescence).

Helping Your Child Communicate about Pain

Children who can communicate verbally are often able to talk about pain or discomfort. They may, however, use very personal or idiosyncratic language. For example, saying "My stomach hurts" may, for some children, mean many different things—not literally that it is the stomach that is hurting. On the other hand, many children will mean exactly what they say.

Other children may have an unconventional way of saying they are in pain. Sometimes they may say a phrase that they first heard when they were sick. Clearly, language of this type would be very difficult for a doctor to understand correctly without your help!

Other children may have some language but cannot communicate in detail or use conventional gestures that otherwise might help localize pain. Use of visual aids and other communication supports may be helpful. For instance, you could show your child a doll or a picture of a girl and ask her to indicate where on the doll it hurts—this will work for some children but not for others.

Some excellent resources are provided in the Reading List. Picture books (for example, the series from the Royal College of Psychiatrists in Great Britain series) have been specifically developed both to review (in advance) what happens when the child (with a disability) goes to a doctor (or to the hospital) and to help her communicate about what happens there. Other books were designed for typically developing children but also can be quite appropriate. Without too much effort, you can also make your own picture books (using photos of your child, the doctor, and doctor's office).

If your child is verbal, it is important to work with the speech-language pathologist to make sure your child has some words she can use to communicate pain and feelings of discomfort. And if your child is nonverbal, you and the SLP should try to figure out a way she can use PECS (Picture Exchange Communication System), manual sign language, or other adaptive aids to communicate that she's in pain. Finally, if your child doesn't seem to understand the meaning of the words "pain" or "hurt," you need to teach her that concept somehow, such as by saying "Ouch, that hurts" every time you sustain a minor injury, or pointing out when your child must be hurting.

Common Medical Problems in Children

Children with autism and PDD can develop any of the medical problems that typical children can develop. Because of their communication and developmental difficulties, it can be harder for a parent or a medical professional to recognize that a child with autism is sick. It can also be harder to diagnose the problem.

Infections

Infections occur when viruses or bacteria invade the body; the body's natural defenses (the immune system) then become active in fighting off the infection in various ways. In some cases, particularly with bacterial infections, the doctor can supply medicine (antibiotics) that help the body fight off infections. These medicines may help shorten the length of an infectious illness or its severity. For viral infections, fewer medicines are available, although immunizations can be given to prevent some viral illnesses in the first place. (We talk about immunizations in Chapter 3.)

While infections can involve any part of the body, the most commonly seen involve the ears, eyes, nose, throat, sinuses, and skin, and the respiratory, gastrointestinal, and urinary tracts. Most infections are caused by a virus and will get better by themselves without antibiotics. Examples include colds, chickenpox, and most GI viruses.

Infections can be harder to diagnosis in children with autism because the child is less likely to complain of pain or discomfort. The infection may present itself only as a

What to Do When Your Child Has a Fever

Children frequently get fevers when they are sick. It is often a parent's first clue that their child has some kind of infection. Fever by itself is not necessarily bad. Some children tend to have higher or more frequent fevers than other children. The height of the fever does not indicate how serious the infection is, although the height of the fever is important. Discuss this issue with your doctor and ask if there is a specific fever at which you should always call.

We treat fevers for several different reasons. An important reason is that a child will often feel better and act more like herself when the temperature comes down. In addition, fevers can lower the seizure threshold. That is, if your child has seizures, she may be more likely to have one when she has a fever. Most pediatricians recommend acetaminophen (Tylenol®) or ibuprofen (Motrin® or Advil®) to bring down a temperature. Many children greatly prefer one of the newer thermometers that measure the temperature in the ear or on the forehead from the temporal artery instead of an oral or rectal thermometer. Temperatures taken this way are generally pretty accurate and make for less stress if your child doesn't want anything like a thermometer in her mouth. Do not use mercury thermometers (which are no longer available on the market due to the risk of children ingesting mercury if the thermometer breaks).

dramatic change in your child's behavior or as a fever. Observing your child and keeping track of the events leading up to the time she goes to the doctor helps the doctor understand the way the illness developed and may help determine the cause of the illness.

Infections unfortunately are a part of growing up. Fortunately, however, many steps can be taken to reduce the frequency and severity of infections in children with ASDs. For example, teaching your child (and other family members) to wash their hands well (with soap and water) or use a handkerchief or Kleenex when coughing can help. You can teach these skills in a very explicit, step-by-step manner—using yourself as an example, picture cards, and other visual aids. You can also try to reduce your child's exposure to large numbers of people with infections in schools and daycare centers. In addition, a number of infections can be prevented through immunization, as discussed in Chapter 3. The sections below discuss common childhood infections that cannot yet be prevented through immunization.

Gastrointestinal Infections (GI "Bugs")

A gastrointestinal (GI) infection is any infection in the stomach or intestinal tract. Often this leads to stomach ache, vomiting, diarrhea (or all three). It can be referred to by several different names—gastroenteritis, GI bugs, or intestinal flu. GI bugs are easy to pass around, and sometimes poor toileting skills, especially if there are large numbers of people in a school or a group setting, may result in gastrointestinal disease occurring in an entire grade or school group at the same time. Usually the diagnosis of gastrointestinal illness is not difficult because the vomiting or diarrhea is quite obvious.

Finding the cause of a GI infection may take some time. Most of them are caused by viruses and are self-limited and will be over in a week or less. If they last longer or there is diarrhea with blood in it, your doctor will probably start to look for a specific cause for the illness. As mentioned earlier, most are caused by viruses, but some are caused by bacteria or parasites.

The treatment for most GI infections generally consists of dietary changes and encouragement of fluids to avoid dehydration. Usually doctors recommend clear liquids and avoidance of dairy products. A BRAT diet (bananas, rice, apple, and toast) is recommended by some doctors for younger children, or a generally bland diet for older children. Avoidance of fatty, fried, or spicy foods is recommended. A few bacterial GI infections such as Shigella and Campylobacter are treated with antibiotics, but others such as Salmonella and E. Coli 0157 are not. In fact, a patient may be made worse by treating these infections with antibiotics. Parasitic infections are most commonly treated with antibiotics.

The most important aspect of caring for a child with vomiting and/or diarrhea is the prevention of dehydration. If your child shows signs of dehydration, contact your doctor immediately. Signs include unusual lethargy, dry mouth, lack of tears, and decreased urination. It is always better to check in with your doctor if the vomiting or diarrhea occurs more than a few times and have him help you assess whether dehydration is starting. If the dehydration worsens, your child may require a visit to the emergency room to have fluids given intravenously.

The best way to prevent GI infections is to foster good hand washing routines in children after the use of the bathroom and for caretakers involved in diapering or toileting to be extra careful about washing their own hands. Keeping sick children out of daycare or school until their vomiting or diarrhea has completely stopped is another important way to prevent the spread of gastrointestinal infections.

A parasitic infection with pinworms (Enterobiasis) can also contribute to behavior change because it can cause intense rectal itching. Pinworms can be hard to detect unless the doctor knows of the severe itching it is causing and instructs you to look for the pinworms in the peri-anal area late at night or first thing in the morning before your child gets out of bed. They are minute but visible and can be seen to move. Your doctor may give you a kit with a small plastic paddle in it to touch to the area with the pinworms. They will stick to the paddle and your doctor can look under the microscope to identify them or send it to the lab to have it looked at. Sometimes people just put a piece of scotch tape over the area with the pinworms and they stick and can be taken to the doctor for inspection.

Urinary Tract Infections (UTI)

Urinary tract infections occur when bacteria infect the urinary tract. These infections are much more common in girls than in boys. Poor hygiene and inadequate cleaning after going to the bathroom can make this kind of infection more likely. Children need to be reminded to wipe from front to back. Irritation of the perineum from soaps or bubble bath may make UTIs more likely for some children, as can constipation.

The most common symptoms of a UTI are pain on urination, increased frequency of urination, and urgency (which means feeling like you have to go immediately). Fever, general irritability, abdominal discomfort, and low back pain may also develop. At times, vomiting and diarrhea are the only clues. If your child develops new onset of daytime or nighttime wetting after she has been routinely dry, you should look for a UTI.

A child with autism or PDD with a urinary tract infection may not complain of pain on urination as other children might. A fever or new onset of bed-wetting or daytime accidents may be the only clues. Your child may suddenly be going to the bathroom more often than usual. Sometimes a change in behavior—such as increased irritability— can be a clue. In an infant, the only apparent symptoms of a UTI might be a high or persistent fever.

It can be a challenge to obtain a urine specimen from a girl with an ASD. Ideally, you should wash your daughter's perineum with soap and water and then collect a specimen directly into a sterile container. If your child doesn't want you holding a cup under her while she is on the toilet, try sterilizing a bowl from a potty seat with boiling water and having her urinate on the potty and then transferring the urine into another sterile container. Having your child take a bath first may make it unnecessary to wipe her first if she resists that.

If your child has repeated UTIs, your doctor will probably want to do some testing to see why it is happening. The younger your child is, especially under three years, or the sicker your child is with the UTI, the more likely the doctor is to do further testing. This usually involves an ultrasound of the kidney and urinary tract or a more invasive test called a voiding cystourethrogram (VCUG). This procedure involves placing a small catheter into the bladder and injecting some dye to see where it goes. Some children have what is known as reflux, which means that some urine from the bladder goes back up towards the kidneys instead of it all going directly to the outside. Some children may need to be sedated for this test.

A UTI is treated with antibiotics. If your child is not too sick, she will be treated with oral antibiotics for approximately ten days. If she has a high fever, and especially if she is vomiting and can't hold down oral antibiotics, she will need to be hospitalized for intravenous antibiotics. If your child has severe or repeated infections, she might be kept on antibiotics for a long time to prevent recurrences.

Respiratory Infections and Sinus Infections

Colds are infections that affect the upper respiratory system (head and neck). Infections of the lower respiratory system (lungs and bronchi or tubes that bring the air to the lungs) are called pneumonia and bronchitis. Sometimes the sinuses (airspaces in the skull behind the face) can become infected—this is called sinusitis.

In general, you do not need to bring your child to the doctor if she has a simple cold (with only a cough and a runny/stuffed nose). There are, however, some times when you should bring her in to see the doctor—or, at a minimum, talk to the doctor's office about it. For example:

- **You suspect she has strep throat.** You may look into her mouth and see that the tonsils are very large and red, sometimes with white patches on them, or she may act as if her throat hurts. Most pediatric offices can now do a quick test for strep infection while the patient is in the office. This involves quickly swabbing your child's tonsils with a Q-tip. You may need to hold her still for this or help to open her mouth so that it can be done.
- **You suspect she has a sinus infection.** If she has continued congestion beyond seven to ten days, mucus is very thick and discolored, her breath has begun to have a foul odor, or you think she has a headache, she may have a sinus infection. Sinus infections can usually be diagnosed by the history and physical exam. At times your doctor may recommend X-ray studies.
- **If your child has a persistent cough, she should see the doctor.** The doctor may order X-rays to evaluate this symptom.

Middle Ear Infections

Infections of the middle ear (otitis media) are one of the most common problems for which children are taken to the doctor. They occur when the fluid in the middle ear— that is, on the other side of the eardrum from the ear canal—becomes infected. Most children have at least one ear infection by the age of two, and many have more. As your child gets older, you can expect the frequency of these infections to decrease. Ear infections are also common in children with autism spectrum disorders. Given the potential of ear infections to interfere with hearing, prompt treatment and control is important.

Anything that makes your child more congested—such as an upper respiratory infection or allergy—will make an ear infection more likely to occur. They can also occur in someone who is otherwise perfectly healthy.

The signs and symptoms of an ear infection will vary with your child's age and with her ability to communicate. Ear infections can cause fever and pain as well as impaired hearing and disturbed balance. As a result, some of the common symptoms of an ear infection are: irritability, especially when your child is lying down, poor feeding, trouble sleeping, inattention, and increased oppositional behavior. The signs can include pulling at the ears or hair, or banging the head against the floor, crib, or bed. Poor balance and falling can also indicate a middle ear problem. Sometimes the eardrum breaks and you will see pus or bloody fluid coming out of the ear. Fevers can at times be the only clue that your child has an ear infection, although not every child will have a fever with every ear infection. Occasionally, the only symptom of an ear infection is a cough. Some children never have any symptoms from an ear infection and it is discovered at a routine health check.

Your pediatrician will make the diagnosis of a middle ear infection by looking into your child's ear and looking at the eardrum with a special instrument called an otoscope that lights up and magnifies the area. Sometimes the doctor will need to remove wax from the ear canal to see the eardrum. This can be done by flushing the wax out with water or picking it out with a plastic curette. The doctor will probably need your help in holding your child still to look in the ear. If your child moves around, the examination of the ear is more likely to be uncomfortable. If your child can't hold still, you may have to try putting some special drops in the ear so that the wax can be more easily washed out at another visit. (Do not try to attempt to remove ear wax any other way or you may injure your child.) Giving your child the chance to get acquainted with the doctor (and his instruments) while not ill makes it easier to examine her when she is not feeling well.

Occasionally, it is impossible to clean the wax out enough to see the eardrum and make the diagnosis of an ear infection. Your doctor might consider giving you a prescription for antibiotics if your child has a history of ear infections and he is pretty sure from your child's behavior that she has another one. If this is done, your doctor is going to want to know if the symptoms are gone and your child is feeling better in one to two days. The sicker your child looks, the less likely the doctor is to treat her without seeing the eardrum and knowing the exact diagnosis. Doctors always worry about under-treating or mistreating a more serious infection if they do not know the exact diagnosis.

Ear infections can be caused by either viral or bacterial infections. The doctor cannot tell by examining the ear which is causing it, but it is more common for it to be caused by bacterial infection. These are the types of infections that antibiotics can cure.

We treat ear infections with antibiotics for several reasons. First, to make your child more comfortable and to correct whatever other problems the infection has caused, such as decreased hearing or poor balance. Second, to prevent any more serious infections from developing such as mastoiditis (an infection of the mastoid bone behind the ear) or meningitis (an infection of the covering of the brain). These complications are fortunately very rare. In fact, recently there has been more of a problem with the overuse of antibiotics and the development of bacteria that are now resistant to the commonly used antibiotics. Because of this, your pediatrician may recommend giving your child medicine such as acetaminophen (Tylenol®) or ibuprofen (Motrin® or Advil®) for pain relief and then waiting and watching for a day or two to see if the ear infection will clear up without antibiotics. If it doesn't improve on its own, or if your child is very uncomfortable when the ear infection is diagnosed or appears quite ill to your doctor, he will probably prescribe antibiotics right away.

Sometimes parents note improvement fairly quickly after starting antibiotics and take this as a sign that the infection is cleared; this may not be the case. It is important to take antibiotics for the full length of time prescribed, even though your child should feel better in one to two days. Most of the antibiotics are taken for ten days, but a few are taken for only five days. Rarely, a single shot of antibiotics is used. If the ear infection does not clear up on the first antibiotic, your doctor will need to prescribe another. Unfortunately, as mentioned, with more widespread use of antibiotics these days there are now bacteria that are resistant to many of the antibiotics. Rarely, children need to see an ear specialist (otolaryngologist or ENT) to have the fluid in the middle ear cultured to see which bacteria is present and what antibiotic it is sensitive to. Your child might also be referred to an ENT if she has chronic ear infections.

Chronic Ear Infections. If your child has frequent ear infections, or if fluid remains in the middle ear after an infection for three months or longer, your child may need to have pressure equalizing tubes surgically placed in the eardrum to restore hearing or prevent infections.

There are times when enlarged adenoids contribute to the problem of recurrent ear infections by blocking the Eustachian tubes and making it hard for the middle ear fluid to drain out. In such cases, their removal will be recommended along with the placement of pressure equalizing tubes. The tonsils are not usually removed unless they have also been infected repeatedly or are causing other problems such as sleep apnea.

The decision to have surgery to put in pressure equalizing tubes will be made only after weighing the risks and benefits involved. Your child will require general anesthesia and usually a short stay in an outpatient surgery center. In some areas, a hospitalization may be required. You will want to have an anesthesiologist and an ENT surgeon (otolaryngologist) who are experienced with children. For children with language and communication problems, often the risk is worth the greater potential benefit of improved hearing and fewer infections. However, decisions are always made jointly by you and your doctor.

Swimmer's Ear (Infection of the Outer Ear)

Children with autism should be taught to swim for many reasons. It is great exercise and (more importantly) helps prevent drowning (see Chapter 7). Children who spend a great deal of time swimming can develop swimmer's ear (otitis externa). This is an infection and inflammation of the ear canal (the part of the ear between the eardrum and the outside of the ear). It can also be caused by local trauma, such as having a cotton tip applicator pushed too far or too forcefully into the ear canal. Usually this is done in an attempt to remove wax, but more often it pushes the wax further in and can injure the sides of the ear canal. If your child has swimmer's ear, she will usually complain of pain (or look as if she is pain) when you move the ear or push in front of it. It may also be painful for her to lie on that ear or to open her mouth wide, which may move the affected area. In addition, her ear may have a discharge with an unpleasant odor.

Swimmer's ear is diagnosed in the same way as a middle ear infection—that is, by looking into the ear with an otoscope. It is usually treated with eardrops—either antibiotics alone, or a combination of antibiotics and steroids to help reduce the inflammation.

Occasionally oral antibiotics are also needed. Sometimes if the infection is very bad, a wick is placed in the ear canal to make it easier for the drops to get into the ear.

If your child gets recurrent swimmer's ear, it is worth trying to prevent it by using special eardrops to try to dry out the ear canal after swimming. There are many nonprescription brands of drops intended for this use. You can check with your pharmacist about which brands he carries. Do not use them if your child has pressure equalizing tubes in her ears, however. Some ENT doctors recommend that children with PE tubes wear specially molded ear plugs while swimming.

Conjunctivitis

Conjunctivitis or pink eye is an inflammation of the outer covering of the eye. It can be caused by either allergies or infection, as well as by irritation or injury. The infections can be either viral or bacterial. As you know, bacterial infections are the ones that improve with antibiotics.

You will know that your child has this problem if you see that her eye looks red, with or without drainage. With bacterial infections, the drainage is usually thick and either yellow or green. If you wipe it away, more will appear. In the morning, there may be crusting along the edges of the eyes and the lids may at first seem stuck shut. With viral infections, the drainage may be thinner and is less likely to be discolored. There may be no drainage at all with allergic conjunctivitis. However, with allergic conjunctivitis, both eyes will be affected and usually itchy. There are other causes of red eyes, so you should check with your healthcare provider if you notice this in your child.

The treatment varies depending on the cause of the conjunctivitis. Bacterial infections are treated with antibiotic eye drops. Occasionally oral antibiotics are used if there is also an ear infection or if it is impossible to get drops into the eyes. When conjunctivitis is due to allergies, it is treated with antihistamines, taken either orally or as eye drops. These will hopefully help decrease or prevent the itching and keep your child from rubbing her eyes.

Allergies and Asthma

Many children have allergies. Allergies occur when the body reacts in an unusual way to common substances in the environment. Common allergens (things that cause allergies) include cat and dog hair, feathers in pillows, household dust, dust mites, pollens, and sometimes medicine or even foods.

Mild or moderate allergies can be annoying to the child. Symptoms often take the form of a runny nose, itchy red eyes, rashes, or cough at certain times of the year. You should suspect an allergy if your child develops a symptom such as a runny nose which never turns into a full-blown cold but doesn't go away in a week or two either. If it happens at the same time each year, that is even further evidence of an allergy. Other allergies can be severe and even life threatening and can involve difficulty breathing or dangerous drops in blood pressure. For example, some children have a sudden and severe reaction to peanuts that requires immediate treatment.

Allergy symptoms differ depending on which system of the body is involved. For example, eczema happens when the allergic response is in the skin; hayfever (allergic rhinitis) is an allergic response in the nose; allergic conjunctivitis, in the eyes; asthma, in the lungs; and diarrhea and vomiting, in the gastrointestinal system. More general reactions (involving multiple body systems) include hives and anaphylaxis.

Children can become allergic to almost anything. Many children have allergies to substances that are found outdoors such as trees, grasses, and plants such as ragweed. Some children have serious allergic reactions when they are stung by an insect such as a bee or wasp. Sometimes the allergies can develop after the child has had no trouble with a particular food or medication for years. Sometimes allergies go away on their own after several years. Food allergies seem to be becoming more common, although the reason for this is not clear. Some parents believe that allergies to certain foods or other things may worsen their child's autism. (See Chapter 16 for a discussion of this controversy and some of the diets that are sometimes used; see Chapter 6 for a list of common food allergies in children.)

Some children develop asthma because of their allergies. In asthma, the allergic response is in the lungs and breathing passageways rather than the nose. Asthma is the most common chronic disease of childhood. Some children have a nagging cough while others may have mild wheezing or more severe difficulty breathing as a sign of their asthma. Asthma can be caused by allergies in some children, but others may have it without allergies. Asthma is becoming an increasingly common problem in children. If your child has episodes of wheezing or periods of difficulty breathing, you should contact your pediatrician.

Diagnosis of Allergies

In understanding allergies and asthma, a careful history of the problem is crucial. For example, a parent may be able to figure out which food is causing hives by keeping a food diary of what foods are eaten and when the rash appears. It may be important to look at the home, school, or work environment to identify actual or possible sources of allergy. A blood test can frequently identify a food allergy.

Seeing an allergist for further blood tests or skin tests to identify the cause of the allergy can be helpful. You may want to ask the allergist ahead of time whether any of the procedures will be painful. For instance, if blood drawing is planned, then putting a topical anesthetic cream on your child's arms ahead of time may reduce the pain. There are different types of skin testing. Usually, what is called prick testing is done first and it is not particularly uncomfortable. Later, the allergist may recommend intradermal skin tests. These are uncomfortable and you and the allergist will need to discuss how important they are and how to help your child handle the situation. The skin tests can be helpful in identifying allergies to animals, dust mites, trees, grasses, molds, and other environmental allergens.

Treatment

A child with mild allergies may have a stuffy nose whenever she wakes up or goes outside, but may not be bothered enough to need medication. Mild allergies often require minimal treatment unless the child is very sensitive or unless the symptoms are sufficiently annoying as to disrupt educational programming. Moderate allergies result in more significant distress; sometimes this may be of short duration but quite severe in intensity, or it may be a longer-term problem which is a chronic irritant to the child. For example, her eyes may be so itchy or watery or her lids so swollen that she is rubbing them constantly and cannot focus on anything else.

There are three basic methods of treating allergies: 1) avoiding the thing that causes the allergy, 2) treating the symptoms of the allergy with medication, and 3) desensitization.

Avoiding Allergens in the Environment. Whenever possible, this is the best treatment. If a certain food is known to cause an allergic reaction, it should be avoided. If something in the home is the cause of the trouble, many things can be done to try and prevent the problem. For example, if your child is allergic to feathers, you can replace the feather pillow with a polyester one.

Treating with Medication. If the allergen cannot be removed, as for example when your child is allergic to trees or grasses, then she will need to be given medication to treat the symptoms that are bothering her. Antihistamine medications taken by mouth are the most commonly used. They prevent cells in the person's body from releasing chemicals that cause the allergy symptoms. Singulair® (montelucast) is a newer medication that can treat mild to moderate asthma and also allergic rhinitis (nasal allergies). Antihistamine eye drops can also be used, although they can be difficult to get into most children. They just treat the eye symptoms of allergies such as itchy, runny eyes or lid swelling. Steroid nose sprays can also be helpful, but, like the eye drops, can be difficult to get into children without a fight.

In the past, most allergy medications caused drowsiness, which was often not a welcome side effect. Today, the newer antihistamine medications avoid some of the problems with drowsiness. Several antihistamines are now available that only have to be taken once a day. There are liquids and pills that melt in the mouth. Some, such as Claritin®, have recently become over-the-counter medications. Others, such as Zyrtec® and Allegra®, are still prescription only.

Always check with your child's doctor before starting a new medicine, especially if your child is already on some medication. Unfortunately, any of these medications can cause unwanted side effects in some children. Sleepiness is the most common problem, but some children will experience the opposite effect and become hyperactive. It's important to be aware of possible behavioral changes when starting any new medication.

Desensitization Treatment. Sometimes desensitization may be indicated if the allergic reaction (such as to a bee sting) is very severe, or if no medication has been able to stop the symptoms. In this treatment, a program of shots is given to reduce the child's allergic reaction. This may require weekly shots for months or years. Your child would have to be having major problems before you would want to consider this option.

Treating Asthma. The treatment of asthma will depend on whether or not it is caused by allergies and by the severity of the asthma. If your child is allergic to something that can be removed from the environment, such as a pet or feather pillow, it is easily treated. If there is nothing that can be changed in the environment, then medication will be needed. Some children only have the problem intermittently and they are usually treated with a medication called albuteral—either in an inhaler or in a nebulizer machine. They only take it when they are having a problem. For example, some children only wheeze when they have colds or with exercise. In these cases, the medication is only used when the child has a cold or before any exercise is planned.

If your child has frequent symptoms the doctor will probably recommend the use of daily medication. Often inhaled steroids are recommended. There are many other medications that are now available and your doctor will have to decide what is appropriate for your child. If your child has severe asthma, your doctor may refer you to either an allergist or a pulmonary specialist.

Being Prepared for Allergic Reactions

If your child has had a serious allergic reaction, you and all daycare or school personnel should be prepared in case it happens again. Caregivers at home, daycare, or school should be alerted as to what your child is allergic to, the symptoms to watch for, and what to do if your child gets exposed to the allergen or starts to have symptoms of an allergy.

Life-Threatening Allergic Reactions

At times children can have very serious and even life-threatening allergic reactions. These reactions are most likely after insect stings or after eating certain foods that your child is known to be allergic to. Peanuts (and any food that contains peanuts or peanut butter) and shellfish are some of the most notorious causes of severe allergic reactions.

A life-threatening reaction may start with hives, which are raised areas on the skin that are usually red, occasionally white, and are very itchy. Next, your child may develop swollen lips, a swollen tongue, or serious difficulty breathing. You may hear a change in her voice or hear wheezing coming from the chest or see that she is struggling to catch a breath. Her blood pressure may drop dangerously low and she may look pale and as though she is going to faint. She may actually faint if the reaction continues. Severe allergic reaction (anaphylaxis) can result in death if not immediately treated. You should therefore call 911 and get your child immediately to the nearest emergency room if you think she may be having a severe reaction.

If your child is known to have serious allergies, talk to your doctor about possible emergency treatments to have available. An antihistamine such as Benadryl® should be available to give by mouth and a shot of epinephrine (adrenaline) should be available. A brand called EpiPen® (either Jr. or Regular) is the most frequently used. Your doctor will need to order this for you and show you how to use it. Young children will need for this to be given by an adult. Some adolescents can learn to use it themselves and carry it with them. Someone in charge of your child's care when you are not there will need to know what she is allergic to and how to recognize an allergic reaction. They will need to know how to administer the EpiPen, if it is needed.

Any time your child needs the EpiPen, it is also critical to call 911 and get your child to the hospital for emergency care, even if she seems better after the shot. The effects will wear off and you want to be where further treatment can be given if it is needed. If your child has serious allergies to medicine or other things, you should consider having her wear a MedicAlert® bracelet so this information is always immediately available in case of emergency when you are not present.

If the reaction in the past was not life threatening, you may want people to wait and watch for symptoms if your child is exposed accidentally at school. For example, if your child developed a rash but nothing more serious when she ate a certain food, you may want them to just watch her carefully if she accidentally eats some of the food again. On the other hand, if she had a more serious reaction with throat swelling and difficulty breathing, you may want them to give diphenhydramine (Benedryl®), use the EpiPen, and call 911 even without waiting for any symptoms.

Skin Disorders

Skin conditions can be especially problematic in children with autism spectrum disorders. The itching, pain, or appearance of skin conditions can be very irritating or distracting, and children with autism may react by scratching and picking.

Any skin disorder can occur in children with developmental delays. Some of the most common are eczema (itchy, dry skin), impetigo (infected skin), and acne. Your pediatrician can make suggestions to help you deal with these problems. Sometimes topical medication (ointment or lotion) will be required, and at other times your child may need to take something orally. Medications that help with itching may be all that is necessary at times, while in other situations an antibiotic may be required.

If your child picks at her skin, monitor her carefully. Quickly treat any minor scratches or infections that develop, in order to prevent more serious problems. Keeping your child's fingernails very short can help prevent problems from scratching and gouging. Sometimes gloves are needed to protect the skin. To keep your child from pulling the gloves off, you may have to clip them or sew them to the sleeves of her sweater or jacket. You may be able to buy clips or short elastic straps made for attaching winter mittens to jackets or you may have to make something yourself. A medication such as Benedryl® to control the itching may be the most effective treatment.

Gastrointestinal Problems

Any gastrointestinal problem can occur in children with PDD. The problems that cause the most difficulty are those that cannot be seen and yet cause discomfort. Common problems that are painful include gastroesophageal reflux disease, constipation, diarrhea, and lactose intolerance.

Gastroesophageal Reflux Disease (GERD)

Gastroesophageal reflux (GER) involves the passage of stomach contents back up into the esophagus, throat, or mouth, where it is either silently swallowed or actually spat all the way out of the mouth. It occurs in many people without causing any symptoms, but when it does cause symptoms it is considered a problem known as gastroesophageal reflux disease (GERD). It can start right after birth or it can develop later in childhood. In children, symptoms of GERD include:

- Vomiting, which at times may be severe enough to limit growth
- Esophagitis (irritation of the esophagus), which can cause pain and irritability

■ Respiratory symptoms such as cough, hoarseness, stridor, and wheezing; less commonly, apnea and recurrent pneumonias

Your child may stop eating because of the pain or have behavioral changes such as irritability or loss of interest in food. These types of changes require investigation to understand their origin. A careful history of the relationship between eating and the pain may allow a doctor to diagnosis GERD. Sometimes testing is required. Your pediatrician may refer you to a pediatric gastroenterologist for this testing.

Because testing for GERD usually involves something unpleasant, such as placing a tube into the stomach or making your child swallow barium before an X-ray, many doctors will treat GERD on the basis of the history to start with.

There are now several different kinds of medication that can be used to treat gastroesophageal reflux very effectively. For infants, dietary changes or positioning after meals can be helpful.

Constipation

One of the most common G.I. problems in all children is constipation. This can mean either having infrequent bowel movements or having hard or difficult-to-pass bowel movements. Some children can have such severe pain from constipation that they are admitted to the hospital to be watched for appendicitis. Often constipation makes children lose their appetite.

There are many different causes of constipation. Some of the most common include dietary problems, lack of activity, and behavioral issues such as reluctance to use the toilet. Some medications can also cause constipation, so if your child develops constipation after starting a new medication, talk to your doctor. There are also many medical problems that can cause constipation, so if the problem persists, again, consult with your doctor.

As a parent you may be able see the problem starting to develop by paying close attention to your child's bowel patterns. Watching how frequently she has a bowel movement and how large or hard it is may allow you to correct a problem before it becomes too severe. If your child is too old or independent for you to be directly monitoring her bowel habits, try to be alert to changes such as your child spending increasing amounts of time in the bathroom or complaining of stomach pain.

Dietary changes can help prevent or correct constipation if your child will allow the changes. Some changes that may help include:

■ **Increase your child's intake of fluids.** If it's hard to get your child to drink much, you can try to sneak fluid into her diet with Jello, Popsicles, and other foods with high water content that your child does like.

■ **Increase the amount of fiber in your child's diet.** Adding many fruits and vegetables, especially the leafy green ones, can be helpful, although frequently children have constipation because they don't like these foods. Bear in mind that bananas, apples, or dairy products can constipate some children. Even if your child doesn't like fruits or vegetables, you may be able to get her to eat some by adding ground-up vegetables such as carrots or zucchini to sauces or cookies or making fruit smoothies. It is possible to buy juice boxes with added fiber that will help some children. You may have to ask your doctor where you can order them.

- **Occasionally, your child may require a stool softener** such as mineral oil, docusate (Colace®), or Miralax®.

Trying to successfully adjust the diet of a child with autism to correct constipation may require the input of many specialists. Your doctor may refer you to a dietitian or a gastroenterologist (see also Chapter 6 on nutrition).

Diarrhea

Acute diarrhea, lasting less than fourteen days, is a common problem in all children. It is most commonly caused by infection. Sometimes foods will cause diarrhea, especially large quantities of juice, or intolerance to milk, wheat, or many other foods. (See Chapter 6 for information about milk and wheat intolerances, as well as food allergies.) If your child has severe or persistent diarrhea or if you see blood in the bowel movement, you should see your pediatrician.

Injuries

Accident prevention, as we discuss in Chapter 7, is crucial for parents of children with autism spectrum disorders. However, even with great vigilance on your part, you can't anticipate or prevent everything. And if your child does injure herself, she may have difficulty in telling you, if she has limited communication skills. You may not realize what has happened unless there is obvious bleeding or she has problems moving an arm or leg. As in dealing with illness in general, it may be a detective project to determine that some new behavior is the response to an injury.

We list several books on first aid in the Reading List. Get and read one of these and keep it handy. Taking a first aid course can also be very helpful in learning how to deal with many injuries and emergencies.

There are some basic aspects of first aid to know about. If someone is not breathing or severely injured, you obviously need to call for emergency medical help. Most communities now have a 911 system to make this as easy as possible. The treatment of major emergencies is beyond the scope of this book. Less serious problems that you may have to deal with include stopping bleeding, cleaning and bandaging cuts, removing splinters, and treating minor burns and bruises.

Cuts and Bleeding

Be sure to put pressure on any cut area that is bleeding until the bleeding has stopped. If your child is uncooperative or noncommunicative, this may take more than one person. Press on the bleeding area with a clean cloth or sterile bandage or dressing. Bear in mind that some areas (such as the scalp) bleed much more than others. Once the bleeding has stopped, wash off the cut areas and apply antibiotic ointment to help prevent infection. Having your child take a bath may be easier than trying to scrub or soak an area in a basin of water.

The injured area may need to be wrapped in gauze and even an ace bandage or sock to keep your child from picking at it. Some children with autism may be more likely to leave a bandage on if it has a favorite cartoon character on it or if you put a special sticker or something else that your child likes on the outside. There is a relatively new nonprescription product called Liquid Band-Aid®. You may find that your child is less able to remove this than a regular Band-Aid. If there is *a lot* of bleeding and you can't get it to stop, keep the pressure on but call 911 for help.

Children with autism sometimes may require casts rather than bandages when an injury must be protected from further damage and when the child is otherwise unable to leave the injury alone. On the other hand, sometimes when an injury is minor it may make more sense to avoid extensive treatment. For example, if your child has a cut that ordinarily would require stitches, you and the doctor may decide that a small scar would be a small price to pay, relative to all that would be required for putting in stitches. You should always consider what your child's best interest is and look at both the short- and long-term picture. Many pediatricians and Emergency Department physicians can now close a wound with a special medical glue called Dermabond, which does not require any needles for local anesthetics or stitches.

If your child gets a bad cut, be sure to find out whether she needs a tetanus shot. Tetanus is caused by a bacteria found in dirt, soil, and rust and causes a serious infection. The tetanus vaccine can prevent infection, but must be followed by booster shots. Your doctor's office can tell you when your child last had the tetanus booster. If it was five or more years ago, your child will need another one.

Splinters

Small splinters of less than a quarter-inch will frequently come out on their own and the trauma of trying to remove them may not be worth it. Ask your pediatrician's advice if you're not sure. Certainly, if there are signs of infection, such as an expanding area of redness or a collection of pus under the splinter, then you should have your doctor check the area.

Burns

The first thing to do if your child is burned is to remove the source of the burning so that no further harm can be done. For example, if your child's clothes are burning or have been soaked with hot water, take them off as quickly as possible. Applying cold water or cold compresses can be helpful if quickly applied to the injured area. Call your doctor if there is any blistering or opening of the skin from the burn.

Head Injury

If you see your child injure her head and know that she had even a brief loss of consciousness, she needs to be seen by a doctor immediately. If there was no loss of consciousness or you didn't see the injury happening, you should watch your child closely. Call or see a doctor if your child has a large swollen area where she hit her head, she starts to vomit, she becomes either lethargic or very irritable, or she isn't using all of her extremities normally. If she just isn't acting herself after a long enough period of time to calm down after the injury, you should check in with your doctor.

Summary

Obviously, you want your child to be as healthy as possible. Whenever possible and appropriate, medical conditions should be treated promptly and thoroughly. However, sometimes children with autism may have relatively minor problems for which treatment may not always be appropriate or a priority. For example, if your doctor proposes desensitizing your child because of allergies by using injections over a long period of time, but your child finds shots traumatic, the risk involved may outweigh the benefit. That is, you sometimes have to decide if your child would be better off suffering the symptoms of a minor condition, rather than suffering from the cure.

To the extent possible and appropriate, your child should be involved in discussion about her treatment. Since the medical care of children with autism is not always cut and dried, it is vital that you are able to make informed decisions about your child's care. This is best done by building a strong working relationship with your doctor and the other healthcare providers who are part of the treatment team.

Questions

Q. My child seems to get a lot of colds and infections and runs a fever when she is sick. Is a fever dangerous?

Your question is really a two-part one. A fever by itself is not necessarily dangerous. A fever is a sign of infection, and, obviously, that is something that needs to be looked into. But fevers per se are not necessarily dangerous unless your child has seizures or the fever is very high and could trigger fever-related (febrile) seizures. You also mention that your child has many infections. Has she recently started to go to school or into daycare? Sometimes children who have not previously had many infections will start to get them when they are exposed to other sick children (one of the reasons why you should try *not* to send your child to school or daycare when she is sick!).

Q. My child hates taking medicines. Are there any tricks to getting her to do so?

Here are several ideas to try:
- Give her something that she likes to taste first and then give her the medicine followed by another helping of whatever it is she likes.
- You can mix many medications with foods or drinks that taste better. *But* be sure to talk to your doctor or pharmacist to check on this first.
- Ask your pharmacist if there is any way for him to mix the medicine in a liquid form that might taste better.

■ Parents have told us many different things that worked for their children. One parent mentioned having the child suck on a cold Popsicle—to numb up the taste buds—and then give her the medicine.

Q. Is there anything I can do for the pain from earache before I see the doctor?

You can start with pain-relieving medications such as Tylenol®, Advil®, or Motrin® (you may prefer Advil® or Motrin® at night because they last a little longer). If it is night time, you can raise your child's head using several pillows or have her sit upright to sleep (this puts less pressure on the eardrum). If all else fails, you can try several drops of either warm (but *not* hot) oil or vodka in the ear—to numb the eardrum (but do not do this if your child has PE tubes in the ear or if there is any drainage from the ear). The oil can be any clear oil such as olive oil or canola oil.

Q. My mother-in-law tells me that there are herbal treatments that prevent children from developing ear infections and can be used to treat them. Is this true?

No. Some ear infections are probably fought off by the body even without treatment with antibiotics, but clearly many ear infections need antibiotic treatment. There is no evidence that herbal treatments prevent ear infections or are an effective treatment against them.

Q. Is it OK to give my son over-the-counter medicines for a cold?

Generally, yes, but if your child is already receiving some medications, check with the pharmacist (or your doctor) to make sure there are no problems with taking the medicines together.

Handling Visits to the Emergency Room or Hospital

Hopefully, most of the time when your child has a medical problem, it can be taken care of at your own doctor's office. Sometimes, however, because of the acute or serious nature of the problem, the type of test or treatment your child needs, or the time of day, you will need to go to the hospital or the emergency room (ER).

Hospital stays or trips to the ER are stressful for almost any child. For children with an ASD, going to the hospital is especially difficult because they are exposed to new people and new environments and often to uncomfortable tests and procedures. The problems that children with autism have in dealing with new situations are compounded by the very stimulating environment and the very rapid pace of activity. This is especially true of the ER, which is a busy and active place (the TV show *ER* is a bit overly dramatized for TV, but only just!).

In this chapter, we discuss some ways to make ER visits a bit more tolerable for your child, as well as some important points to keep in mind when preparing your child for a planned hospitalization. It goes without saying that you should read the information about ERs *before* an emergency arises, as you will have your hands full taking care of your child in the event of a real emergency.

The Emergency Room (ER)

Is a Trip to the ER Really Necessary?

Sometimes it will be obvious that you need to go to the ER: your child is having a seizure or a severe allergic reaction, has a broken bone, has a laceration requiring stitches that your child's doctor can't handle, or even is having a dramatic change in behavior that you don't understand. Other times, you may be unsure how urgent the situation is. For example, your child may be ill and there may be subtle differences that can be difficult to understand or to put into words. For example, you may notice more irritability, changes in sleep patterns, weight loss, or perhaps apparent changes in level of functioning.

If you are in doubt, call your child's doctor first, even if it is the middle of the night. Although you may feel shy about doing this, consider the alternative of having to explain your child's problem to one or more unfamiliar healthcare professionals in a fast-paced, busy ER. Unfortunately, doctors, nurses, and other ER staff often have little experience with children with autism and related disorders. Even if they are knowledgeable about autism spectrum disorders, they are not familiar with your child's history. Not surprisingly, the combination of inexperienced staff and an overly stimulating environment can increase your child's anxiety, complicating visits to the emergency room.

There is a trend in our society to over-utilize the emergency room for situations that are not really emergencies. If the situation is not an emergency, remember you can deal with your child's primary healthcare provider more effectively than the emergency room and make for less stress for all concerned!

Communicating about the Problem

In dealing with an emergency, remember that all the doctors, nurses, and other healthcare professionals want to provide quality care to your child and indeed to all patients. As with other areas of medical care, you have an important role in this process. You have to be a persistent and effective advocate for your child when dealing with the ER, just as you do when dealing with the educational and other health systems. You can be assertive and helpful without being hostile and overbearing. It's important that the personnel in the emergency room understand that you are trying to help them help your child.

Obviously, in an acute emergency, the healthcare professionals will do whatever is necessary to manage the situation. That is, if your child is not breathing or his heart is not beating, resuscitation will have to be carried on. This requires the full attention, effort, and energy of all the ER department and you will probably have relatively little role in the process.

More typically, however, the problem is one of an acute illness or injury that is not really life threatening. Many of the same considerations come into play in the emergency room as in other settings. For example, as with school programs, children with autism often do better in situations where there are fewer distractions—a quieter and less distracting room is better than a busy and over-stimulating one. Similarly, although there will be many people around the ER, it will be better if you and your child interact with as few of them as possible. Hopefully, the emergency room staff will pay close attention to the information that you can give them. Keep in mind that it's easy to overwhelm them with information. The most important things to tell them are that your child has autism or a similar disability and that you are the parent and know the child's medical history. Use of a MedicAlert® bracelet can be helpful (in case you are not around).

If there are important issues such as allergies to medications, information relevant to the current emergency, or chronic healthcare problems, you should communicate this very quickly and briefly to the ER department. The doctors and staff will also want to know the name of your primary care physician. Your child's doctor or one of the staff can be very helpful to you as well. For example, she could call ahead to let the emergency room staff know you're coming or talk with the staff to alert them to what works best for your child.

The doctors and healthcare providers should be thoughtful and considerate in dealing with you. Except in a life-threatening situation, they should introduce themselves to you as well as to your child. If someone comes into the room without doing this, you should take it on yourself to introduce yourself to them. It's important to realize that the ER staff may be misled by your child's appearance. Indeed, Leo Kanner in his original report on autism noted the "attractive appearance" of many children with autism. This may, at times, lead ER staff to overestimate levels of functioning. If you notice that this seems to be happening, let them know. Obviously, if it's possible, your child should answer questions about his injury or illness. More typically, however, you will be the person to do this. Again, your primary care provider may be able to provide information by phone or in person that will help the emergency room staff.

In a non-life-threatening situation, you can usually be present to assist the staff in working with your child. Your presence will generally help calm your child and you can also tell the doctors whether there are any "tricks of the trade" in examining him. For instance, you may know that your child particularly hates having his ears looked at and recommend that the doctor save this part of the examination to the very end. You can also try to do favorite activities with your child to help comfort him.

Physical Examination

Unless your child's injury or illness is quite obvious, ER staff will need to do a physical examination to pinpoint the problem. Your child may have to partially undress for this. He may be more comfortable if the ER staff allows him to stay in his own clothes and to lift parts of them up for the examination rather than undressing and changing into an unfamiliar gown.

In deciding where to look for the problem with your child, the ER doctors should be very aware of the types of problems that often cause behavioral difficulties and acute behavioral change in children with autism and PDD. The doctor should be sure to look at your child's mouth, to look for abscesses, inflammation, tooth or gum disorders, emergent wisdom teeth, and so forth. It sometimes may take a while for your child to feel comfortable having his mouth looked at. Ear infections may be another source of difficulties, so the doctor will, at some point, have to look at your child's eardrums. Particularly in nonverbal children, problems in the mouth and in the ears can often result in acute behavioral change. A child may, for instance, suddenly begin hitting himself on one side of the head.

If your child has breathing problems or allergies, the doctor should listen to his chest and consider the possibility of pneumonia or other chest problems. The doctor will listen to the heart to be sure your child does not have an unusual heart rate or murmurs. She will want to examine your child's abdomen by gently feeling different parts of his belly. The doctor will be looking for signs that indicate an acute infection, such as the point tenderness in the right lower part of the abdomen that occurs with appendicitis or other problems. The doctor also may wish to do a rectal examination to see if your child is losing any blood in the digestive system and to be sure that constipation or bowel impaction is not causing the trouble. You should explain that such an exam may be very difficult for your child and that it should only be done if it will provide information that is critical to finding out what is wrong with him and cannot be gotten in any other way.

Particularly if your child has recently fallen or had another injury, the doctor will also be alert to the possibility that he might have a broken bone. She will examine your child's arms and legs for swelling of the joints and so on. She will also look for any skin problems, such as rashes, skin infections, or any signs of injury. In addition, if your child has seemed to lose abilities over a short period of time, the doctor will want to do a careful neurological examination. That involves checking the function and strength of many parts of the body, as well as checking reflexes with a reflex hammer. It is hard to do a thorough neurological exam with an uncooperative child, but the doctor will have to do the best that she can.

For girls and women with autism, a gynecological examination may sometimes be needed. It will be very important that the doctor or nurse practitioner know whether your child has previously had a gynecological examination (see Chapter 14).

Lab Tests

Sometimes, even after a thorough search, the physical examination does not show any particular disease or evidence of injury. Often the doctor will then want to order laboratory tests. These may include urine analysis, a complete blood count, blood chemistry, tests of liver function, an EKG, or X-rays. Depending on the circumstance, the doctor may also wish to look for levels of medications your child is currently on. If your child has apparently ingested something he should not have, the doctor may order toxicology screens. These can be either urine or blood tests.

If blood tests are needed, you may want to ask if an anesthetic cream can be used to numb your child's skin before the blood is drawn. Emla® is one brand that is frequently used. It can make blood drawing a much less painful and upsetting process for your child. Unfortunately, the cream is meant to be put on the skin for an hour before the blood drawing in order to be maximally effective. In the emergency setting, this is often not possible.

Occasionally, a new illness will be heralded by an acute change in behavior or level of functioning, and again the doctor will be alert to this. If there is a marked change in your child's level of consciousness or awareness of the environment, the doctor may conduct an LP, or lumbar puncture (spinal tap), in order to check for bleeding or signs of infection around the brain. This test involves removing a small amount of the spinal fluid through a needle placed in the back. Your child will need to be held still for this test. The doctor might also obtain a CT scan of the brain to look for signs of infection, injury, or a tumor. If there are concerns that your child may have had a seizure, he may need an EEG. Depending on the circumstances, this is usually done at a later time.)

Sedation

Sometimes it may be preferable for more invasive tests and procedures such as a vaginal examination, lumbar puncture, or even treatment of broken bones to be done with some degree of sedation. By this we mean that your child can be given some medication to make him less anxious or somewhat sleepy without putting him completely to sleep, as happens with general anesthesia. Medications to sedate your child can be given by the doctors in the ER either by mouth or as a shot in the muscle or through an IV. If general anesthesia is required, an anesthesiologist (a specialist in anesthesia) will be needed and your child will probably need to be taken to the operating room. This can sometimes take a long time to arrange.

It is important that the doctor realize that sometimes people with autism have "paradoxical" reactions to some sedatives. That is, they become more agitated, rather than calm. Consultation with an anesthesiologist may be helpful if sedation is needed. If you know that a particular medicine has been used before with good results—for example, at the dentist's—be sure to let the ER doctors know this. Similarly, if you know that some medicine resulted in a worsening of behavior rather than sedation, be sure to mention this.

Follow-up with Your Pediatrician

If the emergency room staff fail to find a cause for a recent change in your child's behavior or level of functioning, it's important that you, yourself, follow up with your child's primary physician. Understandably, ER staff who are not familiar with your child might not catch subtle changes in behavior or development that your primary physician might note. In other words, in the ER, your child's developmental disabilities might serve to "mask" a serious illness—another reason for you to be an effective advocate for your child.

It's important that your primary care doctor realize that you have been to the ER and that the ER staff communicate results of their assessment and any lab or other studies directly to her. Usually, your emergency room doctors will be in close touch with your own physician or members of the physician's group. There should be good communication between you, them, and the primary doctor. Sometimes your insurance company will only reimburse medical room charges if you've called your doctor first.

Hospitalization

In contrast to visits to the ER, hospitalizations are usually planned in advance. This gives you at least some opportunity to prepare your child and the hospital staff for his stay. Still, as a general rule, it is best for children with autism to avoid hospitalizations if possible—due to the stress of having uncomfortable or painful procedures done in an unfamiliar environment by unfamiliar healthcare providers. This means that whenever possible, tests such as brain wave tests (EEGs), hearing tests, or minor medical or surgical procedures such as having wisdom teeth removed are best handled on an outpatient basis. When this isn't possible, a one-day admission to the hospital sometimes can be arranged so your child does not have to stay overnight. These possibilities should always be explored with your child's healthcare provider.

Sometimes it is impossible to avoid a hospital stay. For example, if your child has to have his appendix removed or if he has an infection that has to be treated by intravenous (IV) antibiotics, hospitalization may be mandatory. If it is possible to anticipate a hospital stay, however, you can at least take some steps to prepare your child.

Choosing a Hospital

The choice of a hospital can be difficult. For simpler problems, a community hospital may be best. These hospitals tend to be smaller with fewer staff members. Often the environment is less threatening and noisy, and if the hospital is closer to home, it is easier for parents, family members, and others to visit.

Sometimes, when problems are more complicated or medical procedures are more extensive, your child will have to be in a larger hospital setting. The strengths here have to do with the number of doctors and specialists available and their expertise. The downside is that often many different doctors are involved in your child's care.

Especially in a larger or teaching hospital, it's important for you to identify which doctor is primarily responsible for your child and work with her to be sure that medical care is well coordinated. Often, your pediatrician or primary healthcare provider will be involved on a regular basis. As in working with your regular doctor, you should never hesitate to ask questions. There may, of course, be times when either the situation is so urgent or the doctor is so busy that she will not have time to discuss something with you at that moment. However, the doctor should always be able to go over your concerns or questions with you later. The hospital staff should help you feel that you work with them as part of the team of people who are helping to provide your child with high quality healthcare.

Preparing Your Child for a Hospital Stay

Depending on your child's level of understanding, he should be informed about the hospitalization in advance in a calm way. It usually is not necessary to go into great detail. It may be helpful for your child to understand a little about what is going to happen. This is a judgment call based on the parents' and the doctor's knowledge of the child.

Particularly if the admission is an elective one, it would be helpful for your child to visit the hospital ahead of time. He should meet the staff, including the doctors, if possible, and even have a tour of the operating room and recovery room facilities. Use of picture books, photographs, and other visual aids may be helpful. School staff might also be able to help prepare your child for the visit.

Many hospitals have what are called *child life* programs in which a trained professional will try to help children understand what is going to happen in the hospital before they get there. This is particularly helpful when your child is going through elective surgery or other planned kinds of procedures. The child life staff member may be able to show your child the room where he will go to sleep, the room where he will wake up, the kinds of materials he will see, and the staff he will meet.

Whenever possible, you should talk to staff about ways to add as much familiarity to the hospital stay as possible. You can bring in a few toys or see if your child can wear his own pajamas. If he has a special blanket or stuffed animal or favorite music, he might want to bring it. Assuming your child likes to watch videos or DVDs, find out whether there is a video or DVD player in the room or whether one can be brought in.

Your child should be accompanied by a family member or another familiar person who is aware of your child's communicative abilities. This person can be a teacher, a staff member, or a family friend, as well as a family member. Having this person around can help the hospital seem like less of a strange place. This person can also help negotiate with hospital staff and try to explain, in terms your child will understand, all that is going to happen. In many hospitals, a parent or family member can "room in" with the child. This option should be utilized whenever possible. Sometimes hospitals will provide staff members called "sitters" to help the family. They can sometimes help keep your child company when no one else is available. If this service is available, it's important that the staff member have some familiarity with children with autism. Ideally, it should be someone who can communicate easily with your child by whatever modality he uses. Sometimes teachers, aides, or other school staff (or friends or family members) can take over this role. If your child is not yet verbal but can use visual aids, you can use them to help him have a sense of what to expect—for instance, by using photographs to make visual schedules or to explain what will happen.

Does Your Child Need to Consent to Medical Treatment?

If your child with autism is in his late teens (the exact age varies from state to state), you need to find out what your state law says about giving consent for medical treatment. Once your child reaches a specific age, the power to withhold or grant consent for medical treatment will ordinarily pass from you, the parents, to your child. This may not be a problem if your child has good communication skills and is likely to understand the need for routine and emergency medical care. However, if he is likely to refuse needed medical care due to comprehension or communication difficulties or because he has an aversion to doctors, you may want to take steps to retain control of medical decision making for him. Usually, this involves you, the parents, becoming the legal guardians of your child. In some situations, it may work well for you to establish some kind of limited guardianship in which you are only responsible for medical and/or financial decisions for your child.

If you have questions about medical consent, talk to your family lawyer or other parents to see what is needed. If possible, discuss the issue with your son or daughter, as well. It is important to do this *before* consent is needed to treat your child!

Preparing the Staff

Preparing the hospital staff is as important as preparing your child for his stay. Hospital staff readily learn to "tune out" all the noises, smells, lights, and myriad activities and stimulations that occur on the hospital floor. They may not understand that a blinking light can be very distracting for a child with autism. Or they may not understand why a loud noise coming from your child's monitor sets him off into a frenzy of activity or aggression. If possible, talk to staff about any potential difficulties your child might have before they occur.

Whenever possible, the hospital staff should know and use your child's routines to help him feel more comfortable in this strange place. So, for example, tell them about your child's self-care skills, his sleeping routines (such as using music, a story, or a favorite object for comfort), and his favorite recreational activities. If your child is not feeling too unwell, school-based activities will also be a good way to help him spend some time and engage in familiar activities. Try to plan these in advance with your child's teacher.

More and more frequently these days, hospitals in the U.S. are set up for patients to have single or private rooms. If your child must share a room with another patient, you and the staff should carefully consider who they put in the other bed in the room. It may be hard for your child to have a fussy baby in the room or someone with many visitors.

Staff should also be educated about any safety measures your child needs. It is a bit surprising, but in fact the hospital can be a somewhat dangerous place. If your child is impulsive or tends to act out behaviorally, are there provisions for his safety? Questions to consider might include:

1. Does he need a room where the windows are protected—for example, so that he cannot be tempted to throw things out or jump out?
2. Does he need an adult in the room at all times?
3. Does he need some of the room furniture to be removed?
4. Can familiar objects be placed in the room to make him feel more comfortable—within reason?
5. If your child is self-abusive, does he need to wear a helmet or mittens?
6. What behavioral techniques help your child avoid difficult behaviors? What techniques are most effective? What techniques are less effective?

Parents can help hospital staff immensely by conveying this kind of information.

Procedures at the Hospital

At the time of admission, whether it is an emergency or scheduled admission, you should review your child's history with members of the treatment team. Also be sure to let hospital staff know whether your child is receiving medications on a regular basis. If he is coming for an elective admission to the hospital, it is easy for you to bring along bottles of medicine. If this is an emergency admission, it would be useful to have a list of medications readily at hand so that you can let the hospital know exactly what medicine your child receives and when. This is particularly important if your child takes seizure medications or medicines to address behavior problems.

Once your child has been admitted, there are several things you can do to make the hospital experience less traumatizing:

Ensure that your child feels as safe as possible in his own room. Some procedures such as blood drawing are uncomfortable, and whenever possible, should not be done in your child's hospital room. A treatment room is preferable so that your child feels as safe as possible in his own room. Everything should be ready in the treatment room by the time your child arrives, so that the procedure can be done as quickly and as safely as possible. You or another caregiver may need to assist with the procedure. If you choose to leave the room, extra hospital staff may be needed.

Make sure your child knows what is going to happen. Before beginning, the hospital staff should explain to your child what is involved in as much detail as he needs. It's important to be honest. Well-meaning lies such as "It won't hurt" cause more trouble in the long run than the truth. If your child can and does ask whether something will hurt, tell the truth. You do not have to go overboard on this but you should be honest and straightforward.

Preparing your child is especially important when he has elective surgery. Here the opportunity for him to meet the staff and to see the recovery room and the operative suite of rooms can be very helpful. With the permission of those involved, you can take photographs (or electronic photographs) which can be put in a book that you can review with your child before (and after) the experience of surgery.

Create a diversion, when possible. Procedures such as lumbar puncture and throat culture may present particular challenges. During uncomfortable procedures, you can sometimes help your child take his mind off the procedure by counting, listening to a favorite story, or talking about his favorite interests. Using rewards both during and after the procedure may also be helpful. One of the things that's very important is for parents to try to stay calm. If you are calm, it's more likely your child will be calm.

Some procedures such as electroencephalograms (EEG), computer tomography (CT) scans, or magnetic resonance imaging (MRI) require a much longer period of time. It may be impossible to get a child with autism to cooperate long enough for these without sedation or general anesthesia. In our research with MRI, we use a mock scanner (i.e., a replica of a real one) for children to use to become familiar with what it feels like to be in an MRI machine. This kind of preparation, if available, may help.

Avoid restraining your child if possible. Sometimes this can be done through careful preparation, but sometimes children cannot cooperate with procedures and have to be restrained. We'd like to avoid this, but when it is necessary, it is better if a number of trained people are available to help things go as smoothly as possible. Although seeing your child restrained can be difficult to watch, he is less likely to hurt himself or others if a number of people hold him still.

Reduce pain as much as possible. Sometimes pain or anxiety can be avoided by pre-medication. Some children with autism may need an anesthetic cream to numb the skin before blood tests and similar procedures; others may be able to tolerate these procedures without the cream if they are in a familiar environment with a familiar caregiver nearby.

Sometimes sedation or general anesthesia may be needed to help your child. Although in some ways more desirable than physical restraint, sedation and anesthesia carry their own risks. If sedation or anesthetic is considered, it is important that the doctor giving these agents (typically an anesthesiologist) is aware of your child's special needs and any medications he is on. Giving your child opportunities to visit the room ahead of time, to see exactly what will happen, and to hear the sounds or feel the materials used decreases the likelihood that he will need sedation.

There are some medications that can provide either mild sedation and anxiety reduction or sometimes more extensive sedation. We discuss these in Chapter 13. We emphasize that it is always important to be careful about sedating a child with autism. Sometimes you can try mild sedatives at home first (or in the hospital), since children with autism sometimes become *more* anxious or excited after they are given these medications. If more extensive sedation or anesthesia is involved, talk to the anesthesiologist ahead of time, if at all possible.

Be sensitive to your child's needs. As with other patients, it's important that hospital staff be sensitive to the needs of your child and your family. Sometimes children (or parents) may overhear aspects of conversations that are not necessarily about them but which may be upsetting to them. Usually it is not good to have "secrets" from your child—often these end up not being secrets at all and they have the potential to backfire in unfortunate ways. Thus, conversations about your child's medical care, current medical status, and future procedures are probably best done outside the room with the parents and doctor first, and then, immediately afterwards, in a briefer and more relevant form, with your child. Of course, all information should be given to your child with tact and sensitivity. Older and more able individuals can and should be involved in discussions of their care whenever possible and realistic.

Surgery

If surgical intervention is being considered (unless on an emergency basis), there should be a careful discussion of the benefits and risks for your child. In considering the benefits and risks, it is important to realize that surgery has the potential for disrupting ongoing programs and causing your child some discomfort, and always has the possibility for complications and infections.

Your child's regular doctor can be helpful to you in balancing the pros and cons of surgery. Sometimes the pro is that the procedure is easier to do when your child is younger or that the problem may become worse as he gets older. Sometimes the procedure may significantly increase your child's ability to profit from educational or other programs. For example, the placement of pressure equalizing (PE) tubes may allow your child to hear better. Other times, such as with appendicitis, surgery is not elective but absolutely necessary.

If your child is having elective (that is, non-emergency) surgery, you fortunately will have time to explore the various options and prepare your child, as much as is possible and appropriate, for the experience. As mentioned earlier, the child life specialist will be able to assist you in preparing your child for the experience. Of course, since you know your child so well, you may also have important information about him to share with the child life specialist. Again, you might want to take some pictures ahead of time to introduce your child to the hospital and the staff. You don't want to be horribly intrusive, but you may be able to take a few pictures during the visit to use in talking to your child afterward. Alternatively, if your child can make use of more verbal modalities, social stories might be helpful.

Anesthesia

If your child will need anesthesia, try to schedule a meeting with the anesthesiologist (a doctor who administers anesthesia) or nurse-anesthetist (nurse who administers anesthesia) to talk to them in advance about your child's special circumstances. These should include his ability to cooperate and understand, any special fears or anxieties you and your child may have, and your child's medical history. Particularly if the procedure or surgery is being done in a one-day surgery center or in anticipation of discharge to home immediately afterward, be sure to listen to the instructions that you are given. For example, usually your child should not eat for some hours prior to anesthesia.

The anesthesiologist will usually talk to you about the kind of anesthesia that she plans to use. Sometimes anesthesia is "local" and only numbs a specific part of the body (such as when the dentist numbs up a tooth before putting a filling in); sometimes it is "general" (when the person is basically put to sleep). Some children with autism may need general anesthesia for even minor procedures because they become so agitated when people try to do anything to them that they cannot be controlled easily. Other children may do just fine with local anesthesia for procedures such as getting a cut stitched up.

Sometimes a small amount of sedation can help a child be able to tolerate local anesthesia. Sedation will make your child less anxious, and the local anesthetic will prevent pain in the area of the procedure. Often before general anesthesia, some sedative agent is given to help your child feel less anxious. The question of what type of anesthesia is something you can discuss with the doctor.

Again, if your child has previously had any unpleasant or unexpected reactions to anesthesia or sedatives, make sure the anesthesiologist knows about it beforehand. He or she can get the details about which medications were used and exactly what happened in order to try and avoid such a reaction this time.

Recovery Room

After a procedure or surgery, your child may be moved back into a recovery room—a special place where nurses and doctors can keep a close eye on your child until they know that things are OK and that he is fully awake. Usually your child should have seen the recovery room ahead of time (assuming that this was not an emergency procedure). It will help if you are around and can stay calm and collected. You should ask to join your child in the recovery room as soon as is practical after the surgery. As always, try to anticipate problems and discuss your child's needs in advance with the staff in the recovery room.

Summary

If you are lucky, your child will never have to go to the hospital. Unfortunately, however, children with autism are just as prone to develop childhood illnesses as other children. Added to that, they are often more impulsive or less safety conscious, increasing the risk for accidental injuries. In addition, if your child has seizures or another serious health condition, an occasional hospitalization or visit to the ER may be necessary.

If hospitalization is unavoidable, remember that you can and should strongly advocate for your child to help ensure that his hospital stay is as stress free as possible. Try to do as much advance planning as you can, such as by pointing out the hospital or emergency room that you would use if you drive by it, or by getting some books about going to the hospital that you can read to your child. Remember, too, that your primary care physician can be your ally in working with the hospital staff to help them better understand your child's special needs and medical problems.

Questions

Q. My son has a dreadful allergy to some antibiotics. My wife and I worry that if he is ever injured and we are not around, he might be taken to a hospital or doctor who doesn't know this. What can we do?

You can do several things. If your child can be persuaded to wear it, a MedicAlert® bracelet can go with him all the time. In any case, your program/school staff should all have a basic record of special medical needs. A copy of this record should travel with your child—to outings, to summer camp, on sleepovers. If your child carries a wallet or purse, you can also put a copy there.

Q. My child has to have some elective surgery. There is a large teaching hospital about fifty miles away and a community hospital in our town. Which one should we use?

This really depends on the nature of the surgery. The advantages of staying in town are pretty obvious, so the question is, are there advantages to the larger teaching hospital that outweigh these known positives? If it is a complicated or specialized surgery, has the staff at the larger hospital had more experience with it? How much of a hassle will it be for you to go to the larger hospital? Can you stay with your child in the hospital? Your child's pediatrician should be a good person to advise you on this. You could also see if there is someone in the Child Life program at the larger hospital whom you could talk to.

6 | Growth and Nutritional Issues

In an ideal world, parents would prepare delicious and nutritious food for their children at every meal, the children would gobble the food up in just the right amounts, and, fueled by the nutrients in the food, the children would grow into healthy, fit adults. Unfortunately, even with typically developing children, this perfect scenario is hard to achieve. For children with autism spectrum disorders, it is even more likely that there will be some problems related to growth and nutrition—often due to idiosyncratic eating habits or overeating, as well as medical problems, at times.

In this chapter, we discuss children's general nutritional needs and how these vary with a child's age. After that we are going to discuss some nutritional issues often found in children with autism and PDD, such as very restricted food choices or unusual preferences for certain textures and color in foods. We will also cover some issues related to growth and weight. In addition, we will describe pica and rumination, unusual behaviors related to food that sometimes occur in autism. Finally, we will touch on lactose intolerance, celiac disease, and allergies, which may be particularly difficult to deal with in children with autism who already have limited food preferences.

Eating a Healthy Diet

A healthy diet plays a very important role in the growth and development of children. For many parents, this issue is extremely challenging, and studies have shown that the great majority of school-age children and teenagers in the U.S. consume diets that need improvement. For example, only 30 percent of children consume the recommended number of servings of milk each day, and as few as 14 percent eat the suggested amount of fruit. Unfortunately, American children receive more nutrients from fortified, sugary foods such as breakfast cereals and flavored drinks than from nonprocessed fruits, vegetables, grains, meats, or protein foods and dairy products. These fortified foods usually have large amounts of added sugar and fat. Soft drink consumption has doubled in the past thirty years. These drinks and other sweetened beverages and baked goods have contributed to an increase of 80 to 230 extra calories per day depending upon the age of the child. Just one hundred "empty" calories that are not needed for energy can result in ten extra pounds per year.

Children need to consume enough energy and nutrients from *wholesome* foods to support growth, fight infections, and fuel their activities all day long. A taller, older, and more active child will usually need more energy calories each day.

Determining Whether Your Child's Diet Is Adequate

Just because you have a child with autism with limited food preferences or other idiosyncrasies related to food doesn't mean that she is *not* getting a good diet. Still, it is important to know what one looks like so you can take steps to improve your child's diet if necessary.

There are five different types of nutrients that everyone needs: carbohydrates, fats, proteins, vitamins, and minerals. The body also needs adequate fluids to stay healthy. The amount of each of these nutrients needed each day varies with age for children. To determine how your child is doing, you should look at the range of foods eaten over several days or a week instead of a single day. The sections below explore two ways to approach the issue of providing adequate nutrients: 1) using the Food Group Pyramid, and 2) counting calories.

Using the Food Guide Pyramid

One way to ensure that you are serving your child a healthy diet is to select food for the day using a guide such as the Food Guide Pyramid that was produced by the U.S. Department of Agriculture in 1992 (see Figures 6-1 on the next page and 6-2 on page 110).This divides all food into five food groups and puts them in different parts of the pyramid according to the amounts, or number of servings of each, that should be eaten every day. These can be used for children and adults of all ages starting at age two years.

The five food groups are:
1. the grains group, including bread, cereal, rice, and pasta,
2. the vegetable group,
3. the fruit group,
4. the milk group, including milk, yogurt, and cheese,
5. the meat and bean group, including meat, poultry, fish, dry beans, eggs, and nuts.

The top of the pyramid includes fats, oils, and sweets. These are found in foods in all of the five food groups, as well as concentrated in foods such as salad dressings, oils, cream, butter, sugars, sodas, jams, bacon, and many desserts.

The number of servings of each food that should be consumed per day are given in ranges in the Food Guide Pyramids. The lowest number of servings is appropriate for young children aged two to six years old, and this is shown on the kid's pyramid. The mid-range of servings is appropriate for older children and teenage girls, and the highest number of servings is recommended for teenage boys. Serving sizes for each food group are included in the kid's pyramid. The serving sizes are appropriate for all ages.

The USDA has recently developed new guidelines which are currently being reviewed. In the future, the pyramid will continue to divide food into five groups plus additional fats and added sugars, but there will be more divisions by level of activity and calories per day. For instance, active teenaged boys will be allotted more servings per day than sedentary older people.

Proponents of lower carbohydrate diets feel strongly that a shift away from the current Food Guide Pyramid is important. They feel that our diets are too high in sugar,

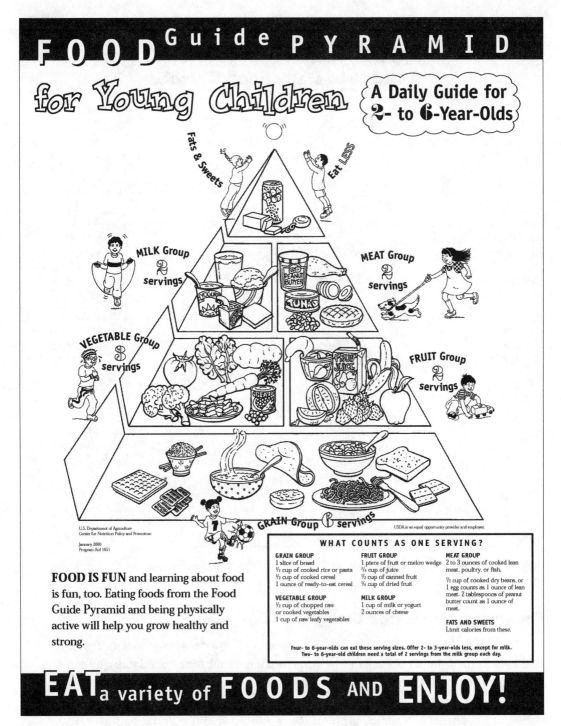

Figure 6-1 Credit: *U.S. Dept of Agriculture (www.usda.gov/cnpp/KidsPyra)*

refined starches, and processed fats and that the majority of children and teenagers do not consume adequate servings of fruits, vegetables, and dairy products. They recommend offering choices from these groups as snacks, as well as serving them as a part of family meals, to encourage a child to enjoy them.

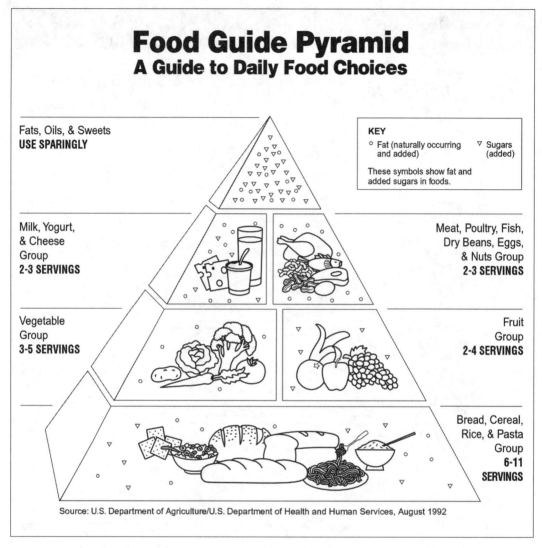

Food Guide Pyramid
A Guide to Daily Food Choices

Fats, Oils, & Sweets
USE SPARINGLY

KEY
○ Fat (naturally occurring   ▽ Sugars
and added)   (added)

These symbols show fat and
added sugars in foods.

Milk, Yogurt,
& Cheese
Group
2-3 SERVINGS

Meat, Poultry, Fish,
Dry Beans, Eggs,
& Nuts Group
2-3 SERVINGS

Vegetable
Group
3-5 SERVINGS

Fruit
Group
2-4 SERVINGS

Bread, Cereal,
Rice, & Pasta
Group
**6-11
SERVINGS**

Source: U.S. Department of Agriculture/U.S. Department of Health and Human Services, August 1992

Figure 6-2 Credit: *U.S. Dept. of Agriculture and U.S. Dept. of Health and Human Services*
(www.usda.gov/cnpp/pyramid.html)

Counting Calories and Eating a Healthy Diet

A second way to make sure a child takes in adequate amounts of necessary nutrients is to look at the amounts of individual nutrients that are needed daily by children of different ages and make sure your child eats the right quantities of each to have a healthy diet. There are recommendations for the amount of overall calories per day, as well as the amounts of carbohydrates, proteins, fats, vitamins, and minerals.

Calories. Calories are a measure of the energy content of food. The number of calories needed per day varies depending on many factors, including a person's age, size, and level of activity. Most young children, from one to six years of age, need between 1300 and 1700 calories per day. That goes up to 1800 to 2000 calories for most school-aged children. For teenagers, the number of calories needed varies considerably depending on the level of the child's activities. Teenage girls need between 1600 and 2200 calories per day, while teenage boys who are very active often need 2800 calories per day, and at times up to 3500 calories. These are obviously approximate numbers and there will be children in each of these groups who will need more or fewer calories. Your pediatrician or a dietitian or nutritionist can help you come up with the right number of calories for your child. They will know whether your child is getting the right amount of calories by checking the growth charts. If your child's weight is appropriate for her height and both are increasing along the same percentile for age, she is getting the correct number of calories.

Cholesterol and Fat. The most recent 2002 Dietary Reference Intakes (DRI) recommend that a balanced diet contain between 20 and 35 percent fat, with less than 25 percent coming from simple sugars. (The remaining 70 percent or so should be split between protein, at approximately 10 to 35 percent protein, and carbohydrates, at approximately 45 to 65 percent percent.) In addition, most health professionals recommend that cholesterol intake be 300 milligrams or less per day for everyone over the age of two.

There has been a great deal in the news in recent years about fat consumption, both the amount and the type. Cholesterol, too, has been the focus of much attention. The reason is that associations have been found between high blood cholesterol and high fat intake and obesity, heart disease, some cancers, and type 2 diabetes. Plant sources of fat

---

Resources on Nutrition and Feeding

These are some of the most helpful publications we know of for parents interested in promoting healthy diets for their children. Additional publications are listed in the Reading List on page 353.

Roberta Larson Duyfee. *American Dietetic Association Complete Food and Nutrition Guide, 2nd edition.* New York: Wiley, 2002.
An excellent resource for basic nutritional information.

Jurgen H. Kedesdy and Karen S. Budd. *Childhood Feeding Disorders: Biobehavioral Assessment and Intervention.* Baltimore: Paul H. Brookes, 1998.
This book is written for professionals, but has good chapters on a number of feeding problems, including over- and under-eating, pica, and rumination.

Joan E. Guthrie Medlen. *The Down Syndrome Nutrition Handbook: A Guide to Promoting Healthy Lifestyles.* Bethesda, MD: Woodbine House, 2002.
Although written for parents of children with Down syndrome, this is an excellent book for parents of children with any developmental disability, covering common problems such as picky eating, texture aversion, and obesity. Also a good resource for helping you plan daily diets.

William V. Tamborlane, M.D., editor. *The Yale Guide to Children's Nutrition.* New Haven, CT: Yale University Press, 1997.
An excellent resource on nutrition. This book includes chapters on nutrition at different ages, common concerns, special problems in nutrition, growth charts, and recipes.

containing mono- or polyunsaturated fatty acids are preferred to saturated or hydroge-nated (trans) fatty acids found in full fat dairy products and processed foods, respectively.

Vitamins and Minerals. The amount of vitamins and minerals needed each day also varies with age. Vitamins are organic chemicals (that is, they contain carbon) that are needed in small amounts in order for many biological reactions in the body to occur. Minerals are inorganic substances (that is, they do not contain carbon) that are also needed in the body in small amounts. They help regulate body processes and give struc-ture to the body. Dietary Reference Intakes (DRIs) include Recommended Dietary Allow-ances (RDA) for children and adults, as well as Adequate Intakes (AI) and Tolerable Upper Intake Levels (UL). The DRIs are set to prevent deficiency diseases and recom-mend appropriate nutrients to reduce sickness or chronic health problems.

Examples of problems with deficiencies include rickets (which can occur due to insufficient vitamin D); iron deficiency anemia (which can occur if there is not enough iron in the diet); and osteoporosis, or weak and thin bones in adults (which can occur if the adult consumed insufficient calcium when young). Inadequate fluoride intake can make dental caries (cavities) more likely. Fluoride is now added to city water in most parts of the country and your child will get enough if she drinks city water or if you use it in cooking. If your family drinks bottled or well water, you should give your child fluoride supplements. The correct amount is important, so your doctor or dentist will prescribe it for your child (see Chapter 10).

Consuming excess amounts of vitamins and minerals can also be harmful. This is why the government has established Tolerable Upper Intake Levels, as mentioned above. For example, vitamin A is needed for normal vision and skin development, but excessive doses can cause bone problems, birth defects, blurred vision, or liver damage. Too much folic acid, a form of folate added to enriched breads and cereals, can mask the anemia caused by B_{12} deficiency, leading to nerve damage if left untreated. Too much calcium taken into the body at one time may contribute to kidney stones in some people and can block the adsorption of the minerals iron and zinc. Iron can also be dangerous in exces-sive amounts.

As we discuss in Chapter 16, over the years many people have suggested "treating" autism with different combinations of vitamins. None of these supplements have been proven to work, however. If your child eats a balanced diet, she probably won't need vita-min supplements (and most children's supplements do not contain a full array of the im-portant nutrients that wholesome foods provide). But, if eating problems such as those described in the next section are of significant concern, a complete multivitamin/mineral supplement may be beneficial. If you have questions, talk to your pediatrician. He or she may suggest that a dietary analysis be performed by a qualified nutrition professional.

Fiber. Fiber is another important ingredient in the diet. In children, it is particu-larly helpful in preventing problems with constipation. Certain kinds of fiber have been linked to lowering blood cholesterol, improving heart health, and preventing cancer. Adults need approximately 20 to 35 grams per day of fiber in their diet. One way to figure out the amount of fiber a child should have in her daily diet is to take her age in years and add 5 and that equals the grams of fiber per day needed. So, an eight-year-old would need 13 grams of dietary fiber per day (8 + 5).

Unfortunately, most Americans do not consume anywhere near enough fiber. The simplest way to increase intake is by consuming bran cereals, which are the most concentrated source of dietary fiber. Other whole foods such as peas, corn, broccoli, lentils, all beans, tomatoes, fresh fruits, nuts, and seeds, as well as whole grain breads, rice, and pasta, are good sources of fiber. Be sure your child drinks plenty of water whenever fiber intake is increased to help prevent constipation. For children with problems with constipation, talk with your doctor. He may want to help you supplement your child's fiber intake. See Chapter 4 for more information about constipation.

Eating Problems

Children with autism and related disorders can have a number of problems with eating and food. These often include:

- unusual food preferences and sensitivities, which can lead to a restricted diet;
- obesity;
- pica (eating nonnutritive substances such as dirt or string); and
- rumination (regurgitation of food that has already been eaten).

In this section, we'll consider some of these problems and potential solutions. Again, keep in mind that this is a general discussion with general suggestions and that when you need specific advice, various professionals (as well as many parents and well-intentioned friends and relatives) will be there to make suggestions!

Unusual Food Preferences and Sensitivities

Children with autism or other pervasive developmental disorders may have unusual eating habits. Some have pronounced likes and dislikes when it comes to food. Sometimes these habits keep the child from having a good diet. Some children are extremely sensitive to certain food textures or tastes or smells. Some children may eat only certain kinds of food (such as foods that are soft and mushy). Other children may resist new foods or may not tolerate foods of certain temperatures. Sometimes children eat the same foods over and over again. We've seen children who would only eat white food, who would only eat cold food, and who would only eat French fries and certain fast foods.

The attempt to introduce new foods at mealtimes can lead to temper tantrums and other difficulties. Occasionally these escalate to the point that the child becomes malnourished, although this is unusual. For example, a few children may eat such a limited range of foods that their physical growth is at risk or they may be at risk for vitamin deficiency diseases. Avoidance of certain foods such as dairy products may affect other aspects of health such as developing strong bones and teeth. These unusual food preferences are not always easy to understand. They may be part of the difficulties children with ASDs have in dealing with change, or perhaps related to oversensitivity to smells and tastes.

Parents of many children with autism report some food sensitivities starting more or less from the moment that solid foods are introduced. It is interesting, however, that we've seen only a handful of children with autism who failed to gain weight appropriately as infants (something called failure to thrive). When problems start early, they often seem to get worse as the child becomes a bit older, so it is worth trying to help your child when these problems first develop.

To some extent, the unusual food preferences of some children with autism spectrum disorders resemble the problems of typically developing toddlers, who often engage in struggles over food. The endless reminders from your mother to eat your peas or broccoli may come to mind! These problems are, however, often much more marked and severe in children with autism. Several things help the typically developing child cope—for example, being motivated to imitate the models provided by family members eating a range of foods or enjoying praise from parents for trying new foods.

Unfortunately, children with ASDs often feel less social motivation and desire for praise. In addition, heightened sensitivities to foods, rigidity, and difficulties with change further complicate attempts to introduce new foods into their diets. These problems can be even more complex when parents are also pursuing dietary interventions (see Chapter 16) that further restrict what the child can eat. For example, some parents restrict the diet so much that their young child may not be able to participate effectively in educational programming because the only foods available to her as reinforcers are unappetizing to her.

The Role of Dietitians

Registered dietitians (RDS) and dietetic technicians (DTR) have had specific training in diet and nutrition. If your doctor suggests a consultation with the dietitian, he or she will talk with you, observe your child, and look at her medical records. The dietitian may be able to identify specific nutritional problems and can evaluate your child's need for special vitamins, minerals, or other diet changes. He or she will also consider any special issues related to your child's appetite, food preferences, medical history, and nutritional needs.

The dietitian can help you design a better diet for your child and may also work on increasing independence in feeding and dietary skills. This can sometimes be done in conjunction with your child's behavioral program. The dietitian may work with other professionals, including your child's doctor, speech-language pathologist, or occupational therapist. Information on diet and accredited dietetic professionals is provided on the American Dietetic Association's website (www. eatright.org).

Helping Your Child Tolerate More Foods

Dealing with unusual food preferences is not easy. Strategies for coping with this problem are quite varied. One approach is to attempt very *gradual* change—very, very gradually introducing new foods. This might work well, for example, for a child who eats only white foods. For this child, you could gradually begin to introduce color into the food. Blenders and food processors can be a real help in this regard. Sometimes unpopular foods can be hidden in other blenderized foods; this may make the texture more tolerable as well. Depending on your child's preferences, it may be possible to add to foods she does like. For example, if she will drink milkshakes, you can try adding different kinds of foods to the shake.

For some children, varying the way in which the food is presented may be the trick. Sometimes freezing pureed vegetables into popsicles may make them more interesting. Or a child who would never eat cooked peas might respond if they were presented in frozen form. Other children might be willing to try dried peas, available in some Asian food stores. The usual rule of thumb is to try gradually introducing new foods. Even though it is a hassle, keep at it, since otherwise the tendency is often for the child to become even more rigid.

If it feels as if you are almost engaged in guerilla warfare to get your child to eat, adopt some of the tactics used in such conflicts! Think about ways to give some otherwise uninteresting food a new "spin." These methods can sound perfectly disgusting, but it is worth experimenting. Try sprinkles, bacon bits, grated cheese, chocolate, or butterscotch sauce on foods. Many typically developing children love to smother foods in catsup or some other sauce, and if this works for your child with an autism spectrum disorder, so much the better!

Sometimes children are delighted to try foods that they have been involved in preparing. This approach can also have payoffs if you need to plan school lunches or snacks. You can try a visual approach to help involve your child in cooking. For example, make up a set of index cards illustrating how to prepare spaghetti and put them in order, in a notebook or on a ring. (Photos might show your child getting the spaghetti box out of your cupboard, getting the pot out, and putting water in it, etc.) For children who can read, the printed words may be sufficient.

You might also try involving your child in grocery shopping to try to spark her interest in new foods. You can consult with your child's school staff about ways to make this a positive learning experience. For example, you can make a visual shopping list ahead of time. Use a digital or instant camera and make photographs of the actual items your child will need in the store. You can put these onto a shopping list using Velcro® tabs. This special list can help your child shop with you in the store while you are doing your shopping. Start with very simple foods and gradually increase the complexity as time goes on. This is a wonderful way to make grocery shopping a positive learning experience for your child and help her take pride in her abilities. You also help encourage adaptive behaviors and important community and daily living skills.

If poor weight gain is an issue, more calories may be added. Adding whole milk to the diet can provide added calories. For children who are lactose intolerant, you can purchase the Lactaid® milk with higher percentages of fat. You may want to try adding a commercial instant breakfast or a product such as Ensure® or Pediasure® that provides both calories and many needed nutrients for the day.

Getting Professional Help

A range of behavioral approaches can also be used to help your child learn to tolerate a greater range of foods. It is important to have the help of an experienced professional in setting these up; some resources can be found in the Reading List. Often a gradual, step-by-step approach is used with carefully selected rewards for more appropriate eating. The specific plan is individualized depending on your child's needs and problems. Praise, time-limited meals, ignoring food refusals, and more frequent "mini-meals" (with limited snacks in between) can all be used in various combinations. As with everything else, it is important to weigh the pros and cons of the various approaches. Children whose limited diets put their growth and development at risk are the ones who will need the most intensive intervention programs.

Various professionals can be helpful to you in dealing with the food preference problem. Behavioral psychologists may help you design a plan for gradually introducing new foods and expanding your child's range of foods. Especially if your child eats a very narrow range of food, it may be worth meeting with a dietitian to review your child's diet and think about ways to supplement it. Often it is the texture, rather than the taste, of food which seems to be a problem. Speech-language pathologists or occupational therapists may be able to work with you in developing ways to help your child tolerate a greater range of textures or help with other aspects of the "presentation" of foods.

Height and Weight

In general, height, weight, and growth are within normal limits for children with autism—even for children who tend to be rather picky eaters. The one interesting exception has to do with head circumference. At least some children with autism spectrum disorders (but not Rett's disorder) develop larger than usual head size. There is some debate about whether they are born with this or whether it develops in the first year or so of life. Some recent research suggests that there may be a growth spurt of the head (that is head circumference) but *not* the body in the first year of life. It is not yet clear what this means, but it may have to do with some differences in the ways in which the brain is being organized. The difference in head size is probably most striking in younger (preschool) children with autism. This observation of "macrocephaly" (big head size) is a relatively recent one and researchers are trying to understand its significance. In individuals with Rett's disorder, on the other hand, head growth decreases in the preschool years.

Every parent wants to be sure that his or her child is growing well and will meet her growth potential. Your pediatrician will keep track of your child's growth at every well child visit. During your child's early years, your pediatrician will measure her length, weight, and head circumference at each of these visits and plot them on standard growth charts. After a year or so, he usually will stop measuring the head circumference. Recently pediatricians have started charting the child's Body Mass Index (BMI) to assess how appropriate the weight is for her height (see below).

The graphs of the height, weight, and head circumference show what percentile your child is in for each of these measurements. The percentile expresses your child's growth relative to other children her age. The 50th percentile for height would, for example, mean that your child is just in the middle for children of her gender and age. Most children will grow somewhere between the 5th and 95th percentile on standardized growth charts for girls and boys at different ages.

Your child's growth potential is largely determined by genetics. That is, tall parents tend to have tall children and short parents tend to have short children. Pediatricians use different methods to predict eventual height. One commonly used formula uses mid-parental height as a predictor. You can calculate this by adding the mother's height in inches to the father's height in inches and then dividing by two. Then for boys, add 2.5 inches and for girls, subtract 2.5 inches. The final number of inches is the estimated height you can expect your child to achieve. (If you are using the metric system, add the parents' heights in centimeters and divide by two, then add 6.5 centimeters for boys or subtract 6.5 centimeters for girls.)

Steady growth is more important than what percentile your child is in. If there is a drop off from previous percentiles, or an unexpected increase from earlier, your pediatrician will be alerted to look for an explanation. An unexpected change in growth may be the first sign that there is some problem with your child. For example, in Rett's disorder the head circumference percentile will slow down after having initially increased as expected. In some instances certain medications, such as Risperidone (see Chapter 13), may lead to weight gain. A careful history of your child's diet and a thorough physical exam will usually provide the explanation for an unexpected change in growth rate, weight gain, or weight loss. In some cases, further testing may be required.

Overeating and Weight Gain

Excessive body weight is now a very common problem in our society. We tend to eat foods that are high in calories and don't engage in the degree of physical work that our forefathers did. This is of concern because obesity is a risk factor for many chronic diseases, such as heart disease and type 2 diabetes. The overweight child with autism often becomes even less likely to exercise and a vicious cycle sets in, which only adds to the weight problem and makes it even harder to manage the child physically.

Although the word "obese" is often used interchangeably with "overweight," it is important to understand the distinctions. In plain language, someone who is "obese" is more overweight than someone who is "overweight," and is also at greater risk for weight-related health problems such as diabetes or mobility problems. Obesity is often defined in terms of Body Mass Index (BMI), as discussed on the next page.

Children with autism and related disorders can be at risk for obesity for several different reasons. Often a lack of interest in team sports and in physical activity means that children with autism may not burn enough calories. For other children, food functions very effectively as a reinforcer to the point that the child lives for snacks and treats. Other children seem never to reach the point of feeling full and eat and eat until interrupted. Occasionally, some medications used for emotional or behavioral difficulties (such as risperidone) may actually stimulate the appetite and lead to weight gain. They may also reduce levels of physical activity further, compounding the problem (see Chapter 13).

Sometimes the overweight problem results from children having unrestricted access to food. This may happen in school or adult programs. It may be more difficult to control food intake in a private home when other members of the family want to have their own access to food. Occasionally a husky adolescent or young adult may become aggressive if food or snacks are denied. There can also be medical problems that are unrelated to autism and PDD that cause increased weight. You should talk to your child's doctor about any sudden or unexpected increases in weight. For example, an underactive thyroid gland can produce both behavior changes and weight gain.

The pediatrician may have specific suggestions and strategies to suggest if your child gains too much weight. These can include increasing activity levels, decreasing calories taken in, limiting use of foods as rewards, and limiting access to food— particularly high calorie food. Generally, when children are overweight, the idea is not to try to help them lose weight. Instead, the strategy is usually to try to stop or slow their weight gain while they "grow into" their weight. A dietitian may also help you think about ways to help provide your child with a healthier diet, as we discussed earlier in this chapter in the section on general nutrition. It's important to balance carefully the degree of weight control desired and the effort it will take to achieve this goal. If the amount of overweight is relatively minimal, it may not be worth the effort.

Determining Body Mass Index (BMI)

Body Mass Index (BMI) is a measure of weight relative to height. Your child's pediatrician or other healthcare provider should be sure to monitor your child's weight and height and Body Mass Index (BMI). The formulas for calculating BMI are:

- weight in pounds ÷ height in inches ÷ height in inches x 703. For example, for a 75 pound child who is 50 inches tall, BMI would be 21 (75 ÷ 50=1.5; 1.5 ÷ 50=.03; .03 x 703=21.09), or:
- weight in kilos ÷ height in meters ÷ height in meters

Your child's pediatrician will have growth charts that show what BMI is appropriate for boys and girls of different ages. If a child's BMI is in the 85th percentile for age, that child is considered at risk for obesity. If she is in the 95th percentile or greater, she is considered obese. BMI should be followed closely because we know that the older a child gets and is still overweight, the greater the chance that she will become an overweight adult. An obese child at age seven years has a 40 percent chance of becoming an obese adult, while an obese adolescent has an 80 percent chance of becoming an obese adult.

Undernourishment

Inadequate weight gain or even weight loss in children with autism is usually caused by eating too little of the right kinds of foods due to unusual food preferences, as described above. Rarely, this occurs because of very restricted diets that children are put on. In addition, some medications such as Ritalin® and other stimulants may make children feel less hungry and contribute to difficulties gaining weight. If weight loss occurs, your pediatrician will need to do some testing to rule out medical explanations as the cause.

A hyperactive thyroid gland is rare, but when present can cause behavior problems and poor weight gain or weight loss. Serious liver or kidney disease can also cause undernourishment and poor weight gain, as can celiac disease (see below). Food allergies (which we'll discuss shortly) can cause chronic diarrhea and result in poor weight gain or weight loss. In addition, unrecognized infections and other chronic health problems can lead to undernourishment. These cases are very rare and are usually diagnosed earlier because of other symptoms. They are not any more common in children with ASDs than in other children.

Unusual Eating Behaviors

Eating Nonfood Substances (Pica)

Some children with autism spectrum disorders eat nonfood substances. This is known as pica. Some eat dirt, paint chips, string, or anything they find on the floor. Other children chew on materials or keep them in their mouths without swallowing them (or sometimes swallowing them by mistake). Still other children may be tempted to eat the leaves of plants (some of which are poisonous). Some may even eat their own feces. These behaviors can be a problem with any toddler, but can be a more persistent problem in children with developmental delays. It is unclear why pica is more common in children with autism spectrum disorders, although it probably reflects more general problems with cognitive development. (Pica also occurs in children with mental retardation who do not have autism.)

Eating nonfood items can lead to various medical problems such as obstruction of the bowel. It can also increase the child's risk for lead poisoning, depending on what is eaten. In addition, there is a risk for infection if children put dirty and unclean items in their mouths. As we talk about in Chapter 7, many other substances (and plants) found around the house can also be poisonous.

Various strategies can be used for dealing with inappropriate eating and mouthing behaviors. The choice of strategy depends on your child's age and developmental level, your ability to restructure the environment to prevent the problem, and the nature of the trouble. Sometimes children really like the experience of moving their mouth and/or chewing. If this is the case, you can try several different things. For very young children, a pacifier may be helpful. For somewhat older children, increased access to foods that are crunchy or chewy may help decrease the desire to chew on other things. (You can try chewing gum, but avoid excess sugar.) An OT might also be able to suggest appropriate nonfood items for your child to chew on, such as rubbery "chew tubes." Occasionally children engage in these behaviors when the environment is too complicated for them—that is, they use chewing as a stress reducer. You can see if reducing the level of environmental stimulation helps with the problem. Occasionally, using an electric toothbrush (sometimes several times a day) can help deal with the child's apparent need for oral simulation (this also has advantages for dental care).

Various professionals may be helpful in reducing pica. The speech-language pathologist or occupational therapist may help you think about new ways to cope with the problem and give your child alternative behaviors. A psychologist or physician with experience in developmental disabilities may also be helpful in suggesting behavioral interventions to try. Sometimes you can find a substitute or alternative behavior such as eating ice chips (with or without flavor). Sometimes your reactions to the behavior may be an important part of what keeps it going. You may need to learn to ignore the behavior if it is not endangering your child's health, and instead give her plenty of praise and attention when she is not chewing on nonfood items.

If you are worried that your child may have eaten something poisonous, consult with your pediatrician. For example, if your child ate paint chips, she may need a blood lead test if the paint came from an old house (see below). Depending on what your child eats, she may be at risk for other diseases, such as intestinal parasites. If you see your child swallow anything that won't dissolve, such as pennies or a pin or other sharp object, call your pediatrician or take your child to the hospital. If your child is having any difficulty breathing, you should immediately assess whether the Heimlich maneuver is appropriate and then call for emergency assistance.

Lead Poisoning

If your child eats or mouths nonfood items, it is essential to take precautions against lead poisoning. The most frequent source of unexpected lead in the United States is from indoor house paint that was used before it was banned for health reasons in the 1970s. It can also come from lead solder used to connect water pipes in older homes. If you live in an older home, you should have both the paint and the water checked for lead. Painting over lead paint will prevent a child from eating loose paint chips. If the original windows are still part of the house, there is the possibility that a fine dust with lead paint in it will fall on toys and other objects in the room when the windows are opened and shut. If your child puts one of these toys into her mouth she will ingest lead. The solution is to scrape the wooden window frames down to bare wood and repaint them with lead-free paint or replace them with new windows.

Elevated lead levels cause different symptoms depending on how much lead is ingested and the age of the child who has ingested it. Usually when children have elevated lead levels, their parents do not notice any symptoms, but they may actually suffer from some subtle neurodevelopmental problems. The Centers for Disease Control considers any lead level of 10 micrograms per deciliter or above to be abnormal and it should prompt a search for the source of the lead. Higher levels, usually of 40 micrograms per deciliter or above, may cause more side effects such as anemia. Extremely high levels of 60 micrograms per deciliter or above may cause worse problems such as behavioral changes, regression of newly acquired skills, and most seriously, acute brain toxicity with seizures and coma. Obviously, higher levels must be treated promptly. It is possible to die from the effects of extremely high lead levels.

Your pediatrician will probably screen your child for lead routinely when she is young. You may want to request a lead level at an older age if you think there has been any possible exposure. If your child tends to mouth everything or to eat nonfood substances, it is worth having your doctor check her lead level with a blood test. If a high lead level is found, various treatments are available, including chelation, which we discuss in Chapter 16 for other reasons. In addition, efforts must be made to discover the source of the lead and remove it.

Rumination

This unusual behavior, fortunately not very common, refers to the habit of regurgitating food and chewing it again. This behavior occasionally occurs in typically developing infants but is most common among people with mental retardation (with or without autism). For the latter group, it may start at more or less any point in time. Problems related to rumination can include damage to the teeth, food aspiration (food passes into the lungs rather than the stomach), and growth problems. To complicate life, gastroesophageal reflux may contribute to the problem at least some of the time.

Various behavioral interventions can be used to deal with rumination, particularly if serious medical complications are present. The assistance of an experienced behavior management professional is really needed to deal with the behavioral aspects of this problem. He can, for instance, figure out what your child "gets" out of the behavior and come up with substitute behaviors to teach instead.

Health Problems That Can Affect Nutrition

Many children with and without autism spectrum disorders have food sensitivities. There is no good research showing that these conditions are more common in children with autism spectrum disorders than in other children, but if certain foods seem to "disagree" with your child, it is certainly worth finding out whether she has lactose intolerance, celiac disease, or a food allergy. If undiagnosed and untreated, these conditions can lead to malnutrition, growth problems, and sometimes serious reactions.

Lactose Intolerance

Some children develop lactose intolerance as they get older. They lack either some or all of the enzyme lactase that is needed to digest the sugar lactose that is found in dairy products. As a result, they can develop gas, abdominal pain, or diarrhea if they consume too much dairy. Any of these symptoms can cause a child to be uncomfortable and fussy.

Lactose intolerance is different from a milk allergy in which a child has an allergic reaction to the protein in milk. A child with lactose intolerance can drink milk if the lactose has been removed from it.

Cutting down on or eliminating dairy products helps. The Lactaid® products available at the grocery story are a good substitute for many people. These are dairy products without the lactose sugar. You can also buy Lastase® pills, which provide some of the missing enzyme and allow some people to comfortably eat small amounts of dairy products. There are tests for lactose intolerance, but often diagnosis can be made without testing by eliminating dairy products for a trial period. If symptoms recur when dairy products are reintroduced, your child is presumed to have lactose intolerance.

Celiac Disease (Gluten Intolerance)

Celiac disease is a disorder of the small intestine. People who have celiac disease cannot eat foods with gluten in them because it damages the lining of the small intestine. This leads to malabsorption of nutrients and poor weight gain or weight loss, as well as fatigue, diarrhea, and discomfort. Other symptoms can also be experienced. The disorder can develop in infants and children, but many times it is not diagnosed (and possibly may not develop) until adolescence or adulthood.

Gluten is found in wheat, rye, and barley, and sometimes oats (if they have been contaminated with wheat). These substances are found in a wide range of foods. Treatment for this disorder requires avoidance of all gluten in the diet. This usually requires the help of a dietitian or nutritionist, at least initially. Some people with gluten intolerance will also have a lactose intolerance because of the damage that the gluten has done to the small intestine. This will improve as the intestine heals. We discuss gluten-free diets in Chapter 16.

If there is a suspicion that your child may have celiac disease, the pediatrician can do a blood test to assess the likelihood that your child has the disorder. To definitively diagnose celiac disease, however, a biopsy (sample of tissue) needs to be taken from your child's small intestine while she is either sedated or under anesthesia. The sample is then examined under a microscope. Testing needs to be done *before* your child starts on a gluten-free diet, or her intestine may heal before biopsy can confirm that it has the damage typical in celiac disease.

Food Allergies

We discuss allergies in detail in Chapter 4. In addition to allergies to nonfood substances such as dog and cat fur, ragweed, and goldenrod, some people have allergies to certain foods. Food allergies are seen in many children, who often "grow out of them" as they get older. Peanut and nut allergies, however, often last a lifetime. Eight major types of foods cause most of the food allergies:

1. peanuts,
2. tree nuts such as almonds, walnuts, or cashews,
3. cow's milk,
4. soy milk,
5. eggs,
6. fish,
7. shellfish,
8. wheat.

The symptoms of food allergies can vary between people and with different foods. Rashes, especially hives, are often seen. Vomiting and diarrhea are common. More serious reactions involve swelling of parts of the body, such as the lips and tongue, and narrowing of the throat and airway causing difficulty breathing. Wheezing can occur and the situation can be life threatening. If the reaction involves a drop in the blood pressure this can also be life threatening. (See Chapter 4 for information on life-threatening reactions.)

Most commonly, allergic reactions can be avoided once you know what your child is allergic to. An antihistamine such as Benedryl® should be given and you may need to use

Special Diets at School

If your child with autism has food sensitivities or allergies that can lead to serious health consequences, your best bet may be to pack her lunch every day. That way you can be reasonably sure that she will not eat something that will cause diarrhea, a stomach ache, or a life-threatening reaction. (If your child also has unusual or limited food preferences, packing a lunch may actually be your *only* bet.)

If your child does sometimes buy lunch in the cafeteria, however, you should be aware of what the National School Lunch Act (NSLA) says about special diets. Under the NSLA, which was issued by the United States Department of Agriculture (USDA), public schools must provide special diets for:

- students on an Individualized Education Program (IEP) who have a physician's statement of need, and
- students with a food allergy or medical condition requiring a special diet who are not on an IEP, with a physician's statement of need.

The physician's statement of need must be kept in the student's file and must include the following information: 1) the student's disability (e.g., autism and peanut allergy, or autism and celiac disease); 2) the major life activity affected by the disability (e.g., learning or caring for herself); and 3) the foods to be omitted or substituted. Usually, this statement should be written on the doctor's stationery or prescription pad and signed by the physician, but check with your school to see if they have any other requirements.

To be safe, provide a copy of the physician's statement and list of safe and unsafe foods to the office staff, your child's teacher(s), and the food service staff, as well as the school nurse.

Note: If your school does not provide school lunches to any students (because it is too small, doesn't have a cafeteria, etc.), it cannot be required to provide a special diet to your child.

an EpiPen® to provide adrenaline in an emergency situation. If your child has a serious food allergy, you should discuss emergency treatment with your child's doctor. You should also alert the school and any individuals who work with your child about her allergy. It may be wise to educate everyone who works in the school cafeteria, including cooks and lunchroom aides, about foods your child must not eat. Consider having your child wear a medical ID bracelet such as the MedicAlert® bracelet (see the Resource Guide).

Summary

Children with autism spectrum disorders can have a variety of different eating problems. Some have food sensitivities, others have limited food preferences, and still others may eat nonfood substances. Occasionally children with autism have problems with overeating, which, when combined with limited physical activity, can lead to obesity. Certain medications, particularly some of the major tranquilizers, may also encourage weight gain. Sometimes if food problems are really substantial, a dietitian, nutritionist, or another professional (occupational therapist or speech-language pathologist) may be needed to consult with you about your child's diet or eating problems. Your child's doctor usually will be the first person to talk with about these issues. Some medical conditions may cause weight changes; you should talk to your doctor about sudden or unexpected increases or decreases in weight.

Although helping your child achieve good growth and nutritional habits may be complicated by her autism, this goal is no less important for your child than for any other child. Indeed, it may even be more important for your child, since her ability to live independently as an adult may depend in part on her learning to eat a healthy diet and avoid any foods that trigger allergies or food sensitivities. If you are concerned about your child, find the professionals who can help you. You cannot and should not have to figure out how to solve your child's food problems alone.

Questions

Q. How can I tell if my child is growing adequately?

Your pediatrician will weigh and measure your child at every well visit and plot these values on growth charts. Your pediatrician will look for steady growth. Most children will grow along a curve somewhere between the 5th and 95th percentile for their age.

Q. My child is on a medication that makes her eat all of the time. How can I tell if she is gaining too much weight?

In addition to measuring your child's height and weight, your pediatrician can calculate a Body Mass Index (BMI) and plot that on a growth chart. If your child's BMI is at the 85th percentile for her age, she is at risk for obesity. If she is at the 95th percentile or greater for her age then she already has a weight problem.

Q. How much milk does my child need?

Milk is important because it provides calcium. A child between 4 and 8 years old needs $2\frac{2}{3}$ glasses of milk and an older child needs approximately 4 glasses of milk per day, if she doesn't get calcium from any other part of her diet.

Q. My child is allergic to milk. How can I get enough calcium into her?

She can drink soy milk if she is allergic to cow's milk but not soy milk. Otherwise, you can give her calcium supplements. There are over-the-counter calcium supplements made for children.

7 | Safety and Your Child

All children have accidents and injuries. The occasional hurt or "owie," broken bone, bump, fall, cut, or scrape is part of growing up. This would be true even if your child did not have a pervasive developmental disorder. However, children with autism and related conditions probably are at increased risk for accidental injuries for several reasons. To begin with, most children with autism spectrum disorders take longer to understand important safety concepts (such as that hot things are dangerous). In addition, they may be more impulsive. Younger children with autism, in particular, seem to have an unusual combination of poor judgment and good motor ability. Other children with autism spectrum disorders (such as Asperger's disorder) may have poor judgment and poor motor ability.

The unusual sensory interests sometimes seen in autism and related conditions (see Chapter 11) can also lead to trouble. For example, your child may not mind the taste of something that most of us would find bitter, or he might be interested in potentially dangerous things that vibrate or twirl, like the wings of a bee or the blades of a fan. Children with autism can also surprise you. The child who is otherwise fearful of new things or situations may seem driven to explore a new construction site, or the child who is otherwise afraid of the water may be preoccupied with a neighbor's swimming pool. Likewise, the child who is usually fearful of things and has been once stung by a bee may not seem to learn from that particular experience. For all these reasons, you should take extra care in trying to prevent problems before they happen.

Your child's developmental age, as well as his size and strength, will greatly influence what he will find enticing and appealing and what he can reach, carry, move, or pull over on himself. All of these factors will influence the kinds of accidents and injuries he may have.

This chapter will include some general information on safety and try to focus on issues specifically related to children with PDD. It is not meant to be an exhaustive discussion of all aspects of safety in children. There are many good books devoted entirely to that topic. Several are mentioned in the Reading List.

We discuss some of the different places in which children spend their time and the different types of accidents and injuries they can have; this is not a complete list, but should give you a sense of the kinds of things to think about. Since many injuries and accidents happen at home, we'll start with general household safety.

These dangers are also often encountered in the daycare or school setting. We'll then discuss separately auto safety, water safety, general outdoor safety, fire safety and burns, choking and suffocation, bites, and poisoning. We'll also discuss self-injury in children with ASDs. In the end, we will explain how to be prepared to deal with these types of problems if they occur despite your efforts to prevent them.

Table 7-1 | Accidents and Injuries

1. Injuries are the leading cause of death in children and adolescents in the U.S.
2. Fatal injuries are just the tip of the iceberg: For every fatal injury, another eighteen children end up in the hospital and over two hundred are treated in the emergency room.
3. The good news (and sad news) is that most of these injuries are preventable.
4. In autism, the available data suggests that children with autism are at increased risk for serious injury and even death due to accidents such as drowning and suffocation.

General Household Safety

Here again, an ounce of prevention is worth a pound of cure. Take sensible precautions as you would for any child. This is especially true for younger children with autism, who have a knack for finding dangerous situations or places. Even for normally developing youngsters, you cannot always anticipate what they will get into.

Typical Precautions

Some of the precautions you might take with small children without disabilities make good sense. Remember, however, that children with autism may be older and larger before they recognize dangerous situations, so you may need to keep these precautions in place much longer than you would for a typical child. Safety steps to take include: cover electrical sockets, lock cabinets that contain poisonous cleaning supplies and paints, put in door latches and stair gates, store knives, scissors, and other sharp objects out of reach. Check the obvious hazards—things like open stairwells, areas where your child could easily fall, sharp objects protruding from walls or floors, etc. Be sure windows are secured and that your child cannot fall out of them. Use window guards on windows, particularly for rooms at the second story and higher. And of course, if there are any guns in your home, be sure they are unloaded and locked away out of all of your children's reach. The absolute safest way to avoid gun accidents is not to have guns in the house.

You also want to keep your home safe from fire or poisonous gases. Matches, flammable materials, candles, and electrical cords can all be dangerous in the hands of a child. Do not run your car in the garage and do not try to use your barbeque inside the house. You should have a smoke detector and a carbon monoxide detector as well as a working fire extinguisher on each floor of your home. Be sure your child cannot turn on the stove himself. Also be sure that your furnace or any wood burning stove or other heaters are working properly. Know what number to call in your area if you have a fire emergency. In many places it is 911.

Special Precautions

To provide a safe environment for your child, you should check your home on a regular basis. Going room by room, think about how things would look from your child's height and point of view. What looks colorful and interesting? What would be tempting to pull at? Something that looks unappealing and unappetizing to you may look delicious to your child. This is even more of a problem when some medications may look, and, indeed, even taste like desirable candies. Remove dangerous objects that your child could get hurt with and block access to places where he could get injured. It is also a good idea to be on the lookout at schools and daycare facilities for obvious dangers so that you can point them out to teachers and others responsible for providing a safe environment.

It's simple to check for obvious hazards, but a little more challenging to be aware of things that are not so obvious, such as poorly fitting screens that are easily jarred loose and might present a temptation to your child. You know your child best and should take precautions based on his idiosyncrasies. However, here are some areas where parents of children with ASDs often need to take extra care:

Preventing Falls. Falls, such as down the stairs or out a window, are mostly a problem for younger children, but some older kids with autism may misjudge a distance or a height and have an unexpected accident. If your child likes to move chairs around and climb, be sure that he can't climb onto a windowsill and then fall out of the window. Make sure all windows have screens that can't be easily dislodged. You may need to block the space in front of windows if your child is a good climber. Gates can be used to protect children from falling down stairs. You may need to fasten the gate to the wall if it is at the top of a staircase. Pressure gates may give way if a bigger child pushes into it.

Keeping Your Child from Wandering. If your child has a tendency to wander outside by himself, there are special locks for outside doors. These make it harder, hopefully impossible, for your child to open the outside door on his own. Some people use deadbolt locks; some use a regular lock or hook and eye type lock as well very high up on the door (well out of the child's reach). You do not want to lock the door with a key and take the key away because of other safety concerns. You need to be able to get out of the door if there is a fire. If your child has a tendency to wander, for example, in a shopping mall or department store, think about helping him learn to wear a MedicAlert® bracelet. The bracelet can have your child's name, your name, and phone number or just the phone number if your prefer; you may want to state that your child has autism. Your pharmacy or doctor can help you get such a bracelet. In Chapter 8 we talk about how you can monitor your child at night.

Mouthing Objects. If your child mouths objects, as many children with autism do, you should be sure that lead-based paint was not used at home or in school. Lead based-paint has not been used for indoor paint in this country for several decades, but some people still live in houses with old paint. (See Chapter 6 for information on lead poisoning.) Also ensure that medications and other things your child might mistake for food are always kept out of reach and in a secure place. You may need to avoid toys with small pieces past the usual recommended age of three years if your child likes to mouth things.

Your Child's Bedroom

You should make sure that your child's bedroom is especially safe because he will spend time in there alone. In fact, children often spend more time in their room than any other place. Often it is best to keep this room sparsely furnished. You may want to put your child's clothes in open plastic baskets instead of a heavy dresser or store them in another room. Also keep his books in another room instead of in a bookcase in his room. This way, your child cannot climb on tables, bookcases, or dresser drawers and have them fall over on him. An alternative is to bolt the furniture to the wall to prevent it from tipping over. If you have decorations on the wall, be sure they are safe or out of reach.

You may need to put a bell on your child's bedroom door or use an intercom to alert you when he is leaving the room, especially at night. Sometimes parents find a loose latch on the door is the only way to keep their child safely in his room at night. Another option that can work nicely is to use a Dutch door; you can then lock shut the bottom half of the door and keep the top half open so you can either see or hear your child.

If your child with autism shares a room with an older sibling, be sure that none of the older child's belongings present a safety hazard. If he shares a room with a younger sibling, be sure, particularly at night, that both children are safe.

Supervising Your Child at Home

Many children with autism or PDD will require safety supervision longer than other children. They may mouth objects or eat unusual items until an older age than children without any disabilities. Their judgment about which places are safe and what might be hot or sharp may not be as good as you would like, and you may need to keep safety measures in place longer than for other children in the family. Many children with autism, particularly young children, are not safe unless someone is watching them all of the time.

The best ways to provide a safe environment will vary with your child's age and surroundings. For younger children and for many older children with PDD, you will need to either:

1. have someone keep an eye on them constantly,
2. take them along when you need to leave the room briefly, or
3. have a safe area where they can be left alone briefly without any risk of harm. A crib or playpen may be a safe place for a younger child. Your child's bedroom can be a safe and secure place to leave him briefly if he can't get out on his own. You want to make sure your child is safe wherever he is—both inside and outside, at home or daycare, in the car or school bus, at school or a sitter's or outside in any play areas.

Auto Safety

Many children are hurt each year in car accidents. You can minimize the chances of injury by following National Highway Traffic Safety Administration (NHTSA) recom-

Teaching Your Child Safety Concepts

As your child gets older and acquires more language, you (and the school) should make a point of teaching safety concepts. You can use picture schedules and visual cues to help children who are just learning language. Topics to teach include ideas like what things are dangerous (hot objects, electrical outlets), how to cross the street, and, as children get older, the appropriate use of household items that have some potential for being dangerous (electrical appliances).

Keep in mind that there is some (relatively slight) potential for "overdoing" this teaching—that is, you could end up making your child frightened of certain situations if you make them sound too dangerous. Focus on concepts important for your child's safety in the real world. Use explicit teaching at whatever level is appropriate to your child. If a situation makes *you* very anxious or frightened, think about having someone else work on this with your child (or work with you first) so that your own anxiety is not part of what your child learns.

Teach *generalization* of safety concepts—don't, for example, let your child learn to cross the street only in one spot. Given the tendency of children with autism toward rigidity, you should work very specifically on generalization and teaching "the big picture."

mendations. They suggest using the child safety locks on the back doors of your car to keep kids from opening the doors from the inside. They also recommend that parents use a window lock to prevent children from being able to open the windows themselves. And, most importantly, they recommend that children under twelve sit in the back in age appropriate safety restraints. That means infants from birth to twenty pounds and one year of age need to be rear facing in a car seat appropriate for their weight. Children from one to approximately four years old should be in a safety seat facing forward. Older and larger children (starting at forty pounds) can be in a booster seat.

In deciding when to switch your older child to a seat belt, the NHTSA website advises, "Use vehicle lap and shoulder belt for children who have outgrown a booster seat and can sit with his or her back straight against the vehicle seat back cushion, with knees bent over the vehicle's seat edge, without slouching, and feet on the floor (approximately 4'9")" (www.nhtsa.dot.gov). Recently there has been a move to keep children in booster seats until they are older and bigger. This is thought to be safer than switching to a regular seatbelt at age four years. Many local fire and police departments provide a free inspection to be sure that you have the car seat or booster seat installed properly.

If your child does not like being restrained, you will need to be sure that he cannot undo the safety belts or restraints. You may want to have another person sit next to him in the back seat to keep him safely buckled up. There are also some products available that can make it harder for your child to unbuckle his seatbelt. For example, there's something called the Childproof Seat Belt Guard® (http://childproofseatbelt.com; 631-474-5851), which consists of a plastic tube that slips over the end of the buckle so that only someone with longer fingers can undo the buckle. You might also consider the Seat Belt Alert® by Child Safety, which makes an alarm sound if your child unbuckles his seatbelt.

If your child gets out of his car seat or seatbelt, be prepared (as soon as you can do so safely) to make a point of pulling over and stopping the car so you can get him back into the car seat or seatbelt.

If your child rides in a bus or van to school, be sure someone supervises him getting properly seated before the ride home. Some children with autism spectrum disorders need an aide on the bus to be sure they don't undo the safety restraint and get out of their seat.

Water Safety

Some parents may find that their child enjoys being in the water, and that this has a calming effect on him. However, you need to be careful that your child is never left alone in the water, not even briefly. This is especially true of any child with seizures. Drowning can occur at home in the bath or outside in a pool, even a small child's pool.

If you use an inflatable or small pool, it is safest to empty it each time after you are finished with it for the day. If you have a larger pool that remains filled, you need adequate gates, locks, and covers to keep your child from trying to swim on his own. Keep a life preserver nearby. A safety alarm that lets you know when something, or someone, has hit the surface of the pool is a worthwhile investment. Teach good safety around the pool—no running, no diving into shallow parts of the pool. Also keep in mind that if you have a pool, you'll also have pool chemicals around that need to be inaccessible to your child.

It is a *very* good idea to have your child learn to swim. Most importantly, he is less likely to drown if he knows how to swim. Furthermore, swimming is a great sport—it provides good exercise, offers opportunities to learn some self-care skills (such as changing clothes), and can be a good way to meet other children and adults in a more controlled and less threatening situation. Unlike team sports (which are highly social), swimming can be a bit more of an isolated activity that you can do in the presence of other people.

Outdoor Activities

Going to the playground can be a great way for your child to get exercise and meet other children. Even when more interactive play is a challenge, the opportunity to be in a new environment and play alongside other children is important. Whenever you visit a new playground—even a school or public playground—take a look around to be sure the area is safe. Look for worn play equipment that is unsteady or ready to break, sharp edges, or exposed nails/screws. Don't let you child mouth play equipment.

For some children, a fenced-in backyard can be a wonderful place for outdoor activities. Again, keep safety in mind, particularly when you put in play equipment. For example, if your child is a fearless climber, you might want to limit the height of playground structures so he won't be tempted to jump. If your child likes to play in the backyard, be sure there are no poisonous plants (see below). Even when an area is fenced in, keep in mind the potential for your child getting out. If possible, try out different types and heights of fencing before you invest in a fence, to make sure you're not wasting money on something your child can scale with ease. Never assume that your child can't get out of a fenced-in area!

Be sure your child is appropriately dressed for the weather. Some children with autism don't like the many layers of clothes worn in cold weather and are at some risk for frostbite if they stay out for any length of time. Conversely, during hot weather be sure your child drinks plenty of fluids and does not become overheated. Some medicines may make it more likely that your child will have trouble tolerating the heat, and a few may increase the risk for serious heat-related disorders. (See Chapter 13.)

Plants and Flowers

Poison ivy, poison oak, and poison sumac are members of a group of plants that often cause reactions in people who come into contact with them. It is the oil or resin of the plant that causes this reaction, which can be mild or quite severe. These plants can pose a problem for children who like to explore and are given opportunities for unsupervised time in an area which the parent thinks safe (e.g., a fenced backyard). Usually a rash develops a day or two after the child is exposed. This rash can be quite a nuisance and can last for days to weeks. It is not contagious, however. For some children with autism spectrum disorders, the rash can set off a whole cycle of itching and scratching, and can lead to skin infection.

Avoiding the plants is the first line of defense. For children who understand it, you can teach the "leaves are three, let it be" rule—because the leaves of these plants come in clusters of three. You can also use actual photographs to teach your child, if this is appropriate. Be sure your own yard does not have poison ivy in it. Also be aware that some pets play in poison ivy and can pass the oil on to humans who touch them.

If your child has been exposed, wash the skin using soap and water. Be careful to do a good job and don't just rub the area (which can spread the oil). Lotions (such as Calamine) and antihistamines (such as oral Benadryl®, not the cream) may help with the itching. If the itching is a real problem or if the poison ivy is quite severe (with blisters and/or swelling or covering a large area of the body), talk to your doctor right away, as there are some prescription medicines that can help. Try *not* to let your child scratch. Also be sure to clean under your child's fingernails (since the oil may stay there unless you clean thoroughly). Also keep in mind that your child's clothing may have been exposed to the oil, so wash everything with soap and water.

In addition to the plants that can cause rashes, there are also a number of plants and flowers that are actually poisonous if ingested. If your child is at all likely to mouth or eat nonfood items, the safest course is not to grow these plants in your house or yard. See the table on the next page.

Table 7-2 | Poisonous or Toxic Flowers and Plants

Common House Plants and Flowers That Are Poisonous or Toxic

- Philodendron
- Dumb Cane
- Peace Lily
- Amaryllis
- Foxglove
- Monkshood
- Lilly-of-the-Valley
- Aloe

- Caladium
- Elephant Ear
- Narcissus
- Daffodil
- Oleander
- Larkspur
- Poinsettia
- Chrysanthemum

Wild Flowers and Plants That Are Poisonous or Toxic

- Nightshade (various varieties)
- Henbane
- Hemlock
- Morning Glory
- Mountain Laurel
- Mistletoe

- Jimson Weed
- Hellebore
- Buttercup
- Castor Bean
- Rhododendron
- English Holly

NOTE: This is just a partial list

Preventing and Treating Accidental Injuries

Burns

Burns can occur in many places. The kitchen stove and oven and fireplace are the most obvious places, but you also need to make sure that your child cannot reach hot liquids such as coffee or soup on kitchen counters or in other rooms. Irons need to be out of reach and hair curlers or straighteners need to be put away safely. You also want to prevent hot water burns in the bath by keeping the water heater temperature at 120 degrees Fahrenheit (49 degrees Celsius) or below, and by testing the water temperature before your child gets into the tub or turns on the water. Also be sure all outlets are covered up and that your child cannot put any objects into the outlets or remove the covers.

Outdoors, barbecues and gas grills should not be left unattended. It is important to realize that they can burn your child even some time after the fire itself has been extinguished and the gas turned off. The same caution applies to wood burning stoves, which can remain hot even if they don't look hot. When your child is outside in warmer weather, be sure he has on sunscreen. You may need to send some along to daycare or school. In many states, schools now require a signed permission slip from a parent to put on sunscreen.

If your child is burned in some way, immediately remove the source of the burn. For example, if a hot liquid spills on your child's shirt, immediately remove the wet clothing and then rinse the area with cold water to wash off any remaining hot liquid. Cool compresses after that can be helpful. A first-degree or superficial burn looks like a sunburn that does not blister. There may be some swelling. Applying cool compresses and giving pain medication when it is needed is probably all you will need to do.

A second-degree or partial thickness burn involves blistering of the skin and is quite painful. A third-degree or full thickness burn is deeper and more serious. For either second- or third-degree burns, you should contact your child's doctor immediately to determine if your child needs to be seen and treated with something other than cool compresses and pain medication.

Choking and Suffocation

Choking and suffocating are problems for children of many ages. Children should be taught to sit while eating and to chew well and not to talk while eating. Small, hard foods such as nuts are some of the most dangerous and frequently inhaled (aspirated). Grapes and pieces of hot dogs can also be dangerous for little children.

Both home and school staff should know about first aid for choking. For example, if you are doing ABA with your child and rewarding him with bits of food, people should know what to do if he starts to choke.

Bed covers and pillows can be a problem with younger children. They may get them over themselves but not be able to remove them. Even older children have to be watched to be sure they do not put a plastic bag over their heads or choke on a piece of a broken balloon. Older brothers' and sisters' toys are often the source of small pieces that can cause choking. Again, keep in mind that if your child shares a bedroom with a brother or sister, you must be sure that no small toys or other choking hazards are available to your child with an autism spectrum disorder.

Some children with ASDs like being in closed spaces. Make sure there isn't anything around the house that your child can climb into and then get trapped if the door closes, such as the washing machine or dryer or an old freezer or refrigerator in the garage or basement.

It is a good idea for all parents to take a CPR and First Aid course. This should cover what to do in situations such as choking. For children over one year of age, parents should know how to do the Heimlich maneuver.

Bites

Animal or Human Bites

Children with ASDs sometimes get too close to animals and run the risk of being bitten. You will usually want to clean the bite area very well and put antibiotic ointment on the area. Some areas become infected more easily than others, especially the face and hands, and bites there may necessitate oral antibiotics.

Call your doctor for advice if your child has a bite that has broken the skin. You will also want to be sure your child is up to date with his tetanus shots, and that whatever animal bit your child is up to date on its shots, especially its rabies shots. If a stray animal or a wild animal has bitten your child, it may need to be quarantined for ten to fourteen day to be sure it is not rabid. Sometimes your doctor will recommend starting shots to prevent rabies until information is available about the health of the animal. If the animal is not caught and therefore is not available for testing for rabies, your child may require the full series of rabies shots. Rabies is a fatal disease that can be prevented with shots but is not treatable once it develops.

Human bites are also important to treat because they can become infected, just like any other breaks in the skin. If your child bites you, another child, or himself, antibiotics should be started if the skin is broken. It can be embarrassing to admit to a doctor that your child bit someone, but you shouldn't risk an infection by not contacting the doctor. Similarly, if another child bites your child and the skin is broken, you should contact your doctor about the need for antibiotics.

Bites are frequently not stitched closed because of concern for infection unless they are very large or on areas of the body that are of cosmetic concern. The best way to deal with bites of all kinds is to try to prevent them. Careful supervision of children can prevent many bites.

Insect bites

Insect bites can be the source of several different kinds of problems. Mosquitoes and ticks can transmit illnesses such as Lyme disease, encephalitis, and Rocky Mountain Spotted Fever. Spider bites can also sometimes be a problem; there are a few spiders that are actually poisonous and can cause serious local reactions, injury, and even death. More commonly, spider bites are uncomfortable and may cause itching and scratching, which can lead to infection. Some children are highly allergic to bug bites such as bee stings, and can have serious—even life threatening—allergic reactions. More frequently, the problem is that the bite leads to skin irritation and scratching, which can set off a negative cycle of more scratching and sometimes even self-injury.

Bug repellants are useful for preventing many insect bites, as is appropriate clothing, such as long-sleeved shirts and long pants. Repellants with DEET® are the most effective. Be sure to wash off repellants at the end of the day. Also be careful not to get them in your child's eyes and don't put any on your child's fingers if he chews or sucks on them. Checking for ticks after your child has been outside can help prevent Lyme disease and other tick-borne diseases.

Usually bug bites are painful and irritating but not a serious problem. However, if you know your child has a serious allergic reaction to bites, you need to be prepared to provide immediate treatment and get medical assistance (see Chapter 4 for a discussion of EpiPens®). For bee stings that are not serious, pull the stinger away with a credit card or dull blade of a clean knife, or use a piece of sticky tape. (Pulling it out with a tweezers is not a good idea since that may inject more venom into the bite.) Then clean the site of the sting with soap and water and put ice or a cold compress on it. You can make a paste of baking soda and water and give Benadryl® if itching is a problem.

Bites and Stings at the Ocean

If your child loves the ocean, you should know which marine animals can be dangerous. Jellyfish, Portuguese-man-of war, and some sharks and fish can sting or bite. You can teach your child what animals to leave alone and what animals he can pick up. Again, pictures can be useful for children who can use them; depending on your child's age and cognitive abilities, you might want to teach him not to pick up *any* sea creatures.

Stingers of ocean animals (jellyfish, anemones, Portugese-man-of war) can be scraped or wiped off, as described above. Be careful when removing these that you don't get stung yourself. Bites and other wounds at the beach are treated in different ways depending on their severity. If you are a frequent beach visitor, know about the animals (and plants) that live in or near the ocean.

Poisoning

Poisonings can occur at many ages. Harmful household cleaners and detergents as well as medications, both prescription and nonprescription, and paints and solvents are common sources of poisonings. Cosmetic products and household plants can also be poisonous if eaten. Be sure to know if any of your indoor or outdoor plants are poisonous. (We list some of the more common ones in the table on page 132.) Other common household poisons are listed in the box below.

Table 7-3 | Common Household Poisons

Kitchen
- Dishwasher detergents
- Drain cleaners
- Ammonia
- Oven cleaners
- Glass cleaners

Bathroom
- Thermometers containing mercury
- Toilet bowel cleaners
- Medicines (over the counter and prescription)
- Deodorizers

Laundry Area
- Detergents
- Bleach

Basement or Garage
- Automotive materials
- Brake fluid
- Gasoline
- Rat/mouse poison
- Lighter fluids/charcoal starter
- Paint thinner/remover
- Antifreeze
- Windshield cleaner/deicer
- Insect killers
- Glues
- Paints
- Kerosene

Other Areas
- Cigarettes
- Furniture polish
- Alcohol
- Moth balls/cakes

To guard against poisoning:

- Keep prescription (and nonprescription) medicines in safe and secure spots with child-resistant caps. (Be aware, however, that even child-resistant caps are not 100 percent effective.)
- Be aware that unfinished alcoholic drinks are potentially dangerous poison if they are consumed by younger children.
- Keep in mind that even a medication or vitamin that you regularly give to your child can be harmful if your child decides to feed himself too many of them.
- Keep poisons in places where your child can't reach them. This can be different places at different ages. Child-resistant latches on cabinets offer some protection, as do child-resistant bottles, but don't underestimate your child's ability to get into things. Substances that are quite poisonous should be kept under lock and key.
- Keep things in their original containers so you know what they are.
- For children who can understand its meaning, use Mr. Yuck stickers and put those on things that are poisonous.

Depending on the poison, sometimes it can cause *more* damage to bring it back up by vomiting. For this reason, the American Academy of Pediatrics now recommends that parents *not* keep syrup of ipecac in the house. Be sure you have the Poison Control Center number near the phone or programmed into your phone. (The national number—which can put you in touch with your local center—is 800-222-1222). When you call the Poison Control Center you should have some basic information:

- Your name and phone number
- Your child's name and age
- Your child's weight
- The name of the product or plant or whatever your child ingested, the amount you think he ingested, and when it was ingested

Also keep important phone numbers ON or VERY NEAR the phone in case of emergency:

It is also important to recognize the warning signs that your child may have gotten into something. These include finding open containers of medicines or cleaning supplies near your child or stains on your child's clothing, or your child suddenly becoming sick (vomiting, seizures, abdominal pain, and so forth). If your child is sick, call 911 first, then poison control. Listen to the poison control people, or your child's doctor, or emergency workers—don't decide what to do on your own! Again, remember that preventing poisoning in the first place is the most important step.

Important Numbers to Post on the Phone

- 911 or local police and fire dept. numbers
- Pediatrician's name and phone number
- Local hospital's emergency room number
- Poison Control Center number

Be especially careful when you have visitors who bring medications or cigarettes with them, or when you go to other people's homes who do not have young children and therefore have not childproofed their homes.

Self-Injury

Besides protecting your child from an unsafe environment, you may occasionally have to protect him from his own self-injury. Although self-injurious behavior is relatively uncommon, when it occurs, it may be so severe that it can cause significant physical injury or may interfere significantly with the child's educational program. Self-injury is most common among children with the most significant degree of developmental delays and seems to increase around adolescence as well as during times of stress.

Self-injurious behaviors can range from repeated scratching and gouging of the skin and eyes, to self-inflicted bites and occasionally to severe head-banging—sometimes severe enough to break bones. Serious damage can result from either the injury itself, or from the injury becoming infected. Skull fractures occur sometimes, as do other permanent injuries or scars. Occasionally, children lose their vision because of self-inflicted wounds.

Sometimes, self-injuries are connected to a medical problem. For example, among adolescents, self-injury may start only when the wisdom teeth cause difficulties, or sometimes nonverbal children may start to bang their ear because they have a painful ear infection. You and your child's doctor should always consider searching for a medical problem associated with the onset of self-injury. Sometimes these problems are difficult to spot and treat. For instance, occasionally a very minor skin problem or irritation may lead to scratching, which results in infection, which causes more irritation and pain and more scratching.

Various methods, including medicines, protective equipment, and behavioral interventions, can be used to control self-injury. Often multiple methods are used together. When these methods are used, parents, doctors, school personnel, and others need to be involved so that everyone works together in a coordinated way in your child's best interest. We talk about some additional aspects of self-injury in Chapter 12.

First Aid

Despite your best efforts at prevention, you will probably have to handle at least an occasional family medical emergency. Knowing what to do ahead of time will help you act quickly and responsibly in an emergency. To prepare yourself, you should read books on first aid such as those mentioned in the Reading List. In addition, all parents can and should take a safety course that includes CPR for children as well as first aid. You will learn to recognize emergency situations and what to do about them. Many courses will include what to do in life-threatening situations such as not breathing, as well as what to do in cases of seizures, choking, near-drowning, bleeding, burns, and other injuries. As mentioned before, you will want to keep a list of important numbers near your phone for yourself or a sitter to use in case of emergency. You may even put labels with these numbers on them on the phone itself.

It can be very useful to have a first aid kit set up in your home before you ever need it. You may want to put everything into a portable container such as a tackle box so that you can take it with you on trips, or show it to a babysitter before you go out. Label it as your first aid kit and put it out of reach of children but where others can easily get their hands on it. You want to be prepared for injuries, bites, bee stings, ingestions, allergies, and illnesses. You may also want to have the same list of emergency phone numbers in your first aid kit that you have posted near the phone. Medical supplies to keep in the kit include:

- A cloth or tourniquet to help stop bleeding
- Soap, hydrogen peroxide, or other cleansers to clean the cut area well. Cotton balls can come in handy for cleaning.
- Both large and small bandages, as well as adhesive tape and gauze pads or rolls. You may also want an antibiotic ointment to apply to the cut area. Sometimes gauze wraps or ace bandages can be helpful in covering the cut and preventing your child from getting to the injured area and scratching or picking at it.
- A pair of tweezers for removing splinters
- Gloves
- Scissors
- Thermometer
- A bulb syringe for suctioning the mouth or nose
- Paper and pencil to keep track of things (such as information from poison control)
- Acetaminophen (Tylenol®) or ibuprofen (Advil® or Motrin®) to treat fevers
- A good measuring spoon, dropper, or syringe
- An antihistamine such as diphenhydramine (Benadryl®), in case of allergic reactions to food, medicine, animals, bee stings, trees, grasses, molds, dust mites, etc.
- If your doctor prescribes it because of a severe allergic reaction in the past, an epinephrine auto injector, such as EpiPen® or EpiPen Jr.®, which is a shot of adrenalin to have available in case of future serious allergic reactions (see page 87 in Chapter 4)

Summary

In this chapter, we've talked about some of the steps you can take to help your child be safe both at home and away from home. As we have said repeatedly, prevention is nine-tenths of the battle here. Go through your home looking for potential danger spots for your child. If your child is small, get down to his level on the floor and take another look (the world can look quite different). Keep in mind your child's special interests and strengths as you are childproofing your home. Help others in your household and at school be aware of safety issues.

Even when you can't prevent an injury or accident (which inevitably will happen to every child), you should be prepared to deal with it effectively. Post poison control and other important numbers near your telephone. Read a book on first aid and take a first aid course that includes CPR training. Finally, keep in mind that issues of safety can change for children over time as they become older. Periodically take a look at your home environment to be sure it is still as safe as possible for your child.

Questions

Q. My son has no sense of danger and will go with anyone. Is there any way to help him get a sense of appropriateness with strangers?

The answer here really depends on your child's age and cognitive ability as well as his ability to communicate. For children who are verbal and have reasonably good cognitive skills, there are some general children's books that teach about the problem with strangers (*Too Safe for Strangers* available from *www.FutureHorizons-autism.com* is one of them.) Some of the curriculums developed for schools in teaching about issues of personal space (and preventing inappropriate physical contact) may also be appropriate (see the chapter on adolescence).

Q. My husband's company is relocating. Are there any precautions we should take when we look for a new place to live?

For homes built before the 1970s, be sure that the house is free of lead-based paints. (There are companies that can test the paint to see if it contains lead.) Also test the water for lead (some older pipes were joined with lead solder). Keep in mind the safety concerns we mention in the chapter and look at the house with these in mind. Depending on your child's special needs, there will be a number of things that you will want to do once you move in. For example, be sure that the water is not so hot that a child could be accidentally scalded, check that there are working fire detectors and carbon monoxide detectors, install safety caps on electrical sockets, and so forth.

8 | Sleep and Sleep Problems

Needs for sleep vary considerably over children's development, although parents' needs stay the same! Autism and related disorders pose many challenges for parents and family members. Of these many challenges, problems in sleep are among some of the most difficult to cope with. There are several reasons why sleep problems can be such a problem:

- Parents, who are often already stressed, can become chronically tired and even more stressed by their child's late bedtimes and frequent awakenings during the night.
- Children who do not get a good night's sleep may have more trouble during the day with problem behaviors and with learning.
- Poor nighttime sleeping may result in changes in sleep patterns (such as daytime napping) that can disrupt the family and interfere with school and behavioral interventions.

In this chapter, we'll review some of the changes in sleep that most children go through during development. We'll also talk about some of the problems that children with autism and ASDs have with sleep and discuss some of the reasons why these children might have trouble with sleep. We'll also review some potential resources and solutions. Keep in mind, however, that compared to other troubles, sleep problems can be more difficult than most to deal with and you may need some special help to cope with them. More than half of children with autism will, at some point, have problems with sleep that last over a month and are distressing to them or their parents.

Typical Sleep Patterns

In understanding sleep problems it helps to know a little bit about sleep and how our sleep pattern evolves in childhood. Infants spend much of their time asleep and their level of awareness seems to vary along a continuum from deep sleep to light sleep to drowsiness, up to alertness. During the first month or so of life, the typical baby sleeps about two-thirds of the time. Regular patterns of sleeping and wakefulness are not yet established, but during much of this time the infant has rapid eye movement (also called REM) sleep—parents can see the baby's eye move even while she is asleep. This is the part of sleep when dreaming occurs. As time goes on, the various stages of alertness and sleep become more and more clearly defined. These changes in sleep pattern also reflect other changes, such as in brainwave patterns, and seem to go along with the increasing maturity of the brain.

Throughout life there is a pattern of cycling between deeper and lighter stages of sleep during the night, with awakenings much more likely to occur during lighter stages of sleep. The lighter stages of sleep appear every 50 to 90 minutes (depending on the age of the child). In addition to this pattern of cycling, a pattern of being awake during the daytime and sleeping during the nighttime also becomes established.

A full-term baby will spend about half its sleep time in REM sleep. This percentage gradually decreases with age so that by age five, only about 20 percent of a child's sleep is spent this way. During the first several months there is not usually a pattern of different day- and nighttime sleeping, but at about four months this starts to shift for most babies. Around this time the baby will start to move towards a pattern of doing more sleeping at night, although she still will be asleep during much of the day. The age at which sleeping through the night occurs on a regular basis is quite variable. Most babies will sleep for a six- to eight-hour stretch by six months. Some will do this as early as three to four months of age, and, unfortunately for parents, some much later than six months. Between six and fifteen months, most children start to sleep ten to twelve hours at night. There will also be regular daytime naps.

Problems in sleeping are fairly common in typically developing toddlers. These include a reluctance in going to bed and getting to sleep, waking during the night, and waking too early in the morning. In general, these sleep problems get better with age and some physicians tell parents that "tincture of time" treatment is indicated—that is, that the child will outgrow the problem. For typically developing children, a pattern of daytime-nighttime sleeping like an adult's will usually be quite well established between ages three and four. Unfortunately, this often is not true for children with autism and related difficulties.

Sleep in Autism

For many children with autism and related conditions, the development of more typical sleep patterns can take much longer. Sometimes parents will tell us that sleep has never been a problem. Other times parents will tell us that their child slept pretty well as an infant but then sleep seemed to get more disorganized. For example, as a toddler she might have started to wake up during the night and climb into her parents' bed or demand attention. Also, it seems that many children with autism may not sleep through the night on a regular basis until much later in life. They may stay up late and sometimes cause troubles for themselves and parents as they wander about the house at night. Sometimes the problem is that they wake up early. Or they may be highly dependent on quite specific and precise routines, which sometimes get more and more complicated over time, with any violation of the routine leading to a rough night.

Many parents are up for a good part of the night waiting until the child finally goes to sleep so that they can go to bed. As parents become more tired and stressed, they may have more difficulty coping with their child (and other parts of their lives) in the daytime—which may further contribute to the child's troubles.

There is a small, but growing, body of research on this important problem. It can, however, be difficult to understand all the studies. Often there are major differences in the ways the investigators approached the problem or they studied only very small groups of children, so we don't have a good sense of how "typical" the population of very atypical children really is. Most importantly, very few studies have followed the same children over time; these longitudinal studies would be very important in helping us understand how sleep problems in autism change over time.

As a result of these problems, researchers do not unanimously agree about the true nature of the sleep troubles in autism. For example, some researchers suggest that it is younger children with autism who are most likely to have sleep problems. Others propose that the issue has less to do with age and more with the child's overall level of development. Still others suggest that differences are not strongly related either to the child's age or developmental level. Some argue that perhaps parents of children with special needs may be more sensitive to sleep problems, although recent data suggest that, if anything, sleep problems are much more common in children with PDD.

In a recent study from California, a bit more than 50 percent of parents of school-age children with PDD reported sleep problems (Honomichl et al., 2002). This was confirmed by use of sleep diaries (records parents kept of the child's sleep), as well as by use of a questionnaire. This number is consistent with reports from other researchers. The problems parents noted included difficulties in getting their child to sleep as well as frequent awakenings in their child. In this study, there were some age-related changes in sleep. For example, younger children who did not have sleep problem slept longer than older children who did not have sleep problems. However, in the children who had sleep problems, these age-related changes were not seen nearly as strongly. In this study, parents of children with sleep problems were, as we might expect, more likely to feel stressed and hassled than parents of children who were "good" sleepers. It also seemed that, if anything, parents probably *underreported* sleep problems, most likely because they were used to them! Unfortunately we don't know how representative the group of children was in this study, but it is clear that sleep problems are very common.

We don't know all the reasons why sleep patterns don't become well organized for many children with autism and other developmental disabilities. There have been many theories and speculations, but relatively little research has been done. There likely are very complicated relationships between the developmental problems and a lack of sleep, which tends to cycle on itself by causing chronic tiredness and further sleep difficulties. Lack of physical exercise—which typically developing children often get through social play at a young age—may also contribute. Some investigators have suggested that some of the brain problems that are responsible for the autism in the first place may disrupt the child's sleep. Basic problems in the day-night cycle may also be involved.

Dealing with Sleep Problems—Some General Advice

Fortunately, there are a number of steps you can take to help your child have, and maintain, a more reasonable sleep cycle. One of the strategies that works here, as well as for other behavior problems, is to capitalize on your child's desire for structure and consistency. That is, try to use your child's desire for routine and predictability to help establish a reasonable sleep pattern. This means having a consistent bedtime for your child and a bedtime routine that you follow consistently. The bedtime routine can include activities and preparations such as a review of the day's events, a relaxing bath, a story, or other favorite (but quiet) activity in the bed. The use of visual schedules or stories specifically focused on bedtime may also be helpful here. You can make a bedtime book, or a story board with pictures, that outlines your child's bedtime routine and then turn over a picture as each bedtime activity is completed.

As with other activities, always think about building in some slight variations to your usual routine, since some children with autism become very rigid about everything involved in the ritual of going to sleep. Try, when you can, to vary things a bit to be sure your child has some flexibility when things *can't* always be the same. You may, for example, want to have a couple of different books your child can look at with you before going to sleep. If your child has a favorite object she sleeps with, it is OK to use it every night (but then be careful because you'll need to have it!). While a routine may help your child get to sleep, you don't want to be stuck with too rigid or involved a bedtime routine that takes forever to get just right.

Keep in mind that while your goal is to help your child get to sleep at a reasonable hour, what you can actually control is only that your child is in bed on time. If your child stays up for a while but is quiet in her bedroom, that may be perfectly fine. Try not to teach your child to be dependent upon you for falling and staying asleep. For many parents, the most burdensome part of sleeping difficulties is coping with their child's need for the parent(s) as part of their bedtime routine. When children have this need and have difficulties falling asleep, parents can quickly find themselves sleep deprived. Some parents will end up sleeping with their child, although then the child's tendency to wake up frequently may make it difficult for the parent to get a good night's sleep (not to mention complicating relationships with the spouse).

Give your child the chance to get to sleep on her own and don't "hover" around her. Praise and rewards can be used—again, not necessarily for sleep but for quiet time in the bedroom. If your child needs a bottle or glass of water next to the bed, that is fine. However, be careful *not* to get into the habit of giving her a snack, since this can unintentionally reinforce her getting up.

Pay attention to the environment in the bedroom. Is it one that will help your child get to sleep (and stay asleep) or is it one that will "jazz" her up and make getting to sleep even more difficult? Some children are very sensitive to sounds and the sound of the furnace coming on may, for example, be a source of annoyance to them. Occasionally parents tell us that working to quiet the various noises in the house (dishwasher, laundry, and so forth) helps. Other parents buy a "white noise" machine or similar device to hide or mask other noises that bother their child. (There are various versions available, some with a choice of sounds like rainwater, the ocean, etc.) Determining the right amount of light can also be crucial. Some children cannot sleep with too much light in the room or hall. Others need the light for reassurance. This may vary with the child's age.

Whatever else you do, do not make the mistake of encouraging problematic sleep patterns, for example, by letting your child miss school because she's had a "bad night." This is a surefire ticket to disaster as the problem starts to build and cycles on itself and your child becomes even more likely to stay up at night and sleep in the daytime. When you are tired and stressed and dealing with a tired child, it can be very easy to unintentionally reinforce the behavior that is causing trouble in the first place.

Pay attention to your child's schedule of daily activities. Excessive sleep (naps) during the day can cause trouble with nighttime sleep. If this is a problem, try to restrict nap times or shorten them. Be sure that your child has enough physical activity during the day. In addition to its many benefits for health (and often for socialization), regular exercise will help your child feel tired when the end of the day comes. It can be worth it to hire an active, energetic teenager to engage your child in some vigorous physical activity before dinner. However, be sure not to have too much exercise too close to bedtime or it may prevent sleeping at that time. Try, as much as you can, to help your child establish a regular pattern or cycle of sleep and waking that is as much like yours as possible.

Dealing with Specific Sleep Problems

Difficulty Getting to Sleep

One of the biggest sleep problems that parents face is getting their child to sleep in the first place. Some people spend hours trying to get their child to sleep, while others stay up much later than they like. Several different strategies can be used to deal with this problem. We will discuss a few of these here. If your child has sleep problems that don't respond to these suggestions, look at the Reading List for additional resources (your doctor and other parents can often be good sources of additional information as well).

One of the most important places to start in trying to improve your child's sleep habits is to set a specific schedule for the bedtime routine, including when it will start, what activities will be involved, and when your child must be in bed. The idea here is to use the tendency of children with autism to be a bit rigid in helping you set a regular and predictable routine that your child will want to follow. Even with a good, consistent schedule, many children won't go easily to bed. Many are used to their parent(s) being with them until they fall asleep. Some people recommend gradually distancing yourself from the child in her room. For example, if your child is used to having a parent lie on her bed until she falls asleep, you can start by sitting beside her on the side of the bed instead of lying down. If that works for a few nights, you can start sitting at the end of the bed. Eventually, you can work your way to a chair in the room and then in the hall (but where your child can still see you), and eventually out of view altogether. This method does not work for all children, but has the advantage of not causing much distress.

Another popular method for reducing your child's reliance on you is called "graduated extinction" by some sleep experts. This involves putting your child into bed by herself and letting her cry for a short, previously set amount of time. Usually this is less than ten minutes. After that you go back into the room to reassure your child that you are near and to assure yourself that your child is OK. You shouldn't pick your child up, turn on the lights, or start to play, but just quickly check on her and leave. You can gradually increase the amount of time you let your child cry before you check on her. This method allows your child to learn how to settle herself down to sleep. Some children will start sleeping on their own within a few days to weeks. It does not work for all children and parents. One of the problems is that many parents cannot stand to see (or hear) their child being upset. It might also be a problem if your child is extremely hard to calm down once she gets upset and starts banging her head.

Another method that is less likely to upset the child is referred to as "bedtime fading." In this method, you determine what time your child always seems to get so tired that she finally falls asleep. This is usually quite a long time after the originally planned bedtime, say 1 AM. But once you determine this time, you start to put your child to bed an hour or so later than the time when she will fall asleep quickly (e.g., 2 AM). Then you gradually move the bedtime back to your originally desired time. Usually you move it back about fifteen minutes every few days until you get to the desired time.

Difficulty with Nighttime Awakenings

Many children go to sleep well but wake up during the night and then don't go back to sleep easily or quickly. If your child can fall asleep on her own at the beginning of the night, she is more likely to get back to sleep on her own if she wakes up during the night. Studies of typically developing children show that they frequently wake up briefly during the night as they transition through the different stages of sleep. The children we call "good sleepers" (who sleep through the night) are the ones who settle back to sleep on their own during the night without needing their parents. If the bedtime routine involves the parent holding the child, or lying next to her in bed, singing to her, or providing something to drink, the same interventions are frequently needed when the child awakens at night. If a child gets into bed awake and falls asleep without the parent there, she has a much better chance of getting back to sleep alone during the night.

Sometimes you have to use methods such as graduated extinction (described earlier) to get your child back to sleep in the middle of the night.

Some children with autism spectrum disorders who wake up during the night may engage in body rocking or other kinds of stereotyped movements. If the movement helps your child get back to sleep and doesn't otherwise cause trouble, you probably won't need to interfere with it. Other behaviors may need more specific intervention. For example, some children engage in head banging, which we talk about more later in the chapter. Sometimes behaviors like head banging can be made worse if parents pay a lot of attention to them. At other times the behavior will be sufficiently serious that you have to pay attention to it. In these complicated situations it is very helpful to get some outside advice and perspectives. Both your child's healthcare providers and other professionals such as psychologists may be helpful. Other habits such as teeth grinding (see Chapter 10) may also need special interventions, as we'll discuss shortly.

Early or Late Awakenings

Sometimes noises or too much light will awaken your child earlier than you want. If these environmental factors are contributing to early awakening, they are easy enough to change. For example, put up shades or curtains to keep the room dark. You can also try putting your child to bed a bit later in hopes that she may sleep longer. Sometimes you may want to help your child learn to play quietly on her own in her bedroom until the household is up. As time goes on, your child can have a list of early morning activities to engage in that will help her transition more easily into the day.

Some children have trouble getting up in the morning. Sometimes this is part of a more complicated set of difficulties (such as going to sleep too late). It is important to realize that one of the important goals for your child is to have a fairly normal sleep-wake cycle. We've seen children who are basically up during the night and asleep during the day—not a situation that helps parents nor helps the child get a decent educational program or a good night's sleep. With the occasional, understandable exception, you do not want your child to sleep too late in the morning.

If your child has trouble getting up, then look at ways that you might help her wake up in the morning in a lower key way—for example, turning on a tape recorder with a favorite song or CD, letting a favored pet into the room to wake your child up, and so forth. Again, having a plan with a clear goal and set of graduated steps can be helpful.

Wandering during the Night

Nighttime wandering refers to children who get up and roam (wander) about the house. It is one thing if your child gets up only to go to the bathroom or get a drink; it is much more difficult if she is getting into trouble—for instance, by leaving the house or engaging in behavior that might be dangerous. If your child has problems with wandering at night, you can think about some modifications to the environment to ensure her safety. Possible solutions include:

- Use strategically placed baby monitors. By strategically placed, we mean putting these just outside your child's bedroom so you don't have to listen to every noise that your child makes at night but will know when she decides to venture outside the room.
- You may need a gate at the door to keep a younger child from wandering outside the room (and possibly hurting herself).
- If your older child can get over a baby gate, you may do well with a Dutch door (one with a top and bottom half) where you can lock the bottom half but keep the top part open.

If your child tries to get out of the house, you'll clearly need to take more extensive precautions such as double locking the front and back doors with a key that you keep hidden or rigging an alarm that goes off if the door is opened.

Nighttime Bedwetting (Enuresis)

Bedwetting during sleep (nocturnal enuresis) is common in typically developing children, particularly boys, who are otherwise dry in the daytime. This problem tends to get much better as children get older, although it persists into adolescence for some children.

Many children with autism/PDD have a prolonged period of toilet training, although for others toilet training goes fairly close to schedule. Some children become toilet trained during the day but then wet themselves at night. Sometimes they have never had a period of being consistently dry through the night (what is called primary enuresis) and other times they are able to be dry for a period of time (typically a month or longer) but then lose this ability and start to wet again (secondary enuresis).

Depending on your child's developmental level, nighttime bedwetting may or may not be distressing to your child (but can still be quite distressing to parents). Before trying any of the solutions in this section, consult your doctor. Also keep in mind that your goal is to be sure not to disrupt any progress your child has already made in getting to sleep.

Studies of children in special sleep laboratories suggest that bedwetting usually happens early in the night. Most often there is no specific physical cause for the bedwetting. Limiting fluids in the evenings usually does *not* help children stay dry at night. (Obviously, if your child is drinking a tremendous amount, that may be a problem.) Sometimes children who had previously been dry at night start bedwetting after experiencing some upsetting event. Sometimes this event is quite understandable—for example, the birth of a new brother or sister or a move from one house to another. But sometimes the responses of children with ASDs are very different from those of other children and it may be hard to understand exactly what has gotten your child upset or stressed. If the bedwetting is a new symptom, you should check with your doctor about getting a urine culture, just to be sure that the bed wetting is not due to a urinary tract infection.

Both behavioral and drug treatments are available for bedwetting that begins after the child has been toilet trained. A hormone called DDAVP helps many children and can be taken at bedtime as a pill or nasal spray. It requires a prescription from your doctor. It only works while you take it and the bedwetting problem will continue until your child outgrows it. The drug imipramine has been used for short times for older children and can be very effective. Other drugs are also available. As with any medication, the potential risk of the medicine should be balanced against the potential benefits.

Behavioral methods have commonly used a kind of learning often referred to as the "bell and pad" in which the child sleeps on a special pad which sounds an alarm when she wets the bed. This wakes the child up, and, over time, she learns to stay dry.

It is worth plugging away at problems with nighttime bedwetting, since, over time, many children do become dry. At the same time, if you reach a point where the hassles involved in changing wet sheets every morning are too much for you, keep the option of using large size "pull ups" in mind.

Nightmares and Night Terrors

Occasionally, verbal children with autism complain of nightmares, often associated with specific fears. Nightmares tend to happen in the later part of the night and your child may remember some part of the bad dream. Nightmares may also occur when children are sick. Usually, going to your child and reassuring her that she was just dreaming is sufficient. If your child has repeated nightmares, however, it may be worth trying to understand more about the problem. For example, if your child is chronically having frightening dreams about school, find out if anything unusual is going on.

Night terrors (also called sleep terrors) are different from nightmares. These tend to happen in the first part of the night's sleep. The child arouses but does not awaken completely, seems to be in a panic, and may not be able to explain what has happened. Unlike with nightmares, the child will have little memory of any content of a bad dream. Sometimes night terrors are associated with sleep walking (somnambulism). If your child seems to be having night terrors, be sure to discuss this with the doctor. Very rarely the symptoms of temporal lobe seizures (see Chapter 9) may be similar.

The most important thing to know about sleep terrors and sleep walking is that it is important to keep your child safe. You can use a baby monitor or alarm system to alert you if your child is up and wandering. Sometimes drug treatment is indicated but only if the problem is severe.

Head Banging and Body Rocking

Some typically developing children (roughly 5 percent) bang their heads or body on the crib or bed. This usually starts in very young children (under a year). Body rocking before the child falls asleep is also seen. In typically developing children, these behaviors tend to disappear on their own—sometimes fairly quickly, but at other times they may go on for several years. These movements are likely pleasurable to the child and are a form of self-soothing around the occasionally anxiety-provoking transition to sleep.

Children with autism and related disorders also sometimes head bang or body rock at night. These behaviors may, however, persist in children with autism for a longer period of time and may become part of the child's nighttime sleeping ritual. Often these movements are not a major problem, but sometimes the behavior may escalate over time and pose a threat to the child.

If your child has these behaviors, keep several things in mind. First, make sure your child is safe. Putting pillows or pads around the bed may help. Second, ask yourself if anything seemed to set the behavior off. Did you move to a new house? Was there a change in your child's behavior during the day? Is she having pain anywhere—for example, are new teeth coming in? If you can figure out what set the behavior off, you may be able to think about some potential solutions. Third, consider whether your child might be using head banging for some reason, such as to communicate frustration or get your attention. For example, does your child stop head banging when you come into the room? Does she stop if you can identify something she wants? Behaviors like head banging can be *very* effective at getting parental attention and this, in turn, may reinforce your child's behavior.

There are some strategies that people suggest to try to help with these problems, but unfortunately they don't always work. Try putting a clock with a loud "tick-tock" in the room. Sometimes the rhythm of the sound of the clock will soothe your child. Or try other forms of rhythmical sounds, such as a sound generator to mimic the sound of the beach or of rain falling down. Some parents have used a metronome.

If there are serious concerns about injury, you will need to take additional steps to ensure your child's safety. If the pillows/cushion approach hasn't worked, you can try taking the bed out of the room and putting the mattress on the floor. (This may be particularly helpful if body rocking is the main problem.) Very occasionally, parents have to resort to having their child wear a helmet or some other protective gear so as to avoid head injury. If you are concerned about your child's safety at night, consult a behavior specialist for suggestions.

Teeth Grinding

Like head banging and body rocking, grinding of the teeth (bruxism) is fairly common in typically developing children. In fact, as many as 10 percent or so of typically developing toddlers and preschool children may grind their teeth. In typically developing children, the problem tends to go away over time, doesn't usually cause trouble for the teeth, and usually does not need any special treatment.

In children with autism spectrum disorders, teeth grinding can be more persistent and thus cause more trouble. As with bedtime body rocking, occasionally teeth grinding seems to be stress related; see if you can find any connection to potentially stressful events in your child's life. At other times, it may be more self-stimulatory. Sometimes teeth grinding is more of a problem for parents than the child, but it can cause dental problems, and a dentist or other dental specialist may need to be involved if it persists (see Chapter 10). If your child grinds her teeth, point this out to your child's dentist so he can keep an eye on it.

Medical Issues and Medications

Keep in mind that some medical problems, as well as some medicines, foods, or drinks that have caffeine, can cause sleep problems. If, for example, your child is drinking many sodas with caffeine in them, you may want to switch to caffeine free.

If your child has been sleeping well but suddenly starts having sleeping troubles, it is worth asking yourself whether she is getting sick or is uncomfortable. This is a complicated issue, particularly for children who are not yet able to use words well to communicate. Some children who have gas or intestinal pain may have trouble sleeping. Has your child been started on a new medicine that might be upsetting her stomach? Other medical problems such as ear infections or urinary tract (bladder) infections or gastrointestinal problems (like reflux) may also disrupt sleep. Ask your child's doctor if any physical problems might be causing trouble. For example, sometimes breathing problems cause sleep difficulties. This may be related to very enlarged tonsils and adenoids, for example, or sometimes to allergies. Ask yourself if there are any regularities to your child's sleep troubles. Do they occur during some months of the year and not others? Some children seem to have more trouble in winter; others in summer. Any such regularities might help you understand what may be going on. For example, if your child has sleeping difficulties only in winter after you turn on your furnace, it might be worth checking for allergies to the dust mites that commonly live in air ducts and get stirred up again once the furnace is switched on.

If your child receives medications, ask your doctor or pharmacist whether these might be affecting sleep. Medicine your child is given for other reasons might also help with sleep problems if they tend to make her drowsy. If so, you can ask whether these medicines could be given at night time. These medicines include some of those given for behavior problems (see Chapter 13) and some given for other reasons, such as allergies.

Parents often ask us about medicines that might help their child with autism go to sleep. These, unfortunately, work with variable success. Medicines for sleep problems are best used as a last resort—for example, at a time when you know you are likely to have trouble (on a vacation or when a parent is away) or to deal with an expected situation or crisis. You should be aware that these are, at best, a temporary solution. There are various medicines that can be used. These include a range of different medicines and your doctor would be the best person to speak to about this possibility.

A commonly used nonprescription medication for temporary relief is diphenhydramine (Benadryl®). It is an antihistamine that often makes people a bit drowsy (sometimes that is enough). There are also many prescription medicines to help people sleep. These include other antihistamines, sedatives, and medicines such as Valium® (diazepam) and the related group of medicines called the benzodiazepines. These sometimes help children with autism, for periods of time, although some children get "hyper" on them. One of the problems with these medicines is that if you take them on a regular basis, your body gets used to them and you must take a larger dose over time.

Melatonin has received a great deal of publicity in recent years as a "natural" cure for many sleep problems. It makes people sleepy and also helps to reset their sleep cycles. It is a hormone that is secreted normally by a part of the brain called the pineal gland. Your body puts out more melatonin as it gets darker outside.

There is some research on the use of melatonin to help with sleep problems in children with various disabilities. A few reports mention its use in autism. None of these are large, well-designed studies. The doses given vary over the different studies and none of the studies look at the possible side effects of long-term use. All this being said, some studies report success. Doses mentioned most frequently are between 1 and 3 mg before bedtime, although one author recommends an even smaller dose. Melatonin is not a prescription drug and is sold widely in health food stores. Keep in mind that because it is not a prescription drug, it is not regulated by the FDA. Be sure to discuss the use of melatonin with your child's healthcare provider before trying it.

If your child has significant sleep problems, your doctor may want to refer you to someone who specializes in the use of medicines in the treatment of autism, as sometimes the process of finding the right medicine can be tricky. Occasionally, children with autism will have the opposite reaction to what is expected (or what is called a "paradoxical" reaction) when given a medicine for help with sleep. As a result, it is usually wise to try the medicine at home once or twice before you use it elsewhere (to be sure that it has the desired effect). As with all medicines, there are risks and potential benefits to medications prescribed for sleep problems, and you should discuss these with the doctor before trying the medicine.

When All Else Fails

When you feel you have done a reasonable job in trying to deal with sleep problems but they still occur, ask your doctor about other resources that may be available. A number of professionals may be able to help, including psychologists and physicians who are interested in autism and related conditions, as well as specialists in sleep problems. Many major medical centers have sleep disorder clinics that may be a resource for you. Also consult some of the publications found in the Reading List. There are now several books that address sleep problems in individuals with autism and other developmental disabilities.

Summary

In this chapter, we've discussed some of the most common sleep problems in children with autism and related disorders. Some children with autism have difficulty falling asleep, others with staying asleep, and yet others with waking up early in the morning. Since insufficient sleep at night can add to your child's learning and behavioral problems during the day and also impair your own coping abilities, you should never just accept sleep problems as an inevitable part of autism. Various methods can be useful in helping your child achieve and maintain a good sleep pattern. A thoughtful analysis of what you really want and can hope to achieve plus a sensible plan for getting to this goal will be very helpful.

Reference

Honomichl, Ryan D., Goodlin-Jones, Beth L, Burnham, M., Gaylor, Eriak, and Anders, Thomas F. (2002). Sleep patterns of children with pervasive developmental disorders. *Journal of Autism and Developmental Disorders, 32:* 553-561.

Questions

Q. I've heard that in typical kids, sleep problems can mimic AD/HD. Do you think that can happen with kids with autism too?

Children (or for that matter adults) can become rather frazzled and disorganized if they don't have enough sleep. There is some research on sleep in children with autism that says that they tend to have more trouble getting to sleep and wake up more during the night—which would mean they get less sleep than they need. However, the fact that a child is frazzled because she didn't get enough sleep is *not* the same thing as having AD/HD (see Chapter 12).

Q. My child is on an SSRI due to her anxiety and it has really helped her be more at ease in the classroom and less anxious about new experiences. At first the medicine seemed to help her fall asleep, but now she sleeps really restlessly and she wakes up multiple times at night. Could the medication be causing this? I hate to lose the good benefits of the medication by discontinuing it, but my child is so irritable and inattentive when she doesn't sleep well. How should I resolve this?

Some children taking an SSRI do have trouble sleeping. Sometimes this side effect is not seen immediately; at other times it is part of a broader pattern of agitation and "activation." Talk to the doctor who is prescribing the medicine. Some children will do well with one SSRI and not with another.

Q. I am just *so* tired all the time. Sometimes I can barely keep my eyes open at work and I feel like I have no energy. But I feel as if it's more important for my child with autism to get a good night's sleep than for me to sleep, so I often sacrifice my own sleep to make sure she goes to sleep and stays asleep. My husband lies there sleeping like a rock and I get so resentful sometimes. What should I do?

Talk with your doctor (and with your husband). Using some of the strategies described in the chapter, try to help your child learn to get to sleep on her own—this is the most important thing. It can take time but is worth doing. Take turns so you and your husband share in getting up if you need to. Discuss the sleeping arrangements with your child's doctor. Also talk with other parents. For yourself, try to arrange (at least for the short term) the chance to take some naps during the day to catch up on your own sleep!

9 | Seizure Disorders

Seizure disorders are the most frequently encountered medical complications associated with autism. Seizures are also observed in other pervasive developmental disorders. Because seizure disorders can begin at any time during the child's development and because these disorders can sometimes be difficult to recognize, it is important that parents and professionals alike be familiar with some aspects of these conditions.

What Is a Seizure?

A seizure is a sudden change in behavior, consciousness, or sensation caused by a change in brain activity. Seizures (also called convulsions, fits, spells, or attacks) are caused by uncontrolled and sudden episodes of abnormal electrical activity in the brain. Some part of the brain begins to "fire" or activate in an uncontrolled fashion and this activity spreads to other parts of the brain and is associated with changes in behavior, the motor system, or sensations. Sometimes the person falls down and loses consciousness, but other times he may simply seem to "tune out" for a few seconds.

Often clues about the origin or location of the starting point of a child's seizures are provided by the symptoms exhibited. These may be seen during what is called the aura—this is a kind of warning sign at the start of certain kinds of seizures. It might take the form of an unusual experience or a change in behavior—for example, the child's lip might begin to twitch or he might experience an unusual smell. Depending on the nature of the seizure, more and more brain cells may become involved and the seizure then becomes more widespread (this is called generalization). The seizure itself can take different forms, which we'll discuss shortly.

Following the seizure, there is often a period when the child is somewhat confused or disoriented as his brain recovers from the seizure. This is called the postictal period (meaning after the attack). After some seizures, the child may go to sleep for a time. The various phases of the seizure can be a bit confusing. That is, the seizure itself may last only a minute but the child can be confused or sleep for a longer period.

Many different kinds of seizures have been identified and you will get a quick education about these types below. You may ask yourself whether taking the time to understand the distinctions among the various types of seizures makes a difference—in this case, the answer is yes! Different kinds of seizures are treated differently. That is the reason neurologists make such a fuss about all this and why it is important for you to understand something about it.

What is the Difference Between Seizure and Epilepsy?

If your child has a single seizure, it will be called just that—a seizure. However, if he goes on to have another seizure, doctors will probably diagnose him as having epilepsy. Epilepsy is a chronic disorder of the brain that involves recurrent seizures, and it can be associated with a range of learning, behavioral, and other problems.

A seizure can be observed as an isolated finding. Sometimes, for example, very young children with autism will have a seizure only in relation to a high fever. These so-called febrile convulsions are not technically classified as epilepsy. Similarly, other seizures can be caused by certain drugs or drug withdrawal, alcohol, or an imbalance of body chemicals. In these instances, epilepsy would not be diagnosed, since the seizures are caused not by a chronic brain disorder, but by something outside of the brain. It is important to realize that a single seizure does not necessarily mean the individual has epilepsy.

How Common Are Seizures?

In the general population, about 5 percent of all children experience a seizure by the time they are 15 years old; more than half of these are seizures associated with a high fever (febrile seizures). Febrile seizures tend not to come back after about the age of six, and do not, of themselves, constitute epilepsy. Only a small number of children with febrile seizures go on to develop chronic seizures or epilepsy. Children who are more likely to go on to develop nonfebrile seizures, or epilepsy, are those who have:

1. underlying brain disorders,
2. focal (localized) seizures, and
3. a family history of epilepsy.

Although most children with autism do *not* have seizures, the risk of having a seizure is still much higher than in typical children. As many as 25 percent or more of all children with autism develop epilepsy. The rate of epilepsy in autism is much higher throughout childhood and adolescence than for typically developing children. (See Figure 1-2 on page 14.) This has been known for some time. In the 1970s, it was appreciated that one of the reasons autism was a distinctive disorder was that many children with autism went on to have seizures in adolescence. The rates of first seizure in autism do vary somewhat between studies and over the age groups studied. Seizures are more common in more strictly diagnosed "classically autistic" cases.

Children with seizures but without other developmental problems often do quite well and the seizures may disappear on their own after some time. However, children with autism tend to develop seizures that are not just due to fevers. Their seizure disorders tend to persist and can further complicate the task of intervention.

Types of Seizures

There are over thirty different kinds of seizures. Most of the seizures that are seen in autism, however, fall into a few general categories. The main distinction made now is between generalized seizures (which involve the entire brain from the beginning of the seizure) and partial seizures (which originate in one part of the brain and may, or may not, spread to involve the entire brain). Sometimes children have both generalized and partial seizures.

In the past, people used other terms to talk about seizures and you sometimes may still hear these old terms, particularly grand mal or petit mal. A grand mal (which means a "big and bad" seizure) tended to be used as a term for what people thought of as "big" seizures (for example, where the child fell down). The term petit mal ("small and bad") was used for seizures that seemed less serious. However, these terms were not used very consistently and often confused things for people. Now the major distinction is between generalized and partial seizures. Seizure types are listed in Table 9-1.

Table 9-1 | Common Types of Seizures*

Generalized seizures (nonfocal seizures)

Name	Other names	Symptoms
Tonic-Clonic	Grand Mal	Loss of consciousness, alternating contraction and relaxation of muscle groups, child may fall, may lose bowel and bladder control. Often confused (postictal) after seizure.
Absence seizures	Petit Mal	Loss of consciousness, with staring, eye fluttering, and maybe facial twitching
Atonic	Drop attacks	Symptoms due to loss of muscle tone; child drops and loses consciousness but there are no generalized convulsions. Recovery is rapid.
Akinetic	Jerk attacks Myoclonic	Muscle jerks (usually arms or head), usually very brief; loss of consciousness is extremely brief

Partial seizures

Name	Other names	Symptoms
Simple partial seizure	Adversive Jacksonian Focal motor	Isolated in one part of the body (movement or sensation). Person remains conscious.
Complex partial seizure	Temporal lobe seizure Psychomotor	Abnormal response to environment, variable across people. Seizures start in one part of the brain and then generalize and the person may lose consciousness.

* selective list

Even with this newer classification system, it can be quite confusing when people talk about the different types of seizures. If your child has a seizure disorder, be sure that your child's physician clarifies for you the type of seizure that your child has.

Generalized Seizures

Generalized seizures affect both sides of the brain at the same time. These account for about 40 percent of seizure disorders in the general population and about 70 percent or more of those seen in autism.

Generalized Tonic-Clonic Seizures

Generalized tonic-clonic seizures are what most people think of when they think about a seizure. These seizures affect the whole body. Usually there's no warning before the seizure starts. The child may fall and lose consciousness. The body then stiffens (the tonic part of the seizure) and muscles begin to alternately contract and relax (the clonic part of the seizure). This gives rise to the jerking movement which is typical of such seizures. Breathing may be affected and might even stop briefly as the muscles become stiff. If this happens, the child may turn blue. The seizure may go on for some minutes with a gradual slowing of the jerking. Often the child may lose bladder or bowel control. Sometimes children sleep for hours after such a seizure. The seizure itself, however, usually lasts only a few minutes.

These are the most common seizures observed in autism. In one study of children with autism, 70 percent of the children who had seizures had generalized tonic-clonic type.

Absence Seizures

Absence seizures (previously known as petit mal) include a very brief loss of consciousness. During this time, which may last for a few seconds, the child stares and may have eye fluttering, mild face twitching, or eye blinking. There are no warning signs before the seizure begins. The child does not fall down, and, once the seizure passes, he is back to normal (but usually cannot remember the seizures).

Often this kind of seizure is very subtle and may be missed. The child "tunes in" and "tunes out" very frequently. This is one of the most common kinds of seizure in children in general. Some children with these seizures have several hundred seizures a day. As might be imagined, these seizures can interfere significantly with learning. Often absence seizures stop before a child reaches adulthood.

Absence seizures can be confused with partial seizures since both kinds of seizure can involve staring; the treatment, however, can be quite different. It can also sometimes be difficult to distinguish this kind of seizure from complex partial seizures. Absence seizures are less common in autism than tonic-clonic seizures and represent maybe 15 percent of all seizures in autism. An EEG will determine which type of seizure your child has. See "Evaluating a Seizure Disorder" below.

If your child has absence seizures, it is especially important that teachers and other people in his life know what these look like so they don't think that it's just "autistic behavior" when your child is staring ahead and not listening to them.

Myoclonic or Atonic Seizures

Myoclonic seizures involve jerking of the muscles (the word myoclonic means muscle jerk). You might see your child kick out unexpectedly. He might fall down if, for example, muscles in the leg are jerking and other muscles are moving. These seizures can be difficult to diagnose in children with autism, given the high rates of stereotyped movements, and because not all muscle jerks are due to seizures.

Atonic seizures are also sometimes seen. These are like myoclonic seizures except that instead of a muscle stiffening, there is actually a loss of muscle tone. That is, suddenly the legs or arm may go limp and the child collapses to the ground.

These seizure types account for less than 10 percent of seizures in autism.

Partial Seizures

Partial seizures probably account for about 10 percent of seizures in autism. The partial seizure may include what is called either a simple partial or a complex partial seizure.

In a simple partial seizure, consciousness is impaired (not totally lost), but in a complex partial seizure, consciousness is lost. The features of simple partial seizures vary depending on what part of the brain is involved. You may see jerking of one part of the body. This might be accompanied by a tingling sensation, but as we have emphasized, the child does not lose consciousness.

Complex partial seizures (sometimes known as temporal lobe seizures or psychomotor seizures) are characterized by unusual but purposeless activity. Consciousness or awareness is altered. There is tremendous variability from person to person, but individuals tend to experience similar symptoms each time they have a seizure. Often there is a warning sign of the seizure. This so-called aura tends to be the same each time. For example, the child may always be aware of an unusual sensation immediately before a seizure. During the seizure itself, the child may be somewhat confused or isolated, may make lip-smacking movements, or may appear drunk or drugged. Abnormalities in sensory perception often occur, particularly at the beginning of the seizure. Although the individual is not violent, he may struggle or fight if restrained. Usually after the seizure the child is very confused but has no memory of the seizure. Typically, such seizures last for one to three minutes. These seizures are somewhat less common in autism compared to generalized seizures.

Partial seizures can involve other symptoms such as change in heart rate and blood pressure or extreme emotions. The way that partial seizures develop may provide important clues as to where in the brain the seizure gets its start.

Febrile Seizures

As we have mentioned, febrile seizures are fever related, are most common in young children (under six), and often do not come back. Do not, however, fail to have your child evaluated following a febrile seizure since you need to be sure that the seizure was not due to something else (like a brain infection). After examination and possibly some lab work, the doctor will likely not recommend more extensive assessment for an isolated febrile seizure.

Susceptibility to febrile seizures may run in families. If you have other children with febrile seizures or if there is a history of seizures in your family, be sure to mention this to your healthcare provider even if your child has not developed seizures. You should also know that if your child has had one febrile seizure, he is at somewhat greater risk for another. There is a 2 to 4 percent chance of developing nonfebrile seizures or epilepsy if your child has had a febrile seizure.

In the past, febrile seizures were treated with antiseizure medicines. This is now uncommon since we now know that many children who have had a febrile seizure don't go on to have seizure disorders and there are potential side effects of medicines used to treat seizures.

Evaluating a Seizure Disorder

If there is a possibility that your child is having seizures, you should consult your child's doctor. She may send you to a neurologist or pediatric neurologist (a specialist in diseases of the nervous system, including the brain). You should explain exactly what you are worried about and your child's primary doctor can help you decide how urgent this is. Even before she sends you to a neurologist, she may want to do some tests or get an EEG (brain wave test). Depending on the results, your child's doctor may then want you to see a neurologist.

The neurological consultation will typically include a comprehensive medical evaluation and a review of your child's and family's history. The neurologist or pediatric neurologist will ask for a very detailed description of what appears to be the seizure. For example, how common are the episodes, do they always happen in exactly the same way or at certain times, can they be interrupted, how long do they last, does your child seem to lose consciousness? Did your child have a fever before the seizures? The doctor will want to know how the episode progresses over time. All this information may provide important clues about whether your child is having seizures, and if so, what kind, and maybe even where they start in the brain.

The neurologist will do a physical examination with a very detailed examination of the central nervous system. This neurological examination will include testing your child's reflexes, looking for specific signs of brain dysfunction. Typically an electroencephalogram (EEG) will also be obtained if it hasn't been already (or it may be repeated).

The EEG (brain wave test) is done by pasting small electrodes onto your child's scalp at certain points. These electrodes have wires that connect to a very sensitive machine that picks up and records very small changes in electrical activity. There is nothing painful involved. Still, it is probably best to try to prepare your child in advance for the EEG. Some children with autism do not like the sensation of paste on their head, but others have no problem. Some may have difficulty staying still and may need help (for example, giving them a favorite video to watch). Discuss the logistics of all this in advance either with the neurologist or the person doing the EEG. In general, it is important to avoid sedating your child with drugs since drugs can, themselves, sometimes affect the EEG.

During the EEG, your child might be exposed to some of the conditions in which seizures are most likely to occur—such as going to sleep or watching a flashing light or even hyperventilating. Sometimes you might be asked to bring your child in after a period of sleep deprivation. Sometimes the doctor will suggest a 24-hour EEG. If so, your child may need to stay in the hospital while a computer records the EEG for a whole day to get a good sense of the various changes in the EEG over the day. Two advantages of 24-hour EEGs are that: 1) any unusual behaviors can be noted by the nursing staff and then related to the EEG, and, 2) a longer EEG record is more likely to show abnormalities. The disadvantage is that it is even more of a nuisance to your child and you. Sometimes a special video EEG will be used to observe your child during the possible seizure itself.

The electroencephalogram or EEG is examined ("read") by a neurologist who takes into account the age of your child as well as clinical symptoms. The doctor looks for the rhythm of the electroencephalogram, for differences between, for example, the right and left side of the brain, and whether there is unusual electrical activity suggestive of seizures. Depending on the history and examination, the doctor may want some other tests done as well—for example, an MRI (magnetic resonance imaging) or CT scan to look at the actual structure of the brain. Some of these studies, such as X-ray, involve radiation, but others, such as magnetic resonance imaging, do not. The doctor may also ask for blood tests in order to look for chemical imbalances, infections, and other factors that

Language Regression and Seizures

Recently, reports on television have suggested that some children diagnosed with autism may actually have a rare form of aphasia (language loss) associated with epilepsy. This is called Landau-Kleffner syndrome. The Landau-Kleffner syndrome (also known as "acquired aphasia with epilepsy" or "epileptic aphasia") usually describes a condition in which epilepsy and language loss occur together (or very close together). Children with LKS develop normally for some years and acquire the ability to speak, but then lose their speech (become aphasic, in medical terminology) and develop seizures (either thing could happen first).

Usually LKS occurs in somewhat older children (after age three) with variable degrees of recovery occurring. One of the reasons neurologists are interested in it is a very characteristic pattern on the EEG that seems to show changes in the language parts of the brain.

Because young children with autism sometimes acquire speech skills and then seem to lose them, some professionals have gotten the idea that treating such children as if they had Landau-Kleffner syndrome (i.e., with seizure medicines) might improve their speech. This idea has gotten a lot of attention and has led some doctors to quickly administer powerful antiseizure medicines to any child who has developmental problems associated with language loss. Some doctors will even treat any child with language loss even if they don't show EEG abnormalities.

At present, there are not good data to suggest that children with autism who do not clearly have seizures should be treated with antiseizure medicines. These medicines have a range of side effects which can sometimes interfere with a child's educational program. See below for information about these medications and their side effects.

might predispose your child to seizures. In preparing your child for these tests, many of the same considerations apply as for the EEG. For some of these tests sedation may, however, be an option. You can discuss this with your doctor.

Unfortunately (as with the diagnosis of autism itself), there is no simple test that absolutely tells you whether what you have seen really was a seizure. You have to rely on the experience of the doctor, who will consider the results of the EEG and other tests, as well as your history and description of the event. Perhaps at this point you are saying to yourself, "You mean you can't just diagnose the seizure from the EEG?" Unfortunately, the answer is yes. Some people have normal EEGs even though they have been experiencing seizures; other people may exhibit some abnormality on the EEG but be just fine.

Many different things can be mistaken for seizures. For example, in all children, fainting spells are sometimes mistaken for seizures. And children with autism often have behaviors such as unusual movements or periods of staring that are easy to mistake for seizures. They may be frightened or have very unusual responses to things that the rest of us take for granted. Even if your child has had one seizure, keep in mind that he may not have another. The decision about how extensively you need to investigate the possible seizure is something you and your doctor should discuss.

Observing a Seizure

When observing a seizure, it is better to be a good and careful observer rather than attempt to be a doctor. That is, describe it, but do not attempt to classify it. What was your child doing before the seizure happened? What did he do during the seizure? How long did it last and what happened afterwards?

When a seizure happens, people tend to become very anxious and disorganized. It is helpful if you keep calm. You should help turn the child onto his side. Do not restrain him in an attempt to stop the seizure. Do not force any water, food, or anything else into the person's mouth. People with seizures do not, popular impression to the contrary, "swallow their tongues" and trying to put something in the mouth often ends up causing other damage. During a generalized tonic-clonic seizure, help the child lie down. Be sure that there are no objects in the area that could injure him. During an absence seizure, you should be aware that the seizure has happened. During a complex partial seizure, do not stop or restrain the person unless you really have to. Seizures are usually over very quickly. Let the child resume normal activities as soon as it seems reasonable.

First Aid for Seizures

- Try to prevent injury if the child falls
- Turn the child to the side to prevent vomit from going into the lungs
- Do NOT try to stop the movements of the seizure
- Do NOT try to put something into the mouth
- Do NOT do CPR

When seizures continue for longer than about thirty minutes or happen very frequently, the condition known as status epilepticus may result. In this situation, the person is more or less continuously having seizures. Status epilepticus is a medical emergency. If your child's seizure lasts longer than usual or if he does not regain consciousness, obtain medical help immediately, as this situation is potentially life threatening.

Treatment of Seizures

Typically, epilepsy or a seizure disorder is treated with special drugs. Occasionally, special dietary treatment or surgery may be indicated. Far and away the most common treatment for a seizure disorder, however, is drugs. There are many different drugs which treat epilepsy. Sometimes these are used alone and sometimes they are used in combination, especially if the seizures prove difficult to control.

In considering the use of drugs, the first question you have to deal with is whether or not to treat right away or wait. As with any other treatment, you and your child's doctor (and your child, if possible) should balance the potential risks and benefits of the treatment.

In general, there are two important considerations to weigh when thinking about drug treatment for seizures:

1. the risk for more seizures, and
2. whether the benefits of using drugs will outweigh any possible risks from side effects.

Your doctor will have information on the kind of seizure and the potential benefits and risks of the treatment, as well as of the seizures themselves. Clearly, recurrent seizures complicate the task of providing an intervention program and it is important to consider the implications of treating the seizures on other parts of your child's life and treatment program. All the various medicines used to treat seizures have their own risks and potential benefits.

Risk of Recurrence. As previously discussed, often fever-related seizures in young children do not come back. Even if your child has had a single major nonfebrile seizure, it is possible that the seizure may not come back—particularly if your child's EEG is normal. Many neurologists will not treat seizures unless a patient has had more than one. On the other hand, some kinds of seizures such as absence seizures are notoriously easy to miss, and it is possible that by the time your child is diagnosed, he may already have had many seizures. In this case, the doctor may recommend treatment as soon as the diagnosis is made.

Risks vs. Benefits of Drug Treatment. The overall goal of drug treatment is to control the seizure disorder with the fewest possible side effects and the fewest possible disruptions to your child's learning. In general, these medications are safe, but they have potentially negative side effects. Accordingly, the neurologist must be involved on a continuous basis in monitoring your child's medication. Amounts of drugs used in treating epilepsy vary depending on the individual's body weight, the level of the drug in the bloodstream, and other drugs being taken. The risk of the drugs depends on the type of medicine and the dose, as well as how long your child is treated.

To monitor how your child is doing on seizure medications, the doctor will need to see your child periodically. He or she will do an exam, talk with you (and your child, if possible), and maybe order blood tests. Blood tests are used to determine levels of the medicine in the bloodstream, as well as to assess liver function and blood counts to be sure that the medication is not interfering with other aspects of the body.

Parents who have children with seizure disorders need to be familiar with the medications given for treating their child's seizure. They should know both the specific trade name as well as the generic name of the medication. They should know the amount that is administered. They should pay attention to the size, shape, and color of the pill and be careful to ask the pharmacist if it looks as if the pill has been changed when they pick up refills from their pharmacy.

It is very important that drugs are taken as they are directed and that they are administered consistently. It may be helpful for parents to buy a pill container in which the pills can be arranged by part of the day or day of the week. When doses are missed, ask the doctor how, or whether, to make up the missed dose. Make sure that the doctor prescribing the medication knows exactly what other medicines your child is receiving. Also let her know about significant changes in your child, such as changes in weight or size, since these may affect the dose of medication needed. It is also important that you be aware of possible side effects of the medication. Usually the doctor will describe these in some detail. Sometimes complications occur when medicines interact with each other (a good reason to always use the same pharmacy, since the pharmacist can also be on the lookout for any problems with taking more than one medicine). And of course, always keep medications out of the reach of children!

If you know your child has seizures, you can also talk to your doctor about ways to try to prevent them, as much as possible. For example, since we know that fevers can make seizures more likely, you may want to be careful to use medicines to try to reduce your child's fevers. You might also help your child avoid excessive tiredness, blinking lights, and other factors that may tend to bring seizures on.

Medicines Used to Treat Seizures

A number of different kinds of medications (called anticonvulsants) are used to treat seizures. We summarize some of the more common medicines used here. Additional medicines are also used, so don't feel badly if your child is on a medicine not discussed here.

Always keep in mind that the dose has to be adjusted with the goal of control of the seizures. Ideal control means your child has no further seizures. Sometimes this is not possible (the seizures cannot be fully controlled). Instead, you may be happy with a reduction in the frequency of seizures and willing to tolerate the occasional seizure without too many bad side effects from the medication. Usually the dose of seizure medicines is adjusted depending on the level of the medicine in the blood, although some medications do not require this. Often it takes a while (and various adjustments) to get this dose to where it should be. The amount of time it takes will vary depending on the medicine, but can range from a few days to several weeks. Depending on the situation and the medicine, the doctor will want to balance the gradual increases in dose with the blood level and the degree of seizure control.

Sometimes a second medicine may be added if the first one is working somewhat but not providing as much seizure control as is wanted. Your neurologist and primary care provider should always be your major source of information on medications for your child, but you can be an even more effective part of the treatment team if you yourself learn something about the medications.

Occasionally, children are truly allergic to a medicine and they get a mild, or sometimes a serious, skin rash that can itself be dangerous. These reactions usually happen in the first couple of weeks, so be sure to keep a careful lookout and call your doctor if you see a skin rash (it is better to be safe than sorry). Other kinds of reactions can involve the blood cells and other organs in the body such as the liver. Your healthcare provider will do periodic blood tests to check for these reactions. Behavioral side effects can also be observed. These can include sleepiness and sedation, but children also sometimes become rather hyper and excited. In addition, some of these medicines have the potential for a negative impact on learning.

Common Seizure Medications (Anticonvulsants)

For each of the following medications, we give the brand name (if there is one) and the generic (or general) name. You can talk with your doctor and pharmacist about the pros/cons of brand and generic medicines—the latter are sometimes much cheaper, but may be absorbed differently. Also, your insurance may only pay for generic so you may need to decide if it's worth paying for the brand name out of your own pocket. Keep in mind that the information here is given for your general information and that this is no substitute for talking with your child's primary physician and neurologist about your child. First we will discuss the oldest anticonvulsants and then the most commonly used ones. After that we will list some of the more frequently used newer drugs.

Phenobarbital. Phenobarbital is used for all kinds of seizures we mention here except for the absence (petit mal) variety. This medicine has been around a long time and is one of the best known (and cheapest) of the anticonvulsants. Because it takes a while for the body to break it down, often your child can take a single dose a day. Your child can develop allergies to this medicine—often this first shows itself as a skin rash. You absolutely should have this seen right away, as the medicine may have to be stopped. In recent years, phenobarbital has been used less often than in the past because of evidence that it can have a negative impact on learning and behavior, and because newer anticonvulsants have become available.

Mysoline. Mysoline® (primidone) is another anticonvulsant that is similar to phenobarbital. It is actually broken down into phenobarbital in the body. Like phenobarbital, it is used for partial and generalized tonic-clonic seizures (but not for the absence or petit mal type). Because it is closely related to phenobarbital, many of the side effects are the same and you should be alert to potential learning difficulties as well as allergies. Usually this medicine is started at a low dose and very gradually built up over time.

Dilantin. Dilantin® (phenytoin) has also been around for a long time. It is frequently used for both generalized tonic-clonic seizures and partial seizures. It has a number of different side effects. Allergies sometimes develop and can be quite serious; any child started on this medicine who develops a skin rash should be seen by his doctor right away. Other problems include an increase in body hair, overgrowth of the gums, anemia, poor coordination, and nausea/vomiting. Behavioral difficulties can include slurred speech and confusion. Rarely, severe reactions develop in the liver or bone marrow. An unusual jerking of the eye (nystagmus) is often an early sign that the blood level is too high. Because of the problems with gum overgrowth, good dental care is very important. The overgrown gums can become a significant cosmetic problem.

Depakene/Depakote. Depakene®/Depakote® (valproic acid) is used in treating many different kinds of seizures (tonic-clonic, absence, and myoclonic, as well as complex partial seizures). There is some disagreement about how useful levels of this drug are in regulating the dose; in any event, it can take several weeks for the medicine to begin to work. This medicine does not commonly cause behavioral difficulties as a side effect. In fact, you'll see in Chapter 13 that this medicine is sometimes used as a "mood stabilizer." Physical difficulties include the potential for very severe liver problems (this is rare, but obviously of concern due to its seriousness). It can also adversely affect the pancreas or decrease the platelet count. Your child will need periodic blood work if he is on Depakene®/Depakote®. This medicine also may affect the way the body breaks down other drugs, thereby changing levels of other anticonvulsants or medicines your child is on. Sometimes children have nausea and vomiting or indigestion. Younger children may have some loss of appetite, while older children may gain weight.

Tegretol. Tegretol® (carbamazepine) is often used for partial seizures and generalized tonic-clonic seizures. It is frequently prescribed because it has fewer side effects than many other anticonvulsants. Because of the way the body adjusts to this medicine, it is usually started gradually. Unlike phenobarbital, which you can give your child maybe just once a day, Tegretol often has to be taken several times a day.

There are several side effects that suggest that the drug level is too high. These include double vision or dizziness (often this goes away, but consult your doctor if this develops and especially if it keeps up). Difficulties in walking, unsteadiness, and sleepiness can also suggest a high drug level. Reducing the drug level (in consultation with the doctor) will take care of these problems.

Potential difficulties include allergic reactions and a decrease in the white blood cell count. The decrease in the white blood cell count has to be monitored. Very rarely a severe reaction in the bone marrow occurs (aplastic anemia). Liver function also has to be monitored. As with some of the other anticonvulsants, taking Tegretol with certain other medicines has the potential for causing trouble. For example, this medicine interacts with a fairly commonly used antibiotic (erythromycin). A few of the other medicines that can at times cause problem interactions are some antifungal drugs, some prescription antihistamines, some antacids, oral contraceptives, and even some other anticonvulsants. Again, the doctor prescribing medicines needs to know all the medicines your child is receiving. Let the neurologist know if your pediatrician has given your child an antibiotic and make sure the pediatrician knows what drugs the neurologist has prescribed. Also be sure to use the same pharmacist/pharmacy for all your child's medicines, as the pharmacist can then also be alert to any potential for problem interactions.

Zarontin. Zarontin® (ethosuximide) is most frequently used in treating absence (petit mal) seizures. It does not work for other kinds of seizures. Various allergies to the medication can develop, although these are not common. Generally, behavioral side effects seem to be minimal. Nightmares can develop on this medication.

Trileptal. Trileptal® (oxcarbazepine) is a relatively new medicine now used quite frequently for treatment of partial seizures. As with many other anticonvulsant medications, blood tests to look for side effects are necessary (in this case, loss of sodium from the body). When stopping this medicine, it is important to taper it off gradually. As with many other antiseizure medicines, there may be effects on thinking and movement. An advantage of this medicine is that you can take it less frequently.

Lamictal. Lamictal® (lamotrigine) is one of the newer anticonvulsant medications now available. It can treat a wide range of seizure types. Usually it is tried when either Depakene® or Tegretol® have failed to stop the seizures, or when there are reasons not to use those medications to begin with. For children with an unusual seizure type known as Lennox-Gastaut syndrome, Lamictal® may be the first drug used. The most important side effect to watch for with Lamictal® is a rash. This can be quite serious.

Neurontin. Neurontin® (gabapentin) is another of the newer anticonvulsants that has become available in recent years. It is used to treat partial seizures and frequently is prescribed along with another anticonvulsant. It may be used alone to treat a type of seizure known as Benign Rolandic epilepsy.

Topamax. Topamax® (topiramine) is also one of the newer anticonvulsants. It, like Lamictal®, is frequently used when other medications such as Depakene® and Tegetol® have not worked by themselves. It can be given alone or in combination with other anticonvulsants. It is used to treat both tonic-clonic seizures and partial seizures. Side effects sometimes include behavioral or cognitive changes. Liver and kidney function need to be monitored when children are taking this medication.

Other New Medications. Other newer medications that are used less often include Felbotol® (felbamate), Keppra® (levetiracetam), and Zonegran® (zonisamide). Your physician can provide more information about these and all other drugs that are recommended for your child.

Benzodiazepines. The Benzodiazepines are a group of medicines that have antiseizure properties. These include such well-known medicines as Valium® (diazepam), Ativan® (lorazepam), and frequently Klonopin® (clonazepam) and Tranxene® (clorazepate). Some of these medicines, such as Valium and Ativan, are shorter acting and are used to treat uncontrollable seizures (status epilepticus, see above). The longer-acting medicines such as Tranxene and Klonopin are used sometimes in nonemergency situations. They can be useful for many different types of seizures. Unfortunately, the behavioral side effects often limit their usefulness in children. These side effects can take the form of hyperactivity and excitability on the one hand and sleepiness and sedation on the other. These drugs most frequently are added to other seizure medicines in an attempt to get better control of seizures.

Dietary Treatments for Seizures

For hundreds of years, it has been observed that fasting seems to make seizures less common in people with epilepsy. As this was studied, it became clear that you could also achieve the same effect not by fasting but by consuming a high-fat diet with very little sugar or starch. What happens in the body is that without sugar to digest, the body forms chemicals called ketones, which appear in the urine. The diet is called "ketogenic" because it generates these ketones. The idea is to give just enough protein and fat to allow for growth but with as little sugar and carbohydrate as possible. Although we still don't know exactly how this diet works, we do know that it can sometimes help control seizures but takes a lot of supervision. You *must* do this diet in consultation with a supervising physician!

The ketogenic diet often is used after multiple medicines have been tried and seizure control has still not been achieved. Given the stringency of the diet, it requires very careful supervision from people who know what they are doing. The diet is not easy to do and not everyone responds with a reduction in seizures. You might consider talking with your neurologist about the diet, particularly if your child has not done well after trials of several different medicines.

Surgery and Seizure Disorders

Rarely, surgery to remove part of the brain is used in the treatment of epilepsy. Usually this surgery is done with adults rather than children, and then usually only as a last resort. One exception would be if it is possible to identify and precisely pinpoint a specific area of the brain that starts the seizures (particularly if this is an area that is easy to get to and can likely be taken out without causing further damage). Another exception would be if seizures are being caused by a tumor or cyst that likely won't be as responsive to medicines.

One surgical procedure that is sometimes considered for children is implanting a device that stimulates the vagus nerve in the neck. This device includes a small battery pack with a wire going from it to the vagus nerve. Stimulation of the nerve can be either preset at a regular interval or initiated during a seizure and may shorten or stop seizures. This is a very specialized technique that would only be tried after other treatments have failed. For example, it may be suggested for children who continue to have seizures even after multiple medications, and possibly diets, have been tried without success.

Alternative Treatments for Seizure Disorder

We discuss alternative treatments approaches in general in Chapter 16, but do want to say a bit in this chapter about complementary/alternative medicine approaches to seizures. Various treatments have been used ranging from massage, biofeedback, Oriental medicine, and so forth. These can (in general) be used in addition to traditional therapies but do not substitute for the traditional therapies. For example, we know that in reasonable doses vitamins are not harmful, but vitamins do not really treat seizure disorders except in the very rare case of severe vitamin deficiency.

Continuing Care and Safety Concerns

It is important that all people with seizures be evaluated periodically. This includes monitoring seizure control and the dose of the medicine, and looking for side effects. Once your child has achieved good seizure control, you may not need to bring him in to the doctor as frequently. Still, you should periodically contact your doctor since things like changes in size and weight of your child may require changes in the dose of medicine. For some children, it is possible to gradually discontinue seizure medicines (under supervision) over time to determine whether they still need them.

Most children, adolescents, and adults with seizures can engage in normal physical activities. At times, you may have to limit certain kinds of activities that could be dangerous if your child lost consciousness or had an impairment in consciousness. As much as possible, try to measure the risks of participating in activities against their possible benefit and take simple, common sense precautions. For example, your child can engage in sports such as swimming, but it's important to have a life preserver and lifeguards readily and immediately available.

Talk with your doctor as well about MedicAlert® bracelets or some other kind of identification that would let others know that your child has seizures. This is probably most important if your child is spending time around people who won't know about his seizure disorder.

What Causes Seizures?

There are many different causes of seizures. For example, babies who are born with congenital infections, were exposed to certain medications in the uterus, or who have had birth injuries and lack of oxygen to the brain may be at increased risk for epilepsy. Other causes include strokes, brain infections after birth, brain tumors, and injuries to the head. Many times, however, a specific cause can't be determined even after the individual is extensively evaluated. These are called idiopathic seizures—a fancy word to say that we don't know the cause.

In autism, it is likely that the same thing that caused the autism causes the epilepsy. Some disorders such as PKU and tuberous sclerosis (see Chapter 1) are sometimes seen in autism and may themselves be associated with seizures. There is also some suggestion that if one of the parents of a child has epilepsy, there is increased risk for the child also to have epilepsy. Similarly, if both parents have epilepsy, the risk increases. In autism, the risk for seizure disorder increases with lower levels of cognitive ability. That is, children with mental retardation that is more severe are more likely to have seizures.

Summary

In this chapter, we have talked about some aspects of seizures and their treatment. Children with autism are at higher risk for seizures than other children. Sometimes the onset of a seizure disorder is very obvious. Other times it may be difficult to notice. Do not hesitate to bring up any concerns about changes in your child's behavior and level of alertness with your child's doctor since seizures can develop at any time.

Many effective treatments for seizure disorders are now available. If you are not satisfied with the care your child is receiving for his seizures, do not hesitate to look for a doctor who can help you achieve reasonable control of your child's seizures.

Questions

Q. My daughter has a seizure disorder and we have now twice had the experience of being called from the emergency room after school staff took her there following a seizure. The seizures take the form of staring spells and do not last long. I think the school is over reacting. What can we do about this?

It sounds like the school is being a bit overly cautious. Discuss this with them as well as with your child's doctor. See if it might be possible for school staff to call you and have you decide, maybe in consultation with your regular doctor, when a trip to the emergency room is best. It is possible that your child could be seen in the doctor's office instead or might just be able to rest in the school health room for awhile before returning to class. If her type of seizure never causes any problems other than staring spells, you may be able to arrange for her to go back to class after the seizure.

Q. A friend told me that all children with autism eventually have seizures. Is this true?

No, about 25 percent or so of children with autism develop seizures. Children with Rett's disorder and CDD also have an increased chance of developing seizures. Seizures are less common in Asperger's disorder and PDD-NOS. For children with autism, there is an increased risk of developing seizures throughout childhood and adolescence—even into young adulthood. Even if your child had an EEG that was normal at one point, he may still, unfortunately, develop seizures later. But clearly, most children with autism don't develop seizures.

Q. My sixteen-year-old son is a pretty high functioning child with autism. He just had his first seizure, but at age five he had a normal EEG. How commonly does this happen?

The risk for developing seizures is increased through adolescence and they do occur for the first time during adolescence with some frequency. Unfortunately, having a normal EEG at one point does *not* mean that the EEG will always be normal. Treating the seizures is important at whatever age they develop.

Q: Our ten-year-old has recently developed seizures. His teacher at school tells us that it is possible to treat these behaviorally without medication. Is this true?

It might be helpful to have your doctor (or your neurologist) talk with the teacher to be absolutely sure the teacher understands the situation and has good information. While an isolated fever-related seizure might not be medicated, it would be very unusual not to try medications for recurrent seizures otherwise. Behavioral treatments are wonderfully helpful for children with autism, but they shouldn't be used to treat seizures! You may want to check with the teacher first to be sure you understand exactly what she meant.

10 | Dental Care

As is true in other areas, an ounce of prevention is worth a pound of cure when it comes to dental care. As much as possible, you should really try to tackle dental care very early in your child's life. Children who have inadequate prevention are at risk for major problems as they get older. For example, dental pain may cause self-injurious behavior, and untreated dental problems can lead to other medical problems—sometimes severe ones. Sadly, some adults with autism we know are only able to have a dental examination and dental procedures under general anesthesia. Your goal should be to try to prevent your child from developing such a fear of dental care.

Children with autism and related conditions are at increased risk for dental problems due to the same symptoms of autism that complicate other aspects of healthcare. These include many of the problems also faced in dealing with going to the doctor's office (see Chapter 3) but may be particularly difficult due to the child's unusual sensitivities (e.g., to the smell or taste or grittiness of toothpaste), difficulties with oral "defensiveness" (an unwillingness to have things in the mouth), or difficulties with attention (making it difficult to sit for a long period in a dental chair). Particularly as they approach school age, many children with autism may not be able to grasp the necessity for all the fuss and bother of going to the dentist. That is, they may not understand the need for long-term prevention of problems—an appreciation of such long-term issues is not usually something children with autism spectrum conditions are known for.

Children with specific diagnoses along the autism spectrum may have additional dental problems. For example, children with Rett's disorder who have problems in eating and swallowing may retain bits of food in the mouth, making cavities even more likely. Children with fragile X syndrome may have specific malformations such as crowding of the teeth.

In this chapter, we'll briefly review how teeth form and emerge and the common problems children have with their teeth. We'll also talk about specific dental problems children with disabilities are more likely to have and the various ways in which these can be treated. Finally, we'll discuss ways to help your child have productive visits with the dentist and to encourage good preventive dental care.

How the Teeth Develop

The teeth start to develop at around the end of the first month or so of pregnancy. While the baby is still in the womb, little tooth buds (which will develop into teeth) form in both the upper jaw (what is technically called the maxilla) and in the lower jaw (the mandible). Ten primary tooth buds (which will form the first or "baby" teeth) form in both the upper and the lower jaw, for a total of twenty baby teeth. Over time, the secondary teeth buds will develop as well; these teeth will eventually emerge after the primary teeth are lost. The secondary teeth are also called permanent teeth since they are not replaced.

The little tooth buds start to harden (or calcify) while the baby is still in the womb. The tooth itself is made up of a hard outer layer called the enamel and underneath that is another layer called the dentin. In the very center of the tooth is the pulp, which contains the nerves and blood vessels.

For most children, teething can begin as early as six months of age as the first primary (baby) tooth emerges; other children may not have any teeth come in ("erupt") until a year of age. Over the next couple of years, all twenty (ten top and ten bottom) teeth come in. The first permanent tooth usually comes in by around age six years. All thirty-two permanent teeth usually coming in by age twelve or so, except for the wisdom teeth (technically the third molars), which usually come in during late adolescence or early adulthood.

Since autism is not usually diagnosed until around two or three years of age, many children will already have some, or all, of their baby teeth by this time. Occasionally, there are still baby teeth that will come in. For children with problems in teething, there are several things you can try. These include pain relievers, teething rings, teething gels, and so forth. Given the communication difficulties in autism, it may be difficult to figure out the nature of the troubles. If you have not yet established contact with a dentist for your child, talk with your child's healthcare provider about ways to relieve your child's discomfort.

Coping with the Dentist's Office

Most children with autism should start seeing a dentist around age three unless problems have been noted earlier. A big part of these early visits to the dentist is to help your child become comfortable with the office and the dentist. It also gives the dentist a chance to get to know you, the parents, and give you information on dental care and on preventive measures such as fluoride. The dentist may also help you think about ways to encourage good dental care (tooth brushing and flossing).

While all this is happening, your child can (within limits and with supervision) get more familiar with the office and its operation. A chance to see and maybe hold the instruments may be helpful. As time goes on, modeling the behaviors needed at the dentist and dental procedures can be useful, with parents and siblings showing the child what to do.

You should be thoughtful and careful in selecting your child's dentist. Good sources of information on potential dentists include your primary physician or other healthcare provider, as well as other parents. Some dentists have special expertise in working with children or individuals with developmental problems. If your child has difficulty working with a regular dentist, it may be worth trying to find a pediatric dentist with special expertise in this area; sometimes these dentists will also work with older individuals who have developmental challenges. You can get a list of pediatric dentists practicing in your state from the American Dental Association (see the Resources at the end of the book).

Just as with visits to the doctor's office, visits to the dentist's office will go more smoothly if your child is familiar with members of the dental care team, the equipment used, and the situation. Sometimes your child may need to visit the dentist's office a number of times before she is ready to actually begin having examinations or dental procedures. The use of picture books in advance of the visit and a visual schedule for procedures may be helpful for many children. Some commercial books are available (see Reading List), and you can make your own as well.

If your child has never visited the dentist's office, it may be worthwhile talking to the dentist on the phone or even arranging for just you and your spouse to visit the dentist beforehand. You can discuss your child's medical and dental history and any chronic problems and also talk about the issues you think may be difficult for your child on her first trip to the office. If the dentist and his staff are agreeable, you can take some photographs to use in producing a picture book or story board for your child.

During the initial visit, the dentist will ask you about your child's medical and dental history. This will include a list of any chronic medical problems your child has, any allergies, and use of any medications. The dentist will also be interested in your child's diet and what you are already doing at home to teach dental self-care.

Some dentists, particularly dentists especially trained in working with children, pride themselves on taking it "slow and easy" with a new patient with autism. They will realize that the new situation has many potentially overwhelming sights and sounds and may be a bit of a push for the child with an ASD. They may try to work out a program for your child in which they gradually do more and more actual dental work. For instance, the first goal may be for your child to just sit in the dental chair and go up and down or sit on your lap on the dental chair. Next, they may work on having your child tolerate the dentist/hygienist looking inside her mouth without touching it, etc. This can take time.

You can also talk to the dentist and the dental hygienist about "tricks of the trade" they may have heard about. For example, some children may not like the texture or taste of certain toothpastes or polishing compounds (sometimes the gritty texture makes for special trouble). A patient dentist will be willing to take the time needed to make your child feel more comfortable because he or she knows that the treatment will be more likely to be successful in the long run.

Occasionally, particularly for more challenging or painful procedures, the dentist may want to use sedative medications or other specific techniques (e.g., laughing gas) to make them more tolerable for your child. Except in cases of emergency, you'll have the chance to discuss these ahead of time. Keep a couple of things in mind when discussing options for anesthesia or medication. In general, don't try something for the first time and expect it to work. Some children with autism get more agitated with anesthesia or pre-medication. In our experience, when pre-medication is going to be used, it may be worthwhile to try a "test dose" at home (or in the dentist's office) and see how your child tolerates it. Similarly, some children may find a long period of local anesthesia upsetting. For these children, shorter-acting local pain killers may be more helpful.

Sometimes the dentist may want to treat your child in a hospital on a day admission or in an outpatient hospital facility where anesthesia is available. The dentist may recommend this for routine examination if he has not been able to do a good exam even after several attempts to help your child be more comfortable. More commonly, this is advised for complicated procedures that involve more extensive dental work such as surgery or sometimes tooth extraction. It can be very helpful to consult with the anesthesiologist before the day of the surgery to discuss your child's medical history, including seizures or other problems she has in addition to autism. Medications that your child takes may influence which anesthetic is used and some medications may need to be stopped in advance of the surgery. Also, it can be very helpful for you and your child to know ahead of time how many people you'll have to deal with, what the recovery room will look like, how much pain to expect, and how you will deal with your child's pain.

Planning Ahead for Dental Visits

Here is a checklist of steps you might want to take before you bring your child to the dental office, to ensure that everything goes as smoothly as possible.

- **As we've mentioned, put together a picture or story book for your child.** If possible, take pictures during initial visits and then go over these periodically at home with the goal of helping your child feel more comfortable with the dentist's office.
- **In advance of your visit, you might want to purchase a dental mirror in a drug store. Let your child see it and play with it.** You can use it to "play dentist" at home and perhaps take turn counting each other's teeth. Likewise, if you use an electric toothbrush at home, it may help your child tolerate the noise and sensations of having dental instruments in the mouth.
- **Alert the staff to your child's special needs when scheduling an appointment.** For example, request appointments at times when waiting may be minimal. If possible, ask if the same room can be used both for the dental exam (with the dentist) and the teeth cleaning (with the oral hygienist). Chances are the office staff will appreciate your trying to work with them to make visits go smoothly.
- **Always bring a couple of things your child will be interested in doing while she's waiting,** since even with the best of intentions dentists often run late.
- **Bring items from home such as your child's toothpaste and/or a favorite toothbrush—this may help her be more comfortable.** It also helps reduce waiting time, since the staff won't have to spend a long time searching for a toothbrush or toothpaste that your child will tolerate.

Preventive Dental Care

More than in almost any other area of healthcare, preventive care here really pays off! Sadly, however, many of the characteristics of children with autism complicate providing good preventive care. As mentioned above, these include:

- difficulties with oral defensiveness

- marked sensitivities (e.g., to the smell, taste, or even the texture of toothpaste)
- difficulties learning from observation and imitation (e.g., of watching Mommy or Daddy brush their teeth)
- difficulties realizing the long-term consequences of poor dental hygiene

Despite all these difficulties, it is really worth investing yourself in good dental care. This is particularly difficult for parents of younger and more challenging children, but, in the end, the effort can really pay off in terms of preventing longer-term problems. Finding and detecting small cavities gives the dentist the chance to slow or stop the decay process. Application of fluorides and fluoride pastes can help to harden the teeth and stop decay.

Tooth Brushing

For children with autism, a variety of factors can complicate establishing good tooth brushing techniques. These include: a dislike of the taste of the toothpaste, the texture of the brush bristles, and the feeling of the brush on the teeth or gums, or just a general dislike of having things in or near the mouth.

Your dentist and his staff, including the oral hygienist, may have some very helpful suggestions. Other parents may also have some ideas. If your child has been working with a speech-language pathologist or occupational therapist, these individuals may also have some ideas to contribute (particularly when the problem has to do with oral defensiveness). Behavioral psychologists can also be helpful in establishing behavioral approaches. Their analysis of the problem may focus more specifically on a gradual process of establishing tooth brushing (breaking the task down into very small, but achievable, progressive steps). A behavioral program will vary a bit depending on the psychologist's sense of what is going on. For example, if anxiety seems to be the major aspect of the problem, the approach may center around getting your child comfortable with the toothbrush. The people who know your child best will be able to give you the most individualized advice for her.

Here are some of the strategies we have known to work over the years in getting children to tolerate tooth brushing. Keep in mind that these are just suggestions and may not be helpful for your particular child.

- **Start early.** Tooth brushing should be started as soon as the teeth begin to come in. You can use a soft brush and try to work quickly. Try to make the situation enjoyable—make it into a game (with its own special song, for example) or have a favorite activity immediately after. Make tooth brushing a regular, routine part of what happens after meals. You do not need to spend a long time doing this—the main thing is to get your child used to the idea.
- **Try different toothpastes.** Talk to the dentist about the pros and cons of the various toothpastes. Also talk about alternatives to toothpastes. Some children won't tolerate the gritty feeling of more abrasive toothpastes but might like the feeling of some of the gel-type toothpastes. Other children may not like toothpastes at all but your dentist might suggest alternatives such as baking soda or some other cleaner. For other children, trying differ-

ent flavors may help. If your child dislikes toothpaste, try brushing without anything—then gradually work up to toothpaste if you can.

- **Talk to your dentist (also maybe to your pharmacist) about ways to give the toothbrush a taste that is interesting to your child.** If your child has favorite foods, try those tastes, or even, maybe, the food itself. (Brushing teeth with peanut butter can be quite an experience—use only a small amount!) Keep in mind that the big goal here is to get your child to tolerate the toothbrush, not necessarily to clean her teeth.
- **If your child won't tolerate the toothbrush, discuss with your dentist— and maybe the speech-language pathologist, occupational therapist, or psychologist—a plan for gradually helping your child learn to tolerate it.** This may start without the toothbrush anywhere in sight. It might be part of the program to help your child—particularly if she is not yet talking—become more familiar with her mouth and how it feels.
- **Try brushing teeth in front of a mirror.** Sometimes children are interested in watching themselves. You can also try tooth brushing as a family activity (occasionally children with autism will get into the swing of this).
- **If your child has trouble tolerating the toothbrush, encourage water drinking immediately after meals** (to try to clean out as much food as possible from the teeth and give the bacteria that cause cavities less food to grow on). You can do this with a bottle for very young children or through a straw or squeeze bottle for older children.
- **Think about other approaches.** Some children like mechanical things and might be willing to try an electric toothbrush or one of the water irrigators (Water Pik® makes these). For some children, this also has the advantage of making them feel more comfortable with the dentist putting instruments in their mouth. If your child tolerates the Water Pik, you can also talk to the dentist about using it to introduce a fluoride mouthwash.
- **Avoid foods that are known to cause cavities.** This means limiting sweets, particularly sticky sweets. Some candies are particularly likely to stick to children's teeth, as are "fruit roll-ups" and dried fruits such as raisins. Keep in mind that many drinks have large amounts of sugar as well. Try to encourage use of other (nonsweet) foods as snacks. For children who receive foods as reinforcers, try to encourage a range of foods.
- **If your child has motor difficulties, talk with the OT or PT about adapted toothbrushes that may give your child more stability and control.**
- **For more able children, "disclosing tablets" (which show areas where more brushing is needed) might be both helpful and instructive.**

You don't want to turn tooth brushing into a daily battle, but try to turn it into a regular and routine habit. As much as humanly possible, try to make sure your child's teeth are cleaned at least once a day—and maybe more. This will help prevent longer-term problems and will also help when you go to the dentist. Don't give up until you come up with a method that works. Children with autism can sometimes surprise parents—the child who you think will have horrible difficulties may do just fine, and sometimes a child who has been having major problems suddenly also can be just fine.

Other Preventive Techniques

Flossing. Flossing can also be started early on for children who will tolerate this (not all will, but it is worth trying). Flossing is needed once the teeth start to touch each other (allowing food to become more easily trapped between the teeth). If the teeth are not close to each other, flossing is less critical. The dentist or dental assistant can help you learn how to do this. Some devices are available to hold the floss for children with motor difficulties. Different kinds of floss are also available, including flavored ones. Discuss flossing with your dentist.

Fluoride. Fluoride is a chemical which makes tooth enamel harder and more resistant to decay. Fluoride in drinking water is now fairly common in the U.S. and can substantially decrease rates of tooth decay. If your family uses water without fluoridation, talk to the dentist about other ways to provide fluoride. Various forms are available which can be applied to the teeth or taken by mouth. Be sure to do this with the dentist's supervision, since too much fluoride can discolor teeth. Keep in mind that if you have a water filter at home, your child may not be getting enough fluoride. Similarly, if you use bottled water for drinking and cooking purposes, check to see whether the dentist wants you to consider adding fluoride in some form to your child's dental care program.

Sealants. Your dentist may advise preventing dental problems by applying sealants (a special plastic which coats the tooth to prevent decay). Discuss the pros and cons of this with your dentist, including the cost and how long the sealants will last. For some children, sealants can make a big difference in reducing cavities.

Medications. If your child is taking medications on a regular basis, talk to the pharmacist and the dentist about possible issues. Some medicines, for example, have high levels of sugar and you may be able to get a sugar-free form.

Common Dental Problems

Tooth Decay

Dental cavities (also called dental caries) are caused by a complex process which involves several culprits including bacteria, diet (particularly sugar and other carbohydrates), and other factors. As the bacteria consume the food left on the teeth, they create an acid which then damages the hard layer of enamel on the outside of the tooth. As time goes on, the cavity gets bigger. If not treated properly, this cavity can turn into an abscess—a dental emergency for anyone (with or without an ASD).

Dental plaque is the term for a mass of bacteria (and their waste products) along with food particles and cells from the mouth. As time goes on, the plaque becomes hard (calcified) and then is called tartar. Both the plaque and tarter which forms from it can cause gum problems and can eventually cause the loss of teeth.

The bacteria that cause tooth decay are transmitted to the child (usually by parents and other caregivers). This makes it important that you set a good example by doing your own tooth brushing (this is also good because it gives you a chance to teach the child about tooth brushing). This also means that you should *not* share toothbrushes.

Dental cavities are less common in children who receive fluoride (either from the drinking water or from special fluoride supplements). Cavities are most common in children, and, fortunately, become less common in adults. Great advances have been made in preventing cavities in recent years.

Children who have lengthy nursing sessions (either at the breast or with a bottle) or who fall asleep with a bottle are at risk for what is called "baby bottle tooth decay." This comes about because of the prolonged exposure of the teeth to milk or other drinks with sugar in them. Some children with autism have difficulty giving up the bottle and may be prone to this type of tooth decay. The only beverage that clearly will *not* cause decay is water. If your child is in the habit of nursing or bottle feeding for what seems like a long time or wants to fall asleep with a bottle, discuss this with your dentist. Sometimes giving your child a bottle of water may be helpful; if you use one of the new flavored waters, be sure there is no sugar.

Filling Cavities

Treatment of dental cavities includes removing the decay and then putting in a filling material or sometimes a crown. When possible, the dentist will use a local anesthetic so your child does not feel any pain associated with the drilling out of the decay. Usually the dentist will want to apply a small amount of surface (skin or topical) anesthetic on the gum before injecting the anesthetic that numbs the nerves to the teeth. Patience and persistence can help here, although some children will tolerate this just fine. A few children will become upset if they have a long period of anesthesia in their mouth. If this is true for your child, talk to the dentist, since there are both longer- and shorter-acting forms available. Keep in mind that some of this you have to learn as you go (and sometimes make up as you go).

Some children get upset with the sounds of the drill. If so, it may help to get noise-canceling earphones and/or to play music through headphones. These are a great way to help children with noise sensitivity. You do, however, need to be sure that your child will wear the headphones, so practice ahead of time.

Reading picture books ahead of time and using other visual aids can help your child know what to expect—this is especially true for the first cavity. It is also usually worthwhile to think about some enjoyable diversions that can help your child cope. Bring along a portable CD player, television, DVD, laptop computer, book, or whatever else will be able to help. With some (usually small) amount of work, you can often set up a small TV or DVD player in such a way that your child can watch a favorite movie while she is in the dental chair. Some children find that watching screensavers on a laptop is very soothing. Do whatever helps *your* child.

In the past, small quantities of mercury have been used in making the fillings (also called amalgams) and there has been some concern that these might be "toxic" to children (see Chapter 16 for information about chelation, sometimes proposed as a treatment). The available scientific evidence does not, however, support this theory. In any case, you can discuss this issue with your dentist, who undoubtedly has a range of materials he can give you to read on this topic.

Periodontal Diseases

These conditions all affect the gums, tissues, and bones which support the teeth. Gingivitis (inflammation of the gums) is the most common periodontal disease, occurring in about half of school-aged children. Like tooth decay, gum inflammation comes about in association with plaque and chronic inflammation. As time goes on, bone loss occurs and eventually the gums may recede and the tooth loosen in its socket. Eventually the tooth can be lost. Other causes of gum disease include viral and bacterial infections.

The best way to prevent and treat mild gingivitis is with good dental hygiene—brushing and flossing. The use of mouth washes will probably not be possible for most children with autism. In some cases, the dentist may want you to apply a special mouth rinse to the gums using a Q-tip to get gingivitis under control.

Some medicines—notably some of the seizure medicines—can cause excessive growth of the gums (see Chapter 9). Sometimes surgery is needed to remove the excessive gum tissue, so monitoring this with your dentist can be very helpful.

Malocclusion and Braces

Sometimes children have some significant problems with the alignment of their teeth. This can lead to problems in how the upper and lower teeth come together (malocclusion) and may increase speech problems or potential for infection.

Malocclusion is fairly common in children and can range from mild to severe. Sometimes the problem is due to crowding of the teeth. Sometimes thumb sucking contributes to the problem. Fragile X syndrome may be more likely to be associated with malocclusion due to tooth crowding. Mild forms of malocclusion may be treated only for cosmetic reasons and thus be a matter for more discussion of pros and cons. More severe forms may require treatment.

In some instances, braces may be needed. In these cases, usually cosmetic concerns are less important than more basic medical and dental concerns. Your child's dentist will refer you to an orthodontist if your child has a malocclusion problem that may need treatment. The age at which orthodonture is started depends on the type of problem. Sometimes children are referred to the orthodontist and just watched carefully to see how the teeth are going to come in. If the mouth does not seem wide enough for all of the teeth that are going to come in, the orthodontist may recommend early palate expansion with a dental "appliance." If it appears that the upper teeth are going to come in behind the lower teeth the orthodontist will want to redirect them before they come all the way down.

Some skeletal malocclusions can be quite severe. For example, if either the upper or lower jaw protrudes much further than the other, it can be quite disfiguring. Less commonly, malocclusions can predispose a person to dental or jaw injuries. The front teeth are more likely to be injured during a fall if they protrude further than they are supposed to. In addition, if the malocclusion is severe and a child's teeth don't meet, others may find her chewing unattractive to watch and her teeth may become damaged.

As with all treatments, the benefits and disadvantages need to be considered carefully before beginning an extensive program such as orthodonture. The discomfort of braces may not be worth the aggravation it causes your child if the only problem is a minor cosmetic one. Limited treatment may be considered to correct a specific problem rather than to obtain a "perfect" bite. Limited treatment may be more acceptable to your child and more realistic. You will need to discuss this with the orthodontist.

Accidents

Given the combination of impulsivity and impaired judgment as a group, children with ASDs are at increased risk for accidents and injury, including injury to the teeth. About half of typically developing children will have some injury to their teeth. Although we don't have precise statistics, our guess is that the rate of injury in autism is much higher. In addition to the problems of impulsive behavior, there are other factors that may increase the risk for dental injury in autism. Sometimes children are self-abusive and may damage their teeth through repeated head banging. Children with seizures or motor problems (as in Rett's disorder, or, to a lesser extent, in Asperger's disorder) are at increased risk for falling. As you might expect, the teeth at the front of the mouth are the ones most likely to be damaged. Sometimes teeth are chipped; at other times they may actually be knocked out or loosened.

As with other accidents, preventing them in the first place is highly desirable. For children at high risk for falls or self-injury, mouth guards can sometimes be used. If an injury occurs, use an ice pack for swelling and be familiar with basic first aid procedures.

Usually your dentist will have a service you can call twenty-four hours a day and if he or she isn't available, someone will be covering. The dentist can advise you on the best course of action. Often if a permanent tooth is lost, the advice is to try to replace it in the child's mouth as quickly as possible. This can be very difficult in an uncooperative child, however, and in such cases is not worth the effort. If you cannot replace the tooth, save it in cold milk. Sometimes even when the tooth is replaced it won't be able to adapt and survive. In this situation, the living part of the tooth (the pulp) dies and the tooth may be removed and replaced with an implanted one (or sometimes with a partial denture). Sometimes you may decide not to replace the tooth.

Wisdom Teeth

Over thousands of years the human mouth has gotten smaller. Sometimes the third molars (wisdom teeth) don't have quite enough room to come in properly and thus cause other problems with tooth alignment and biting. In the past, the wisdom teeth were almost always removed in late adolescence as they came in. In recent years, however, it is more and more common for dentists to recommend leaving wisdom teeth in if they don't seem to be causing a problem. You can discuss this with your dentist. If a teenager with autism starts complaining about pain or starts head banging, it is often a good idea to check the wisdom teeth. This is particularly true for children with more significant communication problems.

Teeth Grinding

Teeth grinding is a form of self-stimulatory behavior that can lead to various dental problems. This phenomenon (also referred to as bruxism) sometimes occurs in typically developing, younger children while they are asleep but decreases dramatically over time and doesn't need any special treatment. In children with autism spectrum disorders, teeth grinding can occur during the daytime. Over time it can lead to grinding down of the teeth as well as jaw pain and malocclusion. Children with Rett's disorder seem to be particularly likely to grind their teeth.

Various treatments are available. Some simple things to try include giving your child more chewy and crunchy foods or using an electric toothbrush several times a day. Occasionally children will grind their teeth when they are in an overstimulating environment, particularly one in which there are too many sounds for the child to cope with. In this instance, reducing the sound or noise level may help. Occasionally, the problem is sufficiently severe that the dentist may have to be involved. He may give your child a grinding guard or mouth guard. Some children are "loud" grinders but don't actually wear their teeth down very much, while others don't make nearly as much noise but do much more damage, so be sure to talk to your dentist if your child grinds her teeth.

Dental Problems and Behavior Change

Occasionally dental problems first present themselves as behavior changes in children and adolescents with autism spectrum disorders. This is particularly common in children who have more difficulties with communication skills and who have had limited ongoing dental care due to their lack of cooperation (sometimes despite the best efforts of parents). This may happen, for example, when a cavity has progressed into a very painful dental abscess. In such a circumstance, the child's behavior may gradually, or more abruptly, deteriorate and self-injurious behavior may develop. The self-injurious behavior usually takes the form of face slapping or head banging and may be quite severe. Sometimes an abscess may be visible on the face as a swollen and puffy bulge in the cheek, but this doesn't always happen. Other painful conditions, such as ear infections, can also lead to self-injurious behavior. Occasionally an older adolescent may develop these problems as the wisdom teeth come in. Younger children with autism sometimes also become self-injurious (although usually in a somewhat less severe form) as their permanent teeth come in.

Sorting out the possible explanations for a sudden change in behavior requires a good bit of detective work. Unless it is clear that the problem is dental, you probably should start with your child's primary physician, who can try to look in your child's mouth and ears. Because pediatricians have a lot of experience in diagnosing problems in very young children (i.e., who don't talk), they are often a good choice in situations like this. If it appears that dental problems are involved and if your child is very resistant to regular office dental care, it may be necessary to use sedation or anesthesia to accurately diagnose and then treat the problem. If your child already has had a positive experience with the dentist (and physician), the task of treating these emergencies will be simplified.

Summary

All children and adolescents have to take care of their teeth to avoid problems with cavities, abscesses, and gum disease. Proper dental care is even more important if your child is receiving a seizure medication, such as Dilantin® (phenytoin), which can cause changes in the gum and mouth. Unfortunately, achieving good dental hygiene for children with autism and other disorders can be difficult, for the many reasons discussed in this chapter.

In the case of dentistry, an ounce of prevention is indeed worth a pound of cure. Overlooking or avoiding dental care because your child resists examination or treatment can lead to many serious problems in the long run, including painful movements of the jaw, tooth abscesses, or gum disease—all of which can affect your child's ability to eat and chew food. Enlist the help of everyone on your child's team who can help make prevention and good dental hygiene a part of her daily life. Occupational and speech therapists sometimes can help your child tolerate tooth brushing or other oral motor activities. The dentist may help you select specific treatments or applications of fluoride to help your child avoid cavities. Although achieving good dental hygiene can be a challenge, it is an important part of your child's medical care and well worth the time and effort you may need to devote to it.

Questions

Q. My child likes to grind her teeth. The dentist is worried about this. What can I do?

This can be a difficult problem to deal with. Occasionally children who are in overly stimulating environments (particularly those with high levels of auditory overstimulation) will grind their teeth—almost in an attempt to "drown out" the other sounds. In this case, it may help to reduce the amount of stimulation your child is getting. Sometimes the use of an electric toothbrush will help. Also, you can try giving your child food that requires a lot of chewing. If all this fails, talk to your dentist about other alternatives.

Q. My child can't seem to get the hang of spitting out the toothpaste. She always swallows it. Should we be concerned?

If she is consuming a large quantity of toothpaste, you should probably switch to one without fluoride in it. Talk with the dentist about this. You can also brush her teeth with a small amount of baking soda or use a wet toothbrush without any paste on it.

Q. Our son likes to chew on things for self-stimulation/calming. Like, he's always gnawing on the ends of his pencils, toys, and chewy-tube things the OT gives him. Is he going to damage his teeth doing this?

He should be all right as long as the objects aren't too hard or too rough. You should periodically have his lead level checked (with a blood test) to be sure that he isn't taking in lead when he chews on things.

Q. Our child won't let anyone else brush her teeth, but she doesn't do a good enough job brushing her own teeth. She's had two cavities so far. What can we do?

This is a difficult situation. You should make sure there is fluoride in your water, and if not, give your child a fluoride supplement, since the fluoride will help prevent cavities. Some children enjoy using an electric toothbrush, which can be more effective at cleaning the teeth and gums. You should try one. Talk to your dentist about other steps you can take such as having special sealants applied that may help prevent cavities.

11 | Sensory Issues in Autism and Related Disorders

Our senses provide us with important information about our environment. Touch, smell, taste, hearing, and sight, as well as sensations of balance, body position, and movement provide us with important cues such as whether something will taste good, or whether an alarm is going off. Most of us learn fairly quickly which sensations we need to pay attention to and which ones we can ignore. For most of us, extraneous stimulation—say, the slight flicker of a florescent light—is something we can quickly learn to block out.

For most children, hearing (especially what others say) and vision become the most important senses—especially for communicating and learning about the world. For children with developmental challenges, particularly children with difficulties on the autism spectrum, the other senses may be just as relevant, if not more relevant. As a result, children with autism may seem to overreact to sensory stimuli and may have trouble filtering out or ignoring less important stimuli. This tendency can lead to higher levels of arousal or feelings of anxiety. Since this can, in turn, affect the child's ability to learn and socially engage, these sorts of sensory issues are very important to address.

In this chapter, we talk about sensory issues in autism spectrum disorders. We'll discuss hearing and vision (and screening for problems in hearing and sight), as well as some aspects of unusual sensitivities and sensory problems that children with ASDs often have. As with other topics, please keep in mind that your child may not have *any* of these problems, although some children have many of them. It clearly is important to make sure that your child is hearing and seeing well so that he can take full benefit of his educational program.

Sensory Differences in Autism

Unusual sensory features in autism were reported by Leo Kanner in his first description of autism. Many children with autism have some unusual sensory responses and interests. Often there seems to be a paradoxical combination of too much sensitivity (some sounds that you might not even notice will drive the child to distraction) and under-sensitivity (the same child may not respond to his own name when it is called). Some children with autism are preoccupied with lights or patterns. Sometimes they bring things very close to their eyes and move them back and forth. Children with autism may also be preoccupied with the feel or texture of things or with other sensory properties. For example, rather than play with the figures in a dollhouse and make up stories about them, they might repeatedly feel the wooden dollhouse furniture or spin the furniture around.

We don't know why all these unusual sensory issues develop in children with autism spectrum disorder. We do know, however, that they can make life more difficult. Sometimes sensory processing differences (usually some combination of over- and under-responsiveness) can be a significant problem for learning and social engagement. For example, at school your child might need to really focus and attend to something, but be constantly distracted because of his hyper-responsiveness to sounds. This can have a two-fold impact on your child's ability to learn. First, because the sounds are unpleasant for your child, he may tune out of the lesson or activity and engage in a behavior such as body rocking or covering his ears. Secondly, your child's teachers or classmates may see such behaviors as odd and "off-putting," and stay away from him, increasing his social isolation.

Various theories have tried to account for these problems in children with autism spectrum disorders, but with only limited success. It is not clear whether the problems have to do with too much (or too little) processing, with anxiety, with difficulties in dealing with change, or with basic aspects of information processing and attention. It is possible that the problems arise, at least to some degree, because of the child's difficulties in dealing with the social world. That is, unlike other young children, children with ASDs may not learn from other people what is, and isn't, so important to focus on. Likewise, they may not learn to respond to overwhelming sensory information by protesting or requesting comfort from a caregiver. As we'll discuss later in this chapter, tests of hearing and vision usually show normal sensory abilities. However, it is interesting that some of the unusual sensitivities and behaviors that children with autism have resemble those seen in some children who have visual impairments or deafness (but not autism).

Sometimes unusual responses to sensations are one of the first warning signs of autism. For example, a parent may notice that her infant won't respond to her voice consistently but becomes very upset if the vacuum cleaner is running. For some children, unusual sensory problems become more dramatic with age. For example, they may spend time looking at their hand, dangling bits of string in front of their eyes, or engaging in body rocking or hand flapping in an apparent attempt to block out more unpleasant stimuli in the environment. For other children, particularly those who have more language, sensory issues may diminish over time. This is probably in large part because language helps them cope more effectively and thus feel less disorganized by the environment. These children may be able to talk themselves through their reactions to the environment. Even higher functioning individuals (with autism or Asperger's disorder) report unusual sensory experiences, however.

Hearing Problems

Probably the most common sensory sensitivities reported among children with autism spectrum disorders involve sensitivity to sounds and noises. Often the parents' initial concern may be that their child is deaf because he doesn't respond to some sounds. At the same time, the child may seem to respond exquisitely to some sounds from the inanimate (non social) environment.

Deafness occasionally is associated with autism. As Chapter 3 discusses, all children can sometimes have some degree of temporary hearing loss due to recurrent ear infections leading to fluid in the middle ear. On the opposite side of the coin, sometimes children with deafness may initially look somewhat autistic but improve markedly when provided with hearing aids or other supplementary aids to their hearing, or when taught to use communication programs such as sign language.

Hearing Tests

Good hearing is a prerequisite to developing the ability to speak. And it is also crucial to the development of good social skills. Accordingly, hearing testing is typically conducted in very young children with autism and related troubles or whenever a child has delayed speech and language skills. It is particularly important if the child seems to respond to no or very few sounds.

Apart from testing for fragile X syndrome, hearing testing is the one additional medical test that is almost always important in autism. Many states are starting to require that a hearing test be done on all newborns before they are discharged from the hospital. This early detection of hearing problems will be very helpful.

Sometimes the pediatrician or family doctor will attempt to assess your child's hearing in her office. Often this is difficult to do adequately. Usually, your child will need the expertise of a professional audiologist—an individual trained and licensed to assess hearing impairment. If possible, the audiologist should be experienced in working with children with developmental problems. Assessing hearing can be difficult even for an audiologist when a child is young or not very cooperative.

Different methods may be used to assess your child's hearing. For very young or more impaired children, something called "sound field audiometry" may be used. In this procedure, your child sits between two loudspeakers in a room. Different sounds are then produced through either speaker and the audiologist watches to see if your child notices where the sound is coming from. Unfortunately, this method is often difficult to apply to children with autism and may not work as well for more subtle hearing losses.

When possible, the audiologist may attempt to do a more definitive test using headphones. Typically, children aren't tested with headphones until around four years of age. Children with autism may have trouble tolerating the headphones at any age, and some may not be able to cooperate or fully understand what they need to do. Depending on your child, you may be able to "desensitize" him or get him used to wearing headphones before he sees the audiologist. Sometimes the audiologist can make accommodations in the environment to let your child become used to the situation and then can use the headphones to test his hearing more adequately.

If your child can wear headphones, the audiologist will play different sounds at different frequencies or pitch and ask your child to indicate whether he heard it. Your child might be asked to drop a block into a bucket each time he hears a sound, or to raise his hand or press a button when he hears something. If your child doesn't understand cause and effect, hasn't learned to imitate, or can't cooperate, this method won't work. Instead, the audiologist will use one of the testing methods in which no response from the child is needed (discussed below).

Generally, the audiologist tries to establish the "hearing threshold"—the softest level at which a tone can just be heard in each ear. The audiologist tests bone conduction as well as the air conduction of sound. A special instrument is placed on the skull just behind the ear to assess how well sounds are transmitted from the bones in the skull to the ear. The audiologist can compare the bone conduction of the sound to the child's air conduction and determine whether the hearing loss, if any, is due to an outer or a middle ear problem or to a different area of the auditory pathway.

Typically, the audiologist will produce what is called an audiogram for your child's hearing. This is a graph showing your child's ability to respond to different sound frequencies. A degree of hearing loss at each frequency is expressed in special units called decibels (dB) which refer to the loudness of sounds. Speech sounds range from 20 to 60 decibels. Generally, people are said to have "normal" hearing if they can hear sounds when they are presented at 15-20 decibels or less. If there is no hearing loss, the lines showing your child's hearing abilities will not dip below the 15-20 dB level on the graph. If there is hearing loss—for example, 40 dB—that means the sounds had to be made that much louder in order for your child to hear them.

The level of loudness that is required to hear the sounds at different frequencies, or pitches, is tested. Pitch is expressed in units called hertz (Hz), with lower numbers of hz indicating deeper pitches and higher numbers of Hz indicating higher pitches. A child needs to hear well at a range of frequencies or pitches from approximately 500Hz to 4000Hz to normally recognize speech. The audiogram will chart the hearing level in decibels needed to hear sounds for each frequency presented at a range of frequencies, usually between 500 and 8000Hz. That is, it will show how loud sounds of different pitches have to be in order for your child to hear them.

Again, audiologists usually consider the normal range of hearing to be below 20 decibels. If the hearing is tested at your pediatrician's office in a room that is not completely soundproofed, a level of 25 decibels may be considered normal. Here is how audiologists usually classify hearing losses:

- 20 or 25 to 40 decibels indicate a mild hearing loss,
- 40 to 55 decibels, a moderate hearing loss,
- 55 to 70 decibels, a moderately severe loss,
- 70 to 90 decibels, a severe hearing loss, and
- over 90 decibels, a profound hearing loss.

When hearing loss is present, it does not always affect all frequencies. Many adults, for example, have hearing losses in the high frequencies (due, perhaps, to listening to music that is too loud) that do not affect their ability to hear speech sounds. If your child does have a hearing loss, it will be important to understand which frequencies (and therefore, which kinds of sounds) are most affected.

Testing Young or Uncooperative Children

Sometimes the audiologist will be unsuccessful in testing your child behaviorally because of his behavioral difficulties. If there is general agreement that your child can hear, the audiologist may request that he return weeks or months later to be rechecked. If there is any suspicion that your child cannot hear, he should be referred for more definitive hearing testing.

Otoacoustic Emissions Test. A relatively new test that is used in many newborn hearing screening programs is called the otoacoustic emissions test (OAE). It can be used with developmentally delayed children because it does not require the child to give any behavioral response. The audiologist places a small probe in the child's ear, which plays sounds into the ear canal. A tiny receiver measures the echo that comes back from the inner ear in response to these sounds. If this echo is normal, the child will "pass" OAE screening. The procedure is painless, but it does require your child to sit still for thirty seconds or so on your lap. Passing this screening means that your child is hearing normally. Failing usually means further testing is needed.

Auditory Brainstem Evoked Response. Another test that is frequently used is called auditory brainstem evoked response. It entails placing three small electrical wires on the surface of the child's head and having him wear headphones. Sounds are played into the headphones and a brain wave is generated each time the child hears a sound. These brain waves are detected by the testing device and eventually graphed on a computer. This test does not require your child's cooperation because he does not have to make a response. It does, however, require him to stay relatively still. He may have to be lightly sedated or otherwise helped to calm down to ensure an accurate recording.

Tympanometry. The audiologist may also perform something called tympanometry. This involves putting a device into the ear to measure the movement of the eardrum. If the middle ear cavity has an unusual amount of fluid or is under pressure, the eardrum won't move in the same way as it does when there is no pressure or fluid. This procedure is not painful, but your child may be frightened of having something placed in his ears. Again, finding an audiologist who works with young children with developmental disabilities is very important in making sure the results are as accurate as possible.

Types of Hearing Loss

There are different kinds of hearing loss:
1. Conductive hearing loss,
2. Sensorineural hearing loss, and
3. Mixed hearing loss.

Children with ASDs can have any of these types of hearing loss.

Conductive Hearing Loss. Conductive hearing loss occurs when there are difficulties in the transmission of the sound as it enters the ear canal through the middle ear and the small bones in the middle ear. This type of hearing loss in children is usually the result of fluid in the middle ear following recurrent infection or other factors.

(For reasons that are unclear, many children with autism have more ear infections than other children.) Children with allergies may be especially likely to have a conductive hearing loss. Impacted wax in the ear canal can also cause conductive hearing loss. Your pediatrician can usually remove the wax.

Children with conductive hearing loss have fluctuating levels of fluid in their middle ears, so sounds may be not be heard consistently. At different times, different sounds may be muffled or distorted in different ways by the fluid. Obviously, when specific speech sounds do not sound the same from day to day, it can be very confusing—especially for children who are just learning language.

Sensorineural Hearing Loss. A sensorineural hearing loss occurs less often. It results from a problem in the transmission of sound further along in the pathway between the middle ear and the brain and indicates that there has been damage to the inner ear or to the auditory nerve. There are many possible causes of sensorineural hearing loss. This type of hearing loss may run in the family, either as the sole problem or associated with certain genetic disorders that also cause other difficulties (such as heart problems). It can be associated with some in utero infections, with very high bilirubin levels in the newborn, with bacterial meningitis, and with the use of certain antibiotics. This kind of hearing loss is generally permanent and does not improve with age.

Mixed Hearing Loss. Some children may have a mixed hearing loss involving both conductive and sensorineural hearing loss.

Treatment of Hearing Loss

Treatment depends on the type of hearing loss and the cause of it. When the hearing loss is due to middle ear fluid, sometimes the placement of special pressure equalizing (PE) tubes will result in normalization of the child's hearing. These tiny tubes prevent the middle ear from having such high levels of fluid by draining the fluid and letting the eardrum function normally. Other solutions to this problem typically include treatment of infections or allergies by your pediatrician, an ENT, or an allergist. See Chapter 4 for more information about middle ear infections.

If your child has a more severe hearing loss, he may require hearing aids or some other amplification device. For some children, an FM system can be used where the teacher wears a microphone that transmits her voice to a device the child carries or wears, enabling him to better pick out the teacher's voice over the background noise. In many states, there are special programs and resources available to children with hearing problems.

Sound Sensitivities

If your child has normal hearing and is bothered by sensitivities to sounds, there are several things you can do. At school, you can advocate for a minimally distracting environment. Some school buildings and classroom seem almost perversely designed to complicate life for the child with an ASD. Concrete block construction and linoleum floors all contribute to an "echo chamber" effect.

Sometimes simple steps can be taken to reduce auditory "clutter" in the classroom. For example, ask that your child's classroom be carpeted, or, failing that, for casters to be put on the bottoms of chair legs, so they won't scrape so loudly when pushed back. Ask for preferential seating for your child, near the teacher and away from noisy air conditioning or heating units. Ask that doors be kept closed when students are walking through the halls. For some children, using earphones to block out extraneous noises may help. Other things that have been tried include special amplifiers that amplify speech sounds for the child (similar to hearing aids) to help him focus on the most important sounds (that is, the teacher's or peers' speech).

Although there is little research on this approach, you can also try to teach your child strategies to cope with problem sounds, such as covering his ears when the school bell rings, or requesting a break when the environment becomes too stimulating. In addition, there are alternative treatments that focus on reducing sound sensitivity (see Chapter 16).

For some children the sounds (and unpredictability) of noises such as fire alarms can lead to tremendous anxiety and behavioral difficulties. You can talk to your child's teacher about this. Reading a picture book or social story about fire drills can help. For instance, if your child is very sensitive to the noise of fire alarms, you could write a story that shows your child pulling out a pair of headphones to muffle the noise as he is leaving the room for the fire drill. If your child is verbal, you could give him a specific script he can use to talk himself through for reassurance. Having a practice run through of a fire drill may also be a good thing to try; we've encountered firemen who were willing to help with this. Often the practice will make it easier for your child when a real fire drill happens.

Visual Problems

Many children with autism have strengths in at least some aspects of visual skills (for example, visual spatial skills of the type used in putting together puzzles). On the other hand, abnormalities are also observed. Some children will spend long periods of time engaged in visual stereotypies (such as flicking a string back and forth in front of their eyes) or may be interested in unusual visual aspects of materials (focusing on minor details of a toy). These visual abnormalities are often related to other behavioral difficulties such as motor mannerisms or odd movements, as well as problems with self-regulation. In addition, many children with autism spectrum disorders have striking difficulties with social gaze—that is, with making eye contact while talking with others.

Children with autism spectrum disorders also sometimes have visual problems. Children born with visual problems sometimes exhibit unusual body movements that may be mistaken for those seen in autism. Clearly, normal vision is important for development and learning.

Eye Exams

If you suspect that your child is not seeing clearly, the doctor should begin by taking a good history of any visual disorders in the family. These could include refractive errors such as nearsightedness or farsightedness, cataracts (a clouding of the lens of the eye), glaucoma (increased pressure within the eye that can cause loss of vision), strabismus (imbalance of the muscles of the eye), and amblyopia or "lazy eye" (a loss of vision in one eye frequently caused by muscle imbalance, a marked difference in vision between the two eyes, or impaired vision from a cataract). The doctor will also ask about prenatal (before birth) problems such as developmental brain abnormalities, infections, or a genetic syndrome, or perinatal (at the time of birth) problems. Prematurity or hypoxia, a lack of adequate oxygen, can also influence visual development.

Early eye exams may be the same for children with autism as for others. Your pediatrician will check the eyelids and the eyes to make sure there is no drooping of a lid, that the pupils react to light, that the size of the eyes is appropriate, that the light reflects normally from the eye, ruling out cataracts or other serious eye disorders, and that your child can fix on an object and follow it, suggesting that some vision is present. Visual testing that requires the child's cooperation and understanding may be hard to perform, however, in children with ASDs.

Most typically developing children can cooperate with vision screening by the age of three or four years. Your pediatrician may have special picture charts that have been developed for children who are not yet reading. They use figures such as a house, an umbrella, or a circle. Children are asked to say which one of these is being pointed to by the examiner instead of naming letters as with the regular adult Snellen eye chart. A nonverbal child can be given a card with pictures of the objects on it and be asked to point to the one shown on the eye chart.

If your pediatrician is unable to test your child's vision, she will probably refer you to a pediatric ophthalmologist. The ophthalmologist can use an instrument called a retinoscope to test your child's vision without your child having to understand and answer questions. (The instrument looks like the otoscope your pediatrician uses to examine your child's ears.) Testing with the retinoscope can determine whether or not your child needs glasses, and, if so, what prescription is needed. Some cooperation is required. Your child will need to sit in the exam chair and allow someone to hold a lens near his eye while the doctor shines a light from the retinoscope at the eye.

If the ophthalmologist is looking for certain kinds of eye diseases, he may need to dilate your child's eyes with drops in order to get a better look. This can be very difficult for a child with an ASD. The doctor may need your assistance in holding your child still or it may require sedation or general anesthesia to allow a good look at the eye. You would only want to go through all of that if there was a high suspicion of an eye problem that couldn't be diagnosed any other way.

Research is being done on a technique known as photoscreening that will hopefully allow a pediatrician to screen a child for disorders that cause amblyopia with a minimum of cooperation. This is important because the earlier it is treated, the more likely the treatment is to work. A child would only have to look at a certain spot long enough for a camera or video system to take images that are then analyzed for factors that cause amblyopia. These include strabismus, significant refractive errors, and the clouding of parts of the eye.

Treatment of Vision Problems

If your child does need glasses, it may be difficult to get him to keep them on. For some children, it is helpful to get bands that go around the back of the head to help the glasses stay on. It is probably worth the extra expense to buy a lifetime warranty when you purchase the glasses. At least that way you can get them repaired or replaced for free if they are broken of lost.

If your child has strabismus or amblyopia, the eye doctor may recommend that one of the eyes be patched part of the time. This forces the child to use the weaker eye, preventing the stronger eye from "taking over" all the visual work. Frequently, it is recommended that the patch be worn six to eight hours a day. Recent research shows that only two hours of patching per day may be enough. An alternative to patching is to put eye drops in the better eye to blur the vision in that eye instead of patching it. This forces the child to use the poorer eye. While it may not be easy to get the drops in, for some children, using drops may be easier than trying to keep a patch in place.

Other Sensory Problems

In addition to having problems with the senses of vision and hearing, children with autism can be over- or under-sensitive to other types of sensations, including touch, movement, smell, and taste. Again, we do not know why these sensitivities are so common in autism, although there are many theories. Below are a few examples of ways that sensory problems may manifest themselves in a child with autism:

- **Movement Sensitivities:** Some children enjoy twirling themselves around; others hate it. Many children like the feeling of swinging in an outdoor swing or hammock. Some children walk in unusual ways, such as on their toes; others may have a peculiar gait.
- **Tactile (Touch) Responsivity:** Some children with autism have tactile defensiveness. That is, they cannot tolerate touching or being touched by things that are a certain texture, consistency, temperature, etc. For example, some children find the feeling of certain kinds of cloth intolerable or won't be able to wear clothes with any labels in them (the labels being a source of consistent annoyance to them). They may find the seasonal change of clothes difficult. For example, going from long sleeves and pants to short pants and shirts. Other children seem less than normally sensitive to temperature change and won't mind being cold in winter or hot in summer. Still other children can't stand to have their hair combed or their face washed.
- **Smell and Taste Sensitivities:** As we discuss in Chapter 6, sometimes these unusual sensitivities extend to food, so certain textures, tastes, smells, or colors of food are avoided. A few children respond dramatically to smells that the rest of us would generally not have a problem with.

Unusual sensitivities to light, touch, and balance (technically what is referred to as proprioception, or the sense of one's body in space) may be very related to self-stimulatory behaviors. For example, the younger child with autism might want to flick a string in front of his eyes, while an older child might want to spin or body rock (both behaviors which stimulate the balance system of the body). Chapter 12 discusses stereotyped (self-stimulatory) behaviors and their treatment in more detail.

Assessing and Treating Sensory Difficulties

Various professionals are often involved in assessing sensory difficulties. As we mentioned above, tests of vision and hearing should be a standard part of the assessment of any child with an autism spectrum disorder. Dietitians and speech-language pathologists may be involved for problems with smell and taste sensitivities. Usually occupational and physical therapists are involved in dealing with unusual sensory responses—particularly those involving the child's ability to feel and have a sense of his body. As a general rule, physical therapists are most involved in assessing motor skills, balance, posture, and movement; occupational therapists may be involved in assessing fine motor movements, self-care, and other adaptive skills. There are a few tests of motor abilities and sensory responsiveness; often an evaluation will focus a lot on "real world" situations and the kinds of responses that cause the child trouble.

Areas evaluated by occupational therapists often include eye-hand coordination, spatial awareness, quality of movements of the hand and body, muscle tone, and sensory integration abilities (see below). Usually there will be a strong focus on functional skills needed by your child in day-to-day activities. Particularly for younger children, there may also be a focus on play.

Occupational therapists can draw on a wonderful range of materials to try to help your child. For example, drawing materials might include chalk, paint, special pens and pencils, and markers—with the idea being to try to find materials that will interest your child or that provide special help for a child with unusual sensitivities. Children who have trouble touching or holding things (tactile defensiveness) may be helped by being introduced to a range of new materials—clay, play dough, sand, shaving cream, bubbles. Difficulties with motor planning can be addressed by breaking down tasks into subparts and working on them. Eye-hand coordination can be worked on with ball play. For children who have trouble having a good sense of their bodies, materials such as a weighted vest might be used to help them stay focused on a task. Specially adapted materials like chairs and tables may also be helpful. Children who spend excessive time spinning or rocking can be helped by providing opportunities for swinging/rocking during movement breaks. By helping to organize the child's sensory experiences, the OT can help him be more attentive and actively involved in learning.

Occupational therapists can also work quite well with other professionals, such as speech-language pathologists, on specific issues such as difficulties with the mouth and eating. The latter are particularly important for children with specific eating and oral-motor difficulties and in Rett's disorder (see also Chapter 15).

Physical therapists tend to focus on body movement and posture problems. They work on the bigger muscle groups in the bodies and focus on problem areas such as balance, stability of the body, muscle strength, and flexibility. Various tests of motor abilities are available. Activities might include swinging or jumping, walking on a balance beam, and other balancing activities. The physical therapist will typically work with you and the classroom teacher to be sure that everyone is working toward the same end.

Sensory Integration Therapy

Sensory integration refers to the process by which we take in, sort out, and organize information from our senses and then use the information to understand and respond to the entire situation. For example, if you wake up in the dark on your first morning of vacation, you may initially feel disoriented. You then become aware that the mattress beneath you is unusually hard and that there is a soft rumbling sound outside the window and a faint whiff of salt in the air. Putting all these sensory clues together, you remember that you are staying at a bed and breakfast by the sea.

Sensory integration therapy (SI) was developed by an occupational therapist, A. Jean Ayres, with the goal of helping people with sensory problems better integrate sensations. It is based on the observation that children with autism and other developmental disabilities often have unusual sensitivities or responses. The hope is that helping the child learn to be more tolerant of different sensory experiences will lead to gains in the child's developmental functioning.

A basic idea behind SI therapy is that repeated experience with the environment will help the child develop better abilities to cope with potentially distracting sensory experiences. Goals include decreasing sensitivity to bothersome sensations, increasing the child's awareness of times when the environment is becoming overwhelming, and helping the child learn techniques for calming himself.

SI treatment may include a "sensory diet" designed to provide the child with a range of materials addressing the child's sensory needs. Massage, stimulation of the sense of balance, joint compression, or a weighted vest might be used. Brushing (using a soft brush) on the arms and legs and back may be combined with other techniques. Some aspects of the intervention can be adapted to include more complicated problem solving for higher functioning individuals—for example, in helping the person be aware of his perceptions and in dealing with overstimulation. You may find a range of therapists trained in SI techniques, including OTs, PTs, and SLPs.

The theoretical basis for sensory integration is not horribly strong. On the other hand, many of the techniques used attract the interest of the child and may help him deal with aspects of the environment that are difficult for him. Particularly when done as part of a broader intervention program, the methods may be helpful in some ways. Children may attend better, sleep better, and have lower activity levels. Evidence for cognitive gains is not, however, very strong.

Summary

Children with ASDs often have unusual sensitivities or responses to the environment. These problems can take the form of either under- or over-responsiveness to the environment, or can include a mix of both under- and over-responsiveness. These can pose difficulties for your child and can complicate the task of providing a good educational program. These sensitivities can also limit opportunities for activities in the community, since peers may be put off by unusual preoccupations and sensitivities. Occupational therapists and other professionals can help you and your child learn to better cope with his sensitivities; there are also medications that can help with some self-stimulatory behaviors linked to sensory sensitivities (see Chapters 12 and 13).

In addition to understanding the unusual sensory responses that children with autism can have, you should also make sure you know about the typical types of hearing and visual problems that any child can develop. It is important to be sure that your child has normal hearing and vision. If anything is wrong, addressing the problem should be a first step in your child's intervention program. As we discuss in this chapter, a range of assessment methods are now available and can be used in very young children.

Questions

Q. My child gets very involved in visual self-stimulation at school. This seems to happen in one classroom in particular. He will look at his fingers and flick them back and forth. Sometimes he looks at things out of the corner of his eye. What can I do about this?

Self-stimulatory behaviors are very common in autism. The kind of behavior you describe is not unusual except for the fact that it seems to happen in one classroom. You might take a look at the classroom. See if it is (from your child's perspective) visually overstimulating. Sometimes classrooms with a lot of visual activity seem to overwhelm children with autism. We've walked into classrooms where there were things dangling from the ceiling and spinning around as well as lots of activity outside the classroom windows. Sometimes there are visual stimuli that no one else realizes are there (in one classroom, a spinning phonograph record was reflecting light in rainbows on the ceiling).

Q. My child likes to mouth things all the times, including dirt and stuff he has picked up off the floor. Can I do anything about this?

In the first place, be sure that the environment is free of lead (lead-based paint can be a source of lead poisoning). Secondly, talk to your child's psychologist, speech-language pathologist, OT, or behavior specialist at school. Some children will do well with a good behavioral intervention program. Sometimes children with autism spectrum disorders have what appears to be a strong need to have something in the mouth. You can try giving your child gum to chew on. Other chewy foods may help, as well, but avoid the "fruit sticks," which do indeed stick to the teeth and can cause cavities. Sometimes very crunchy foods will help the child; sometimes food with fairly intense flavors will help. Occasionally, children respond well to activities that involve blowing or sucking. (Also see the section on Pica on page 119.)

Q. My child seems to body rock a lot. It makes him seem very odd. Is there anything I can do about this?

Sometimes giving your child many opportunities for movement during the day can help. For instance, let him use a rocking chair or swing. Sometimes using seats that have some "give" (such as large therapy balls or cushions) may decrease body rocking. Talk with your OT for other ideas.

Q. Our daughter frequently hums to herself—especially when she's in her inclusive classroom setting. The other kids find this strange (and it is somewhat disruptive).

You mention that your daughter does this in one setting—an important clue in and of itself. Our suspicion would be that she is overwhelmed with auditory input in this setting and is attempting to compensate (by producing her own sounds). See if there is some way either to reduce noise levels in the classroom or help her by giving her a portable tape or CD player so she can play her own music. Sometimes children with this kind of problem also respond well to opportunities to blow on musical instruments.

12 | Common Challenging Behaviors

Behavioral difficulties in autism and related conditions can take many forms. Some children have few, if any, such difficulties. Other children have so many or such severe behavior problems that it is hard to provide a good quality educational program for them. Behavioral problems tend to change over time. For example, what was a slightly problematic behavior in a three-year-old can become a much more problematic behavior in a thirteen-year-old.

In this chapter, we'll discuss some of the behavioral problems and emotional difficulties sometimes seen in autism spectrum disorders. Keep in mind that, when the issue is your child, you'll need to work with people who know her very well. Also keep in mind that we're discussing the entire range of difficulties that can be seen, but your child may not have many or even any of these problems. When considering any treatment, you must always consider the potential benefits as well as the risks of treatment. Several excellent resources for parents are now available on behavioral and drug treatments and are listed in the Reading List at the end of the book.

For purposes of this chapter, we'll group problem behaviors (and emotional problems) into several broad categories covering some of the more frequent kinds of behaviors you might see within each category. Then we'll discuss some general aspects of behavioral and drug interventions. Specific medications and aspects of drug treatment are discussed in Chapter 13.

In an ideal world, there would be a simple one-to-one correspondence between a behavioral or emotional difficulty and a treatment. Unfortunately, things are a lot more complicated than this in the real world. First, it may be difficult to apply the usual diagnostic categories, particularly in a more impaired child with autism spectrum disorder. (This is a general problem for all children with significant disabilities.) Second, people sometimes do not recognize the other difficulties/disorders that are present, or mistakenly assume that having autism somehow protects you from other problems. That is, the diagnosis of autism or Asperger's disorder overshadows an awareness of other difficulties. As we'll discuss later in this chapter, these issues complicate decisions about how best to treat behavioral difficulties—particularly in children who have significant communication problems.

Another complication is that children with autism spectrum disorders often have many different problems. For example, problems with attention may go along with problems with stereotyped behaviors. Sometimes one or the other will seem more important to deal with (for various reasons); other times it can be hard to tell where to start. It is important to decide which problems are the ones to focus on, as well as what the benefits and potential risks of the treatment are. On the other hand, sometimes the fact that the child has several different problems will be very important in selecting a treatment—for example, there may be a drug that might help with both rigidity and depression. Also keep in mind that problem behaviors often seem to travel in groups!

Behavioral Interventions—A Brief Introduction

Although the main focus of this book is on medical treatments, it is important to realize that behavioral and educational interventions are usually the first line of treatment for behavioral difficulties. A whole body of work on behavioral difficulties (applied behavior analysis or ABA) provides a very helpful framework for dealing with behavioral difficulties. The assumptions of ABA are that, like other children, those with autism spectrum disorder learn through experience. Accordingly, the events that precede behavioral difficulties (the antecedents) and those that follow them (the consequences) are important. The antecedents are the things that set off the behavior in the first place. For example, if you ask your child to stop body rocking and put away her toys and this leads to a tantrum, you have a pretty good idea that your child does not want to stop her body rocking or put away her toys. On the other hand, if your response to the tantrum is to let your child continue to body rock, you've given a pretty strong message (the consequence) that your child doesn't need to listen to you.

There are many different approaches to dealing with behavior problems. Generally, however, one of the most important steps is to see if you can observe regularities in the problem behaviors—for example, does the behavior only happen in a certain time or place or following a certain activity? Look at what goes before and what follows the behavior—is the behavior being (unintentionally) rewarded (reinforced)?

Keep in mind that you want to reinforce good behavior. To do this, be sure to praise such behavior quickly and specifically (with praise, tangible rewards, etc.) when it happens. In many ways, the solution to the problem of bad behavior is to get your child to increase good behaviors. Planning ahead is helpful; if you know a situation will be stressful or a problem for your child, have a plan in advance. It is always easier to prevent problems than to have to react to them during a crisis.

Be a careful observer of your child. Often you'll be able to notice subtle behaviors that may be clues that she is going to have difficulties. Use these warning signs to head off problem behaviors—for example, by giving your child something else to do. When you do need to set limits or have consequences, be clear, be specific, and then follow through. Again, being prepared is a big part of the battle! If you have a plan in place, you can implement it rather than feeling confused and overwhelmed. If, for example, your child has trouble at the grocery store, you should make a specific plan before you go. First, you probably should do everything possible to make initial visits a success—for example, by going in to get the child's favorite ice cream. Use a shopping list (with visual cues or actual labels from cans/cartons) that your child can help you complete. If your child has behavioral difficulties, tell her in advance what will happen if she engages in the problem behavior: "Jenny, there is no screaming in the grocery store; if you scream we'll have to leave and can't get ice cream."

It may help to take notes and/or develop a chart where you can list the "ABCs" of problem behaviors—antecedents, the behavior itself, and the consequences. Often, as you pay more attention, you'll start to notice important clues—for example, that the behavior only happens in one place or at one time of the day.

Also take a careful look at the environment. Sometimes what seem to be simple adjustments in your child's environment (for example, moving her from a more disorganized and disorganizing environment to a simpler, structured one) can make for a major change in her behavior. Children with autism respond well to structure, predictability, and consistency, and it is important to be sure that the environment is not contributing to your child's problems.

In addition, pay attention to the function of the behavior. If your child is using some behavior to get your attention, then try planned ignoring. That is, don't acknowledge what your child is doing inappropriately but *do* pay attention when she starts doing something you want her to do. You might even try time outs. Be sure to pair this with lavish and appropriate praise when your child is behaving well. If your child has trouble with the word "no" (as most children do) be careful not to reinforce tantrums or other inappropriate behaviors. Sometimes parents unintentionally encourage this behavior by doing exactly what the child wants.

Sometimes problems will arise because your child is trying to avoid work or other activities. Unfortunately, if you give in, this sends a strong message to your child about how to get out of work. Try instead to get her to engage for a short time in the activity, then praise her and let her do something else for a while. Also try to model and encourage good, straightforward communication.

Some sensory behaviors (see Chapter 11) can be addressed by helping your child find more appropriate ways to engage in the behavior. Your child's occupational therapist may be helpful to you here. For example, if your child has trouble with prolonged body rocking, you might start by trying to contain the behavior to a certain place (e.g., a rocking chair) with set amounts of time for rocking alternated with periods of time for work. (These periods of time can be made progressively longer.)

Many times, children who have major communication difficulties use problem behaviors as an inappropriate way of communicating. To try to minimize communication difficulties in dealing with problem behaviors, keep your own communications clear and simple. Be sure your child is paying attention when you communicate with her. Be exact and specific about what you want. Try to give her appropriate ways for communicating frustration, anxiety, and other difficult feelings. This can be done by specifically teaching an alternative behavior for communicating the same meaning or intention. For example, teach your child a manual sign for "help" to replace the tantrum that occurs when she is frustrated during a difficult task. Your child's speech-language pathologist should be able to suggest strategies or communication methods to help with this.

Keep the big picture in mind. It is often easy to say what you *don't* want your child to do, but what is it that you want her *to do?* Your child's classroom teacher, the school psychologist, speech-language pathologist, and OT or PT may all have valuable advice for you. Sometimes the assistance of a behavior specialist may be needed. Unfortunately, children with autism spectrum disorders are all sufficiently different from each other that you really need to tailor the intervention to your child. Having an outside specialist can be a great help in this process.

Drug Interventions—A Brief Introduction

Although behavioral and educational interventions are often tried first, medications also play an important role in helping children with behavioral difficulties. Sometimes behavioral interventions alone don't do the trick. Other times there may be a real emergency (such as when a child is seriously injuring herself by head banging). For still other situations—for example, depression—medicines may be the first line of treatment. Medicines and behavioral procedures can be used together—often very effectively. We discuss this issue in much more detail in Chapter 13.

There are several times in the life of a child with autism when medications are more likely to be considered. Generally, very young children are least likely to receive medications. Usually their behavioral difficulties are less serious, and can be managed by teaching them more acceptable alternatives to problem behaviors. It is also much easier to physically manage an out-of-control two-year-old than a twelve-year-old. The year or so before children enter puberty is often a time when behavioral difficulties arise. We are not sure why this is, although the various changes they experience in their bodies and changes in hormone levels probably are part of the picture.

For some children, particularly higher functioning children, the advent of adolescence also means that the child is more aware of being different, in some important ways, from other children. This can give rise to feelings of depression and sometimes serious symptoms of depression. Fortunately, we have fairly effective treatments for depression. Even more importantly, the desire to fit in really spurs remarkable growth in some children.

Types of Behavioral and Emotional Difficulties

Behavioral and emotional difficulties in autism and related conditions can take many different forms, but these generally fall into several, sometimes overlapping, categories.

Sometimes the child exhibits so many difficulties that it is hard to sort out exactly what is going on. This is particularly true if—as is understandable for a parent—you are so closely involved that it is hard to get a sense of the "big picture." This is one of the reasons that an outside consultant (a behavioral psychologist or other behavior specialist or a physician) can be helpful. In thinking about behavior problems and their treatment, it is often helpful if you can step back a bit.

Stereotyped Behaviors and Agitation

Stereotyped movements are common in young children with autism and related conditions (although not as common in Asperger's disorder). These seemingly purposeless, repeti-

Table 12-1 | Common Behavioral/Mood Problems in ASDs

Types of Behaviors	Specific Examples
Stereotyped Behaviors	Body rocking; hand/finger flicking; other repetitive behaviors
Self-Injury and Aggression	Injury to self or others
Problems with Rigidity and Perseveration	Resistance to change; compulsiveness; unusual interests; getting mentally "stuck" on a thought, word, or activity
Overactivity and Problems with Attention	High activity levels; difficulties with attention; impulsivity
Mood Problems	Depression; anxiety; bipolar disorders

tive movements can include body rocking, finger flicking, toe walking, and other complex, whole body movements. As discussed in Chapter 15, other kinds of unusual movements are seen in Rett's disorder—for example, hand washing or hand wringing, as well as some other very odd behaviors such as pulling at the tongue. Stereotyped movements may also be referred to as self-stimulatory movements (although this sometimes leads to confusion with masturbation, which is a somewhat different problem—see Chapter 14).

Stereotyped movements are often associated with other behavior problems such as self-injury or sometimes with aggression (particularly if you attempt to interrupt the movements). They also are often associated with behavioral rigidity and difficulties with change. Some degree of agitation or general tendency towards being upset and "on edge" is also often seen; you can feel as if your child is about to explode at any second.

Sometimes infants and very young children who go on to have typical development engage in some body rocking, occasionally even head banging, while asleep. For these children, the problem usually goes away on its own in the first couple of years of life. We also occasionally see typical children and adolescents engage in self-stimulatory movements such as moving their leg rapidly while taking a test. These seem to have an anxiety-reducing function, but are not as all-encompassing as those seen in autism.

In contrast to the stereotyped movements seen in autism spectrum disorders, the unusual movements or tics of Tourette syndrome are different in several ways. Tics tend to occur in bouts, tend to involve the head and neck—particularly early on—and the child doesn't seem to enjoy engaging in them. Movement problems may also be seen in other disorders (for example, sometimes following infections), and occasionally it can be difficult to disentangle the nature of the movements. This is one of the reasons it is good to have a specialist such as an experienced psychiatrist or neurologist involved if your child is making seemingly purposeless movements.

For children with autism and related disorders, some unusual interests and fascinations often come before the more typical stereotyped behaviors. These interests can include lights (and light switches), twirling and spinning objects (such as fans and tops), and fascination with the smell, taste, or feel of things. The child may begin to engage in some form of visual self-stimulation—for example, looking at things out of the corner of the eye or bringing materials up to the corner of her eye. Sometimes the development of an unusual attachment—such as to a ball or string or unusual objects—may come before the more typical stereotyped movements.

Repetitive, stereotyped movements vary over both the short and long term. Often they seem to increase after about age three and then may increase in frequency or intensity (or both) again around five or six years of age. For some children, they may then subside only to return in force around the time they enter puberty—often some months before. These behaviors can show up at times when the child is bored or stressed, as well as overstimulated or anxious. They may also seem to serve as a preferred mode of activity for the child—almost like relaxation. Sometimes these behaviors shade off into more compulsive and ritualistic behaviors (which we discuss shortly).

Parents often ask us when we would intervene with these behaviors and often are eager to try medications. These behaviors are particularly difficult for parents to explain when the child is in more public settings, and parents—and particularly siblings—are often quite distressed by these behaviors. Although these behaviors are difficult to entirely eliminate, many children can be helped to decrease them.

The decision to pursue treatment should include consideration of whether the behavior really interferes with your child's (or family's) life in some way. Low levels of such behavior are often easier to live with and parents and others can work to confine the behaviors to certain places or contexts. Occasionally, giving your child the opportunity to engage in these behaviors can even be used as a reward for appropriate behavior. With occasional exceptions (e.g., when the behavior is putting the child in some danger), we would not generally recommend medications as a first step.

Behavioral Interventions

There are many different behaviorally based approaches for dealing with these behaviors. A whole body of work in psychology has focused on reducing levels of such behaviors by viewing them as learned behaviors. That is, they are not necessarily so much part and parcel of autism, but, rather, responses that the child learns to help her deal with her environment. Many of the effective treatments developed have used this perspective—for example, to see when the behaviors occur, what sets them off, what keeps them going, and so forth. Having understood something about the functions of these behaviors, steps can then be taken to reduce them. For example, if a child has problems with finger flicking or spinning objects, giving her something else to do with her hands may reduce the behavior. Analysis of the environment may reveal that it is too stimulating and that the child is overloaded with information. By giving the child a less stimulating environment, levels of self-stimulation may be reduced.

It is clear that movement and vigorous physical activity can help reduce stereotyped behaviors. Children who engage in high levels of spinning or twirling can benefit from regular exercise. Even getting the child up for short periods in the classroom to engage in vigorous movement such as stretching, jumping, or bouncing can help. One of the problems, sometimes, with more inclusive classroom settings is that opportunities for physical movement and vigorous activity are limited to gym class and recess (times where children with autism often need the most supervision). In addition, students are generally encourage to stay seated in the regular classroom setting. Some modification in the program to allow for breaks for movement and other physical activity can be helpful. Often the OT can be very useful in consulting with you and the classroom teacher about possible activities to try.

Occasionally children engage in auditory self-stimulation—for example, by spending long periods of time humming or making noises. Again, this sometimes happens when the child is overly stimulated (particularly by noises and sounds), and a look at the environment may help clarify what is going on. For children who are overly responsive to sounds, various devices are available ranging from simple earplugs to music devices (a portable CD, Ipod®, or MP3 player) and those that produce "white noise" or certain sounds (such as the sound of the ocean or of rain falling).

Drug Treatments

Various medications can reduce levels of these troublesome behaviors. Usually behavioral interventions are tried first, with exceptions made for an emergency situation. As with any medicine, the potential benefit and risk should be carefully considered. When a major change occurs in your child's behavior, you should also ask your pediatrician to rule out medical reasons. Sometimes behavior problems increase as a child is becoming sick or when she is unable to communicate that she is ill or in pain.

Common medications used to treat stereotyped and similar behaviors include the major tranquilizers, the selective serotonin reuptake inhibitors, and alpha-adrenergic agonists; these are discussed in detail in Chapter 13.

Aggression and Self-injury

Behaviors that involve either self-inflicted injury or injury to others are among the most difficult and problematic behaviors for parents, teachers, and professionals to deal with. Fortunately, this problem is not that common, and, even when it occurs, there are a number of potential interventions. Aggression and/or self-injury tend to occur with other problems (such as rigidity or perseveration).

Self-injury can take many different forms, including head banging, pinching one's self, pulling out hair, poking the eye, biting the hand, and so forth. Aggression against others may include biting or hitting. Behavior that is destructive to property is also often grouped in this category of difficulties. Self-injurious behavior can be extremely distressing for parents to see. It usually does not begin until the age of five or six, although occasionally it occurs in younger children with autism.

The sudden onset of self-injurious behavior, particularly head banging, should prompt a trip to the pediatrician, since nonverbal children sometimes use such behavior to communicate about physical pain. Infected ears are particularly likely culprits in younger children; in adolescents who start head banging for the first time, dental problems such as impacted wisdom teeth are sometimes to blame. (This is another important reason for your child to have regular dental care.) Children who start to poke their eye may have some physical problem or occasionally even a visual difficulty that they can't complain about in words.

Aggression toward others is often (but not always) "provoked" in some way. For example, a child might be interrupted or asked to do something more challenging. Like

Table 12-2 | Drugs for Behavioral Difficulties

Area of Difficulty	Group of Drug	Examples	
		Generic Name	Trade Name
Stereotyped movements	Neuroleptics	haloperidol	Haldol®
	Atypical neuroleptics	risperidone	Risperdal®
	SSRIs	fluoxetine	Prozac®
	Alpha adrenergic agonists	clonidine	Catapres®
Aggression/Self-injury	Neuroleptics	thiothixene	Navane®
	Atypical neuroleptics	risperidone	Risperdal®
	SSRIs	fluvoxamine	Luvox®
	Alpha adrenergic agonists	guanfacine	Tenex®
	Beta blockers	propranolol	Inderal®
	Mood stabilizers	carbamazepine	Tegretol®
Rigidity and Perseveration	SSRIs	sertraline	Zoloft®
	Alpha adrenergic agonists	guanfacine	Tenex®
	Atypical neuroleptic	quetiapine	Seroquel®
Attentional difficulties/ hyperactivity	Neuroleptics	haloperidol	Haldol®
	Atypical neuroleptics	risperidone	Risperdal®
	Stimulant medications	methylphenidate	Ritalin®
Mood Problems Depression	Antidepressants	imipramine	Tofranil®
	SSRIs	trazadone	Deseryl®
Anxiety Problems	Benzodiazepines	lorazepam	Ativan®
Bipolar disorder	Mood stabilizers	divalproex	Depakote®/ Depakene®

Drugs listed are examples only; often other drugs are available within the same class or category of medication. Specific medications, doses, indications, and side effects are discussed in detail in Chapter 13.

self-injury, aggression can be a major problem for parents as well as teachers and school staff. It may take the form of biting, hitting, kicking, scratching, or head butting.

A careful analysis of what seems to set off the behavior is very important. For example, is it a response to frustration, or an escape behavior, or the child's way of saying, "No, I don't want to do this"? In analyzing the behavior, it is also important to look at the context in which the behavior occurs. For example, is it only at school? Only with some care providers? Only during some activities or situations? Only at certain times of the day? Often this information gives important clues as to why the behavior may be happening and what you can do about it.

Behavioral Interventions

The parents of one eight-year-old boy with autism called one of us complaining that their child needed medication to decrease his aggression. Discussion with the parents made it clear that this was a new behavior for the boy. The aggression had started when the child's bus route and driver had been changed. The new route (itself a potential problem) was much longer, there was no longer a bus monitor, and there was another student on board who screamed during the bus ride. The child, who was very sensitive to loud sounds and greatly annoyed by the screaming student, reacted by trying to bite him. In this case, some modifications in the bus arrangements resulted in a quick change in the behavior.

As our example illustrates and as with other behavioral difficulties, a good analysis of potential causes and consequences of the behavior is very important. Did the head banging or self-injury start after the child entered a new classroom or after some aspect of her program was changed? Does the self-injury occur only during "down times"? Is it related to levels of environmental stimulation (either too much or too little)? Some children head bang only at night, while others will engage in this behavior only in very specific situations.

For situations where the behavior is potentially very dangerous, medications may be used much more quickly. For example, occasionally children with autism will bite themselves to the point of causing significant injury and may need medications. Even when medications are used, it is important to try to understand what sets off, and keeps up, the behavior. Other parents and professionals may be sources of good ideas for intervention.

Aggression against others is usually seen in very specific situations. These include: when the child is frustrated and unable to communicate, when favored routines are violated, or when someone attempts to interfere with the child's behavior. Many people have made the observation that such behaviors may represent a very basic (and sometimes difficult to understand) communication—that is, that the child is overwhelmed and unable to cope.

Communication difficulties may make it hard for children with autism to tell people how they feel or when they are being pushed too much. This can happen even with older children who can communicate. For example, a ten-year-old boy with Asperger's disorder went to his P.E. class in school without his usual aide (a stressful situation now made worse), where the children were running sprints and timing themselves using a stopwatch. The regular gym teacher gave him a stopwatch (which he did not know how to operate) and told him to run as fast as he could. The boy put in a great effort, but at the finish line discovered that the stopwatch hadn't worked because he hadn't realized you had to start it. The coach refused to let him run again. The boy threw the stopwatch on the ground, breaking it, and the coach came up to restrain the boy, only to get smacked in the face. The school threatened to expel the youngster for aggression since he should have "used his words" and not hit the teacher. In this case, the multiple difficulties included the stressful situation, the lack of his usual supporter, a lack of any instruction on how to operate the stopwatch, an unsympathetic coach, and a boy who was really trying his hardest to cope. In fact, the aggression toward the coach would not have happened at all had the coach "used his words" at any of a number of points with the boy!

Some children with autism also have problems with destroying property. Again, many different solutions are available, depending on the circumstance. You should *not* feel as if you have to turn your home into Stalag 17. Rather, explore different options, talk with other parents, and, if need be, talk to professionals who can provide suggestions. Again, the help of someone who can stand back a bit and see the big picture may be helpful. One child we know loved tearing up clothes, books, and furniture. His parents coped with this in several ways but most importantly realized that by giving him his own (more-or-less indestructible) room, as well as plenty of physical exercise, they could greatly reduce his destructive behavior.

Drug Treatments

Some of the same medicines used for treating stereotyped behaviors can be used for treating aggression. Again, behavioral methods are, generally, the first things to try, and again, the exception has to do with dangerous behaviors. As with other behaviors, it is important to do an analysis of the behavior to understand when it occurs, what makes it better or worse, how it changes over time, and so forth.

In addition to the medications already listed for treating stereotyped behaviors (see Table 12-2), other kinds of medications used include beta blockers (see Chapter 13) as well as mood stabilizers (some of these are also antiseizure medicines).

Rigidity and Perseverative Behaviors

Unusual interests, ritualistic and compulsive behaviors, and problems with transitions are frequent in children with autism spectrum disorders. These behaviors can take many forms. For example, a child may be preoccupied with turning lights on and off, or opening and closing doors, or feeling water run out of faucets.

Although sometimes hard to measure, these behaviors can be particular sources of difficulty for higher functioning children. For example, children with Asperger's disorder can spend inordinate amounts of time pursuing more facts about their topic of interest. Typical kinds of interests in these children include time, geology, astronomy, dinosaurs, and snakes. Some of the more unusual interests we've seen have included deep fat fryers, telegraph pole line insulators, disasters, and the names, dates of birth, and home addresses of every member of Congress (and of their spouses and children).

Sometimes lower functioning children with autism who otherwise seem to have very short attention spans can spend seemingly endless time on their particular fixation. Regardless of the child's level of functioning, these special interests are a problem if the child spends so much time on them that they actually interfere with her functioning in other areas.

A related set of problems are the "resistance to change" and "insistence on sameness" first described by Leo Kanner back in 1943. These problems often are combined with the restricted interests, since, in some ways, they are two sides of the same coin. That is, by being so fixated on a particular object or topic, the child also avoids being exposed to new situations and learning new things. Teaching staff and parents may find themselves going to great lengths not to provoke the child by keeping her from pursuing her interests, and, as a result, the child's learning may suffer

In younger and lower functioning children, insistence on sameness can take various forms. For example, a child may insist on always taking the same route to school, or always wearing the same clothes to church, or always having pizza on Monday night. Sometimes it seems almost as if the child learns a thing once—the first time—and then cannot tolerate any change. Older and higher functioning children may rely on a set of very specific social routines. For example, one young man one of us knows always opens any conversation with a question from the quiz show *Jeopardy!* This is (kind of) OK for someone who knows him, but does cause trouble for those who don't when he opens a conversation with, "Monica Lewinsky and the category is politics."

The difficulties that children with autism have in dealing with change really speak to a number of much broader issues about their tendency to learn things in whole chunks (what psychologists call "gestalt learning") rather than breaking things down into bits. As long as things stay exactly the same, the child doesn't have to deal with the complexity posed by change. This problem also speaks to the difficulties children with autism have in getting the big picture of social interaction. That is, social interaction presents many significant obstacles if you have trouble dealing with any change, since meaning is always changing depending on who is talking and what they are talking about. Furthermore, the multiple competing cues in interaction (tone of voice, facial expression, gesture, and content of words) which provide important meaning for the rest of us are potential sources of confusion and disorganization for children with autism.

Sometimes, particularly for higher functioning children, special interests and preoccupations can be put to good use. For example, a child with Asperger's disorder who was interested in astronomy led the discussion of space and planets in his fifth grade class. Unfortunately, finding a good use for special interests is not usually so easily done.

Behavioral Interventions

Various strategies can be used to help deal with resistance to change. For children who do not have much spoken language, visual schedules can be quite helpful. As we mentioned previously, a small camera and notebook or cards can be used to help the child see what came before, what is happening now, and what is happening in the future. These visual schedules can be placed on refrigerators at home or on bulletin boards in the classroom and the student's attention can periodically be drawn to them. A whole literature on the use of these schedules now exists (see the Reading List). A second strategy entails helping the child tolerate change through a more gradual process. Again, an entire body of work based on learning theory can be used to introduce change gradually. Another approach is to make the behavior more functional—that is, by helping the child use her interest in a more normal or typical way. The idea is that by helping the child learn to use her behavior in more productive ways, she can be helped to be more functional in daily life.

Other strategies are available for verbal individuals and are especially effective for children with Asperger's disorder. These can include use of:

- scripts and verbal routines (basically a "canned" set of verbalized guidelines a child can use to talk herself through specific situations);
- Social Stories (prewritten stories a child can review to help her practice and rehearse strategies for dealing with potentially problematic situations; see the references by Carol Gray in the Reading List);
- provided "rules" (e.g., you must always ask before you take something) that are simple, functional, and can be written down (particularly helpful to children who read).

Once again, a careful analysis of the nature of the problem behavior can be very helpful. For example, many higher functioning individuals have difficulty dealing with novelty—

which makes them anxious—partly because they have trouble both in recognizing that something is new and in realizing that they are anxious. Explicit teaching and counseling can be quite helpful for these children.

A related issue has to do with compulsive and ritualistic behaviors. The child may have to go through a set series of actions or behaviors when engaging in some activity. One high functioning man with autism we know will, for example, walk three miles out of his way every day as he walks to work to pick up his (same) lunch at a corner market because that market is the one he happened to go to on his first day on the job. A young adult woman with autism we know is very preoccupied with keeping all her clothes neat—every single item has a place in her room and heaven help anyone who tries to interfere with this!

Some ritualistic or compulsive behaviors have some similarity to those seen in obsessive compulsive disorder (OCD)—a condition where people are troubled by obsessions (things they can't stop thinking about, such as the thought that they are bad, or the need to do something) and compulsions (the need to do an activity over and over, such as washing your hands because you are afraid they are dirty). Some degree of obsessiveness and compulsiveness is perfectly normal. It is not normal, however, if the child is washing her hands for fifty minutes at a time (often to the point where they are bleeding) or is so troubled by doing something bad that she is essentially immobilized.

The similarities of more typical OCD-type behaviors to some of these seen in autism (the rigidity and tendency to repeat things) are very interesting, and some of the drug treatments for these behaviors are similar for OCD and autism. A major point of difference is that often children (or adolescents and adults) with OCD will tell you that they *don't like* having to engage in the behaviors. In contrast, individuals with ASDs often find their compulsive behaviors are not distressing—if anything, they are things the child *likes* to do.

Drug Treatments

Various medications may be helpful with this set of problems (see Table 12-2). The most frequently used medications are the SSRIs. The particular advantage of these medications is that they target both the rigidity and compulsiveness as well as the anxiety involved in dealing with change. Sometimes these behaviors respond to other medications, including both neuroleptics and atypical neuroleptics as well as the alpha adrenergic agonists.

Overactivity and Problems with Attention

Problems with attention and overactivity (hyperactivity) are fairly common in children with autism spectrum disorders. These behaviors often occur together, but some children have more problems with one than the other. These problems may include difficulties with listening, disorganization, high levels of activity, and impulsiveness. The child may be restless and on the go more or less all the time. Difficulties with not listening and impulsive behavior can be the source of much trouble, such as bolting into the street. For children with emerging language or no language, it is important to realize that at least some of the difficulties may relate to difficulties with language and communication. That is, if you have language, you can use it to help organize yourself, but if you don't, you will tend to be disorganized.

For higher functioning children with PDD-NOS, autism, and Asperger's disorder who have language, the attention problems (and to some extent hyperactivity) may suggest attention-deficit/hyperactivity disorder (AD/HD)—a commonly recognized disorder in typically developing children of school age. The question as to whether to formally diagnose AD/HD in children with ASDs remains somewhat controversial. One reasons is that—at least for some children—language problems, learning issues, and difficulties with organization and lack of good judgment seem more part and parcel of the autism spectrum disorder. We know, for example, that children with language problems are also likely to have attention problems. Particularly if attention problems are confined to the school setting, it is important to look at the curriculum to be sure it is appropriately matched to the student's needs.

Behavioral Interventions

One of the first questions to ask yourself is whether your child's difficulties with activity and attention are seen in all situations or only at school. If they only occur at school, it is then worth asking if these difficulties are seen in every class or setting or only in some. If only in school and only in some settings, it would be worth paying careful attention to what is going on. Ask questions such as:

- Are the language demands for your child too high?
- Is the academic material over her head?
- Can the classroom environment be modified to be less disorganized?
- Can visual support or augmentative communication systems be used to help your child be more organized (for example, visual schedules, use of visual aids, and so forth).
- Does your child start the day doing well and then seem to "lose it" as time goes on? (If so, fatigue may be a factor.)
- Do different approaches seem to be helpful (giving your child periods for activity interspersed with school work)?

It may be helpful to request a functional analysis (in which a behavioral psychologist or trained special educator analyzes what exactly sets off and follows the problem behavior).

If the problems with attention and/or hyperactivity seem to be happening in all parts of your child's life, some of the same considerations will apply. For instance, there should be a functional analysis and consideration of measures (such as visual cues) to help your child be more organized. A behavioral program may be helpful in both school and home settings, with consistent record keeping and attention to your child's behavior coupled with a system of rewards and positive supports. This effort should involve both parents and teachers so that the system can be applied consistently across your child's day.

Drug Treatments

A number of different treatments have been used over the years to help children with attentional problems. The most commonly used medicines (in all children) are the stimulants (amphetamines, methylphenidate). Some children, particularly more "classically autistic" children, may respond to these medicines by becoming *more* disorganized and active. (This does not always happen and even when it does, the medicine is out of the system fairly quickly.) Other medicines that are used include the neuroleptics, atypical neuroleptics, and opiate antagonists.

Mood Problems

All of us experience changes in our mood during the course of the day, as well as over longer periods. Some of us have periods when we feel low and depressed for long periods of time. Clinical depression is defined by symptoms such as lack of energy, loss of appetite, feeling "down" all the time, and so forth. Others of us have more difficulties with anxiety, including anxiety about certain events or situations or sometimes more general, free-floating anxiety.

Individuals with autism spectrum disorder (and particularly adolescents and young adults) seem to have an increased risk for depression. This is particularly true among higher functioning individuals (with autism, Asperger's, or PDD-NOS) who may, as time goes on, have an increasing sense of being isolated and missing out on many things their typically developing peers enjoy. Recent research also suggests that there may be a genetic basis for some increased vulnerability for depression in the families of children with ASDs.

Symptoms of depression can include the stated feeling of being depressed, as well as difficulties with sleep, appetite, and loss of energy. More verbal children may talk about feeling depressed or express negative thoughts about themselves. Occasionally (and this can be tricky to sort out), children may feel irritable rather than depressed. To complicate things further, some children seem to get more agitated and upset when depressed. Not surprisingly, depression can be difficult to diagnose in younger children with developmental problems and in older children who have significant communication problems.

Occasionally, children with ASDs have periods of depression and then go back to "normal" before becoming somewhat high and "hyper." It has been suggested that perhaps they have bipolar disorder. This is what used to be known as manic-depressive illness and is characterized by pronounced mood swings. Often the individual experiences periods of depression followed by "normal" periods and then periods of elation and grandiosity with rapid speech, giving the impression that she is on a "natural high." The final word is not yet in on whether some children with ASDs truly have bipolar disorder, although marked swings in mood combined with major changes in behavior suggest that this might be considered. It is always important to look at the big picture, since, for example, some of the medicines used to treat depression can cause children to be agitated if they actually have bipolar disorder, not depression.

Recurrent difficulties with anxiety can also be seen in children with autism spectrum disorder. These may include free-floating, high levels of anxiety (sometimes related to difficulties with change), as well as more specific anxiety problems (anxiety in social situations or anxiety around specific things or activities, such as fear of cats or dogs). Sometimes the problem is with panic attacks—that is, the child becomes profoundly anxious and fearful and her heart races. Children with better language skills may be able to talk about some of the symptoms of anxiety, but even when children do not have good language, you may be able to see that they "look anxious." Sometimes the difficulties with anxiety lead to other problems, such as self-injury, aggression, or stereotyped movements.

Some researchers have suggested that anxiety may be part of the autism spectrum disorders. Others suggest that it may come about as a result of repeated frustration and negative experiences. We certainly know that higher functioning children with ASDs complain about feeling socially isolated and victimized. The growing awareness of difficulties in dealing with peers and social situations may lead to a vicious cycle in which anxiety increases and makes it more likely that the child won't join in with peers.

Behavioral Interventions

For typically developing children, counseling, psychotherapy, and play therapy can often be helpful. This is sometimes true for children with autism spectrum disorders, although usually the therapist has to be more structured and problem focused (more like a teacher in some respects). Various behavioral techniques can also be used, particularly for anxiety difficulties. These include teaching the child how to relax through methods such as biofeedback, visual imagery, and relaxation training. If you decide to pursue any of these interventions, you would be well advised to find a psychologist or other professional who has had a fair amount of experience with the technique and who ideally has had experience working with children with autism.

Drug Treatments

Fortunately, depression is usually quite treatable with medication and sometimes with counseling or with both. A number of effective drug treatments for depression are available. These include the more traditional antidepressants as well as the more recently developed SSRIs (see Chapter 13). Keep in mind that it may take some time for these medicines to reach an effective level, and you may not see an improvement for some weeks. These medicines need to be appropriately monitored, including for side effects.

There are also various medications that can be used to help deal with anxiety problems. These include the minor tranquilizers, the SSRIs, and some of the alpha-adrenergic agonist medications (like clonidine). These are discussed in Chapter 13. Careful monitoring is again important. Side effects can include a kind of behavioral disinhibition—that is the child becomes *more* agitated, not less.

For children with mood swings, various medications are available. These are often referred to as mood stabilizers. The dose of these medications can often be monitored and adjusted based on drug levels in the blood.

Summary

In this chapter, we've described some of the more common behavior problems that children with autism spectrum disorders exhibit. Again, we emphasize that many children with autism do *not* have these problems. Sometimes problems come up at certain times in life or in certain situations (the start of a new school, adolescence) and sometimes they go away on their own. It is important to realize that behavioral interventions can be very effective. Medications also have a role in managing behavior problems, but they don't magically take away the child's autism. (See Chapter 13.) Thinking about interventions requires a careful look at the entire situation, including the child's environment and a detailed analysis of when, where, and why the behaviors seem to be occurring.

Questions

Q. **We have a child with autism who engages in severe self-injury. We want to find a specialist who can work with us and the school. What kind of doctor are we looking for?**

Various specialists might be helpful. These include adult and child psychiatrists, adult and child neurologists, psychologists, and developmental and behavioral pediatricians. You should look for someone who has experience in dealing with self-injury. Your primary care doctor may be able to give you names of people. Other good sources of information include school staff and other parents.

Q. **Our adolescent son has developed some significant behavior problems. Our doctor recommended a consultation with a child psychiatrist around medications. Our insurance company has a long list of people who they say are psychiatrists but when we call them they either don't see children, won't see our son, or—in the case of one person who turned out to be a social worker—they weren't even able to prescribe medications!**

This is unfortunately a common problem. Insurance companies often seem to play shell games with long lists of consultants who they claim are available but actually aren't. Sometimes the ones who are available are not very good. Unfortunately, often the doctors who end up on these lists who actually *see* people (as opposed to just being listed) are under tremendous time pressure and will only be able, at best, to spend a short time with you and your child.

Complain directly to the insurance company and see if they will cover an "out of network" consultation. If they give you any grief at all, complain at the state level about your coverage (to the department that monitors insurance in your state). If the insurance comes through your employer, feel free to complain to them as well. If there are really only going to be limited number of visits, think about paying out of pocket to see a qualified psychiatrist who is not on the insurance company's list if you need to—it may be worth it in the end.

Q. **My child has recently started slapping the side of his jaw. He has never done this before and only slaps one spot. What should I do?**

You might want to see your doctor and your dentist—to check his ears and his teeth. The new onset of self-injurious behavior should usually prompt a doctor visit, particularly in a child who is not able to communicate well with words.

Q. My four-year-old has been head banging a lot. I notice that it gets worse when he wants something that I won't give him or when he wants something and we can't understand what it is. (He only has a few words.) He always checks to be sure I'm watching when he starts head banging. The speech-language pathologist wants us to use PECS (Picture Exchange Communication System) but we worry that if we do, he won't use the words he has. What should we do?

Head banging can be a difficult problem to deal with. However, your question gives us several important bits of information. First, your son's head banging seems to have a communication function (he does it when frustrated around not communicating). And second, it clearly seems to be socially related (he checks you out to be sure you're getting his message). You should tackle both fronts. We agree with the SLP: use PECS or whatever it takes to help increase his communication ability. Do *not* worry that this will delay his spoken language. The thinking now is that anything we can do to make a child more communicative will only increase the likelihood that he will acquire more language.

Talk with your school psychologist or behavioral specialist as well. If you start to make a point of ignoring the head banging while simultaneously making a big point of attending to his bids for appropriate communication (including through pictures), the head banging may disappear. We have seen parents who were able to extinguish head banging over the space of an hour. Of course, if your child is obviously injuring himself, you cannot ignore him. There are also some medical problems to consider if head banging starts abruptly (ears and teeth should be checked), but in this case we guess your child will respond positively.

Q. My eight-year-old daughter has a thing about doors. She loves to open and close them. In the past, she liked to turn light switches off and on, but the doors have now replaced this interest. I know it doesn't sound like a big problem, but it drives us a little crazy!

The problems in social development and communication in children with autism also result in major problems in play. The kind of behaviors you describe (repeated doing and undoing) occur in very young, typically developing children who enjoy opening and closing, stacking and knocking down. For many children with autism, these interests become entwined with what Kanner called insistence on sameness—that is the child fixates on one thing.

There are several things you can try. First, see if your daughter can be interested in simple play materials that have doors or light switches (little doll houses, or even make her a special board with a door in it). Look in a toy store for simple cause-and-effect toys and see whether she might be interested in these. If this doesn't work, talk with your behavioral consultant about behavioral approaches you could try. These options include helping her localize her interest in doors—for example, by using five minutes of door opening as a reward after a good lesson. The idea is to get some control over the behavior (in either time or location or both) and go from there. You might also have her be in charge of the doors at home or school. That is, she is the official door opener and closer, but only opens the door when someone knocks.

Q. My twelve-year-old with Asperger's disorder is starting to hit other kids. As far as we can tell from talking with him, he is hitting kids when he thinks they make fun of him. But the teacher says that she thinks the other kids really aren't teasing him—rather, our son mishears something that is said and then gets upset.

Children with Asperger's often have a problem with hearing only *part* of what is said. Putting together the "big picture" of social interaction can be difficult for them. So, it is not unusual that they have trouble understanding humor, sarcasm, irony, and so forth.

The approach to this problem is through several routes. First, talk with your son's speech-language pathologist. She may be able to help him work on understanding some of the situations that have led to trouble and can then coach him on understanding what was keeping him from getting the whole picture. Use of videotapes, Carol Gray's Social Stories, and other explicit forms of teaching can be helpful. In general, the goal should be to help your son observe all the relevant bits of information and then put them together. Explicit teaching is critical here. Another part of the solution is to help your child understand and use strategies for correcting incorrect perceptions (asking for clarification, asking the other child to say it again or in a different way). Finally, it is important to teach your son strategies to use instead of hitting and to teach about his own feelings (the various ways it feels when he is mad and what he can do *other* than hitting).

Q. My six-year-old son used to have a real problem with spinning things or sometimes flicking things back and forth in front of his eyes. This had largely disappeared until this year, when he started kindergarten. He is in an inclusive setting part of the day. It only seems to come up in the mainstream setting, but the teacher says the other kids really notice it.

It is always helpful to ask yourself why a behavior like this might be coming up. For instance, it is possible that your child is overstimulated visually in the mainstream classroom and, as a result, is going back to some older behaviors which help him feel more in control. Visit the classroom and take a look at what is going on. Reducing the amount of time in the inclusive class might help, as might reducing sensory stimulation, as discussed in Chapter 11.

13 | Medications for Challenging Behaviors

Unfortunately, at the present time, there is no medication that can cure a child of autism. However, as we discussed in the preceding chapter, medications are playing a growing and promising role in treating some of the behaviors that often go along with autism. For some children, drugs can significantly help with difficulties with anxiety, moodiness or irritability, attention, stereotyped behaviors, or other emotional or behavioral problems. Decreasing these problem behaviors can often help children be more amenable to educational and other interventions.

When to Use a Medication

In Chapter 12, we discussed the various kinds of behavioral and emotional difficulties common in children with autism and related conditions and briefly mentioned some of the medicines sometimes used in treatment.

In thinking about whether to try medication to help your child, there are several things you should consider:

- Are there alternatives to medication and have these been given a (good) try?
- Are there any physical problems or changes in your child's life that may have contributed to the problem?
- How serious is the problem—for example, does it jeopardize your child's education, or does it put him or others at risk?
- Is it possible that addressing the problem may improve your child's feelings or adjustment to his intervention program?
- When did the behavior/problem start? How long does it last? How severe is it?
- What makes it worse (or better)? Does it happen in some places and not others?
- Is this a longstanding problem or worsening of a longstanding problem or is it really a new problem? Is the problem getting better or worse?
- Is the problem getting better or worse? How is it changing over time?

As we have discussed in Chapter 12, a careful behavioral assessment may be very worthwhile. There is no reason that medications can't be used with behavioral interventions (in some ways these often work quite well together). *But* keep in mind that once you start doing multiple things it gets more and more difficult to understand *why* someone might get better.

Depending on the specifics of the situation, it may make the most sense to try behavioral interventions first and then move to medications if these are not successful or only partly successful. Exceptions would be for problems that are more serious, such as those that pose some risk of serious physical injury to the child or others. For example, an adolescent girl who engages in dangerous self-injurious behavior might well be appropriately treated with medication even to the point of slight sedation. In weighing the risks and benefits of the medication, the risks of slight sedation might well be worth the benefit of preventing serious self-injury. On the other hand, drug interventions may be less effective than behavioral ones for infrequent behaviors that are much less intense and that seem to come up only in certain places or at certain times.

Often children with autism spectrum disorders have more than one emotional or behavioral problem. In such cases, it is sometimes possible to choose a medication that may target both problems. For example, some of the medications we'll talk about can target anxiety and compulsive behaviors.

It's important to realize that all drugs have potential side effects, and, in general, drugs should not be the first thing you try in treating behavior problems. When medications are used, they are usually best combined with behavioral and educational approaches to produce more lasting benefit. The use of medications always requires a careful balancing act between risk and benefit and a consideration of all the causes of behavioral difficulties.

The variety of medications used to treat children with autism and related conditions is growing. Some medications have been used more frequently and have been carefully studied in a scientific way so we know a fair amount about them. For other medications, the information available is based on a small number of children treated with the medication, children treated "non-blind," or single case reports. In the following discussion, it's important to realize that knowledge is constantly increasing, that we are providing you with some general information, and that, in considering medications, it will always be important to review your child's specific needs with his physician.

Ruling Out Pain as a Cause

Sometimes behavioral troubles arise because a child is in pain. This is most common in children with limited communication skills. For example, a child who previously had not had self-injurious behavior might one day start to hit the side of his head. Before beginning medications to control his self-injurious behavior, it would be important for his physician to look in his ears and mouth to be sure that an ear infection, sore throat, or some other medical problem has not triggered the self-injury. See Chapter 4 for more information about determining whether your child is in pain.

Medication Fads and Off Label Uses

Often when a new medicine is first proposed for autism there is great enthusiasm for it. Usually, early reports make it appear to be helpful in many, if not most, cases with few, if any, side effects. An example of such a medication was fenfluramine, which initially, according to a few case reports, seemed to produce significant and dramatic improvements in children with autism. Unfortunately, this turned out not to be the case over time. In general, it is better not to jump on the bandwagon when a new drug treatment first receives attention, but instead use medications that have a proven track record in autism.

Once a medication has been approved for a specific use (or what is called the "indication") by the Food and Drug Administration (FDA), it is available for doctors to prescribe. After the FDA has approved the drug for one use, doctors are free to prescribe it for other uses. This is called "unlabeled use" or "off label use," since it is used for a condition that doesn't show up on the official FDA approved label. Usually the data that support unlabeled use of medication come from case reports and uncontrolled studies (see Chapter 12). Eventually, the FDA (www.fda.gov) may approve the medicine for the new use.

Unfortunately, there has not been much of a financial incentive for drug companies to develop new medicines for autism. Furthermore, until recently, there has been little interest on the part of drug companies in supporting research work for any children. As a result, many of the drugs commonly given to children with autism for behavioral and emotional problems may not have been specifically studied or officially approved by the FDA for use in children with autism (or in any children, for that matter). The end result is that most of the medicines now used to treat autism were developed for other purposes. For example, they may have been developed for another condition such as schizophrenia in adults but then have been observed to work on some symptom in autism. Your doctor may discuss the complexities of all this with you, but you should realize that "off label" use of medications is quite common—really the rule, rather than the exception.

Many medicines have several names, which can be confusing for parents and teachers. The *generic* name of a medicine is usually some form or variation of the chemical name of the medication. The *trade name* (also called the *proprietary name)* is the brand of medication—that is, the name given to it by a specific drug company. The generic name is not capitalized, while the trade name usually is capitalized and often has a ® superscript after it. When a medicine is first developed, it is typically only available under the trade name of the drug company that developed it. As time goes on, the patents on a new drug expires, and then other companies are able to produce it under their own trade names or as a generic drug. This can mean that several different names can refer to exactly the same medicine. These brand name variations and generic versions of the drug are the same medicine and should work just as effectively as the original brand name medicine.

In this chapter, we will be talking about *some* of the medicines more frequently used in treating challenging behaviors in individuals with autism spectrum disorders. A discussion of *all* the medicines would fill this book (and has filled several others listed in the Reading List). Keep in mind that your healthcare provider may want to recommend a drug that we don't discuss here, and that can be just fine. As we've mentioned repeatedly, there is no substitute for working with an experienced healthcare provider.

Research on Medications

Double-blind, Placebo Controlled Studies:
(These are studies of groups of individuals done with careful attention to scientific controls, such as randomly dividing individuals into groups. One group (the control group) might receive a placebo or "sugar pill," while the other group might receive the active medication. Neither the child, parents, nor doctor giving the medicine necessarily know what group the child is in, hence the term "double blind.")

- The data that are collected can be analyzed free from the potential bias that goes with an uncontrolled study.
- In the variation on this method called the crossover design, children might be treated with a placebo for some weeks and then started on the active medicine or vice versa, giving all participants the opportunity to try the treatment being studied.
- Limitations: Although controlled studies are the most effective ways for giving us good information, they are the most costly to do.

Open Label Studies:
(In these studies, the treatment is administered to many people and everyone involved knows what medication is being studied—hence the term "open label")

- Groups of individuals are studied (more powerful than studying just a few people).
- May provide information about who does and doesn't respond and what the side effects are.
- Limited by the fact that the study is open (or technically what is termed "nonblinded") so things like the placebo effect can cloud the results.

Case Reports:
(These are written accounts of individual patients' responses to a treatment; sometimes results are collected and reported with objective, scientific rigor, but sometimes the report may be more casual or even biased, whether intentionally or unintentionally.)

- Often provide the first clues that a drug may be effective for a problem.
- Limited by
  a. concerns about whether the children studied actually had the disorder (e.g., autism) to begin with,
  b. the possibility that lack of good controls and the "placebo effect" may make the medicine look more effective,
  c. the possibility that gains made may not last.

What Is the Placebo Effect?

The placebo effect refers to the many important benefits and effects of merely being involved in research, whether or not the child is receiving the treatment being studied or a placebo (inactive medication). These effects can all can make a major change (for the better) in the child.

Why do children get better on placebo?

- Research involves high levels of clinician, parent, and teacher involvement.
- Every effort is made to provide high quality care during a study.
- Symptoms change over time (often people try something new—such as volunteering for a research study—when things are at their worst and the only way for things to change is to get better).
- More attention and interest may benefit the child.
- The effects of expecting a change for the better can be very important (they can, for example, change how a parent or teacher observes and interacts with the child).

Developing a Treatment Plan

If you plan to pursue drug treatment for your child's behavioral or emotional problems, you should work with a physician or other healthcare provider who is reasonably knowledgeable about the use of these medicines (and their side effects). This doctor (who may be a psychiatrist or child psychiatrist or sometimes a pediatrician or neurologist) will want to meet with you and your child. During this meeting, the doctor will take a history of the problem as well as a more general history of your child. This will typically include your child's birth and developmental history, results of any previous evaluations, your child's medical history, previous drugs used (if any), and your child's response. The doctor will also ask you in detail about the problem you want help with. Your family history may also be important, because conditions such as depression and other mood disorders can run in families. Any history of unusual responses to medication, drug allergies, and similar information will also be reviewed. The doctor will want to spend some time with your child and may want to either see your child in his classroom or talk with school staff (obviously, with your permission).

The doctor will tell you about the pros and cons of various options and develop a treatment plan. Depending on the kinds of medicines that are being discussed, some baseline lab tests (for example, of the blood or urine) might be obtained. Before beginning some medicines, the doctor might want your child to have an electrocardiogram (EKG). For other medicines, periodic blood tests might be needed to monitor the level of the medication or to look for possible side effects.

If the doctor prescribes medication for your child, she should tell you:

- the name or names of the medication,
- what the expected benefit is,
- what the possible side effects and risks are,

- how the medicine is monitored and the dose is adjusted,
- when you should see a change, and what to do when you see a change.

To the extent possible and appropriate your child should be involved in discussing the medicine and the development of a treatment plan.

As part of weighing the pros and cons of the various medicines, the doctor will want to help you understand the potential risks and benefits of medications. The doctor may ask you to sign something to document, for the record, what you have actually discussed. With your permission, the doctor may share this documentation with your child's primary physician so that there is a record of her having discussed the potential benefits and problems of the medicine with you. If appropriate, your child (particularly if an adolescent or young adult) should be involved in this discussion.

Your child's primary care physician should be kept carefully informed about your child's medication(s), if she is not the one prescribing them. This is important because she is likely the healthcare provider who knows your child's medical history best. In some cases, you may see a specialist some distance away for a consultation but your local doctor may be willing to prescribe the medications as long as the specialist is available for back up. Depending on the nature of your child's problems and other aspects of the situation, it may also be advisable to inform school staff such as the classroom teacher and school nurse that your child is receiving medicine. This is mandatory if your child is to receive medicines during the day at school. Schools may have their own requirements about documenting medicine, and the staff may be helpful in documenting how well the medicine is working and in observing side effects.

Understanding Potential Side Effects

All drugs have at least some potential side effects. This is true for medications as simple as aspirin! Sometimes side effects are related to dose and are more likely at higher doses. Other times, side effects may occur regardless of the dose, as is the case with true allergies to medications. Side effects vary from medicine to medicine. In the discussion of medicines later in this chapter, we mention some of the main side effects seen with different groups of medicines. Your child may not have any of these side effects. On the other hand, your child may have some side effects we don't list. Sometimes side effects are seen right away; other times they can take a while to develop. Some side effects might be seen early on but then tend to go away.

All of this means that when you discuss medicine for behavioral or emotional problems with the doctor, you should be sure to get a good sense of the more common possible side effects, as well as the rare but more worrisome side effects. You also should learn what to look for so that you can recognize side effects if they are present. Based on the side effects you report to the doctor, she may want to change the dose, switch to a new medicine, or even add a medicine that will help with the side effects or further strengthen a positive response.

Do's and Don'ts for Parents

Parents play an integral role in working with the doctor to ensure their child is benefiting from medication and receiving the optimal dose. Here are some do's and don'ts to pay attention to, whenever your child starts taking a new medication.

DO:
- Have a detailed discussion with the doctor prescribing the medication about exactly what you can expect: the possible benefits and risks, how long it might take to see results, how the doctor will monitor the medicine, how often you will see the doctor.
- Ask why the doctor favors one medicine over another and what form the medicine is in (pills, capsule, liquid).
- Make sure you understand when to administer the medication and what to do if your child misses a dose.
- Ask if there are reasons to call the doctor right away and how you can get hold of her if there is an emergency.
- Ask how you can help determine whether the medication is helping your child. Is there specific information you (or the school) can collect? What kind of data should you keep and how often should you record it? How can you best record this information and get it to the doctor?
- Be sure your child's primary healthcare provider is "in the loop" and knows why the medicine is being prescribed and what the side effects might be.
- Ask your primary care provider if you need any blood tests or other medical tests before you start the medication. Remember, your child may be much more comfortable having blood taken in a familiar office than a strange place.
- Use the same pharmacy for all of your child's prescriptions. The pharmacist can help you monitor all the medicines your child is taking and may also be able to think about ways to make the medicine more palatable to your child (see page 69).
- Let the doctor and pharmacist know if your child is taking vitamin supplements, herbal treatments, or any other nonprescription remedies that could affect the way medication works.
- Be a careful observer of your child; often you'll notice changes before other people do.

DON'T:
- Pretend to be a doctor (it takes years to complete medical school!).
- Stop the medication without asking the doctor first. Some medicines must be slowly discontinued (tapered) and not stopped abruptly.
- Give up too quickly. Some medicines can take weeks or months to work.
- Stop behavioral or educational interventions when you begin a new medication.
- Try to do a lot of new things at the same time you are beginning a medicine. This complicates figuring out what accounts for any improvement.

Medications Used in Autism and Related Conditions

The following sections provide some basic information on the major classes or groups of medication sometimes used in treating the behavioral difficulties of children with autism and other pervasive developmental disorders. In each section, there is a short description of what we know about how the medication works and what it seems most useful for. The more common side effects of the medications are discussed and we give some examples of medications in this group. Please remember that this is a selective and not an exhaustive list of medications. Also keep in mind that we provide only a short description of potential side effects. If you are considering a trial of medication, you need to have a detailed discussion of the potential benefits and risks **as they apply to your child.** That is, the discussion should take into account all the information relevant to your child such as her medical history, family history, previous response to medications, and so forth.

The Reading List provides some references to fairly detailed books on medications written for parents. You may want to look at these. Some excellent medical books (written specifically for medical professionals) are also available, and some of these are included in the Reading List as well.

With a few notable exceptions (discussed below), most of the information available to us on medications for treating behavior problems is, unfortunately, rather limited. Mostly we are relying on case reports and studies of series of cases rather than on well-controlled, double blind studies. Fortunately, more research is now being done on these medicines and new knowledge will be coming out at an increasingly rapid pace. Although the information we provide here is up-to-date at the time of our writing, keep in mind that new studies are always being done and information may change—another reason to work with a professional who keeps up with new developments!

Neuroleptics (Major Tranquilizers)

Medications most often prescribed to treat behavior problems in autism are called neuroleptics or "major tranquilizers." These medicines were some of the first medicines developed specifically for psychiatry, and, as a result, there is more research on them than on other classes of drugs. (Some newer "second generation" medicines in this group have been developed in recent years and lack some of the side effects of the older medicines in this group. See below.)

These medicines are often used when children have significant problems with self-injury, stereotyped behaviors, agitation, and irritability. They are sometimes used for children with high levels of activity or behavioral rigidity.

The neuroleptics seem to have a major effect on the brain systems which contain dopamine, one of the messengers (neurotransmitters) between nerve cells. All these medications act in some way to block the effects of dopamine in the brain. They also have effects on other chemical systems in the brain. These various effects account for both the desired—or positive—effects, as well as the side effects (negative effects) of medication. The brain chemical dopamine appears to be involved in some way in certain behavior problems in autism—for example, the self-injurious and stereotyped or purposeless repetitive movements. Sometimes low doses of major tranquilizers effectively increase the attention span of children with autism and help them to learn more effectively. This is the opposite of how the stimulant medications used to improve attention in typical children with AD/HD work—that is (in simplified terms), children with AD/HD generally benefit from drugs that increase, rather than decrease, the amount of dopamine.

Usually the dose is started at a very low level and gradually increased. The effects of the medicine are relatively rapid. Occasionally a higher dose may be used to start. This is mostly done in emergency situations.

We'll start our discussion with the newer of these medications (the ones most commonly used today) before we discuss some of the older medications in this group.

Second Generation ("Atypical") Neuroleptics

The atypical neuroleptics are a relatively new group of medicines which have attracted much attention because of their much reduced risk of tardive dyskinesia (a side effect that can occur with the first generation drugs, discussed below). These medicines also seem to be more effective in helping with the social withdrawal and lack of motivation in adults with schizophrenia (which may or may not have much to do with the social problems in autism). Additionally, these medicines seem to help with agitation, temper tantrums, aggressiveness, self-injury, high activity levels, and impulsivity—the same problems that the older "first generation" neuroleptics were used for. One large, double-blind, placebo-controlled study of these medications has shown them to be effective in children with autism.

The atypical neuroleptics are largely replacing the older, "first generation" medications, in part because of the lower risk of serious side effects. Still, there are a variety of side effects, which can include sedation, movement problems, weight gain (with the possible exception of ziprazodone), changes in the electrocardiogram, and, possibly, diabetes.

Table 13-1 | Selected "Second Generation" (Atypical) Neuroleptics

Generic Name	Brand Name	Typical Range of Dose
Risperidone	Risperdal®	0.25 to 5 mg per day
Quetiapine	Seroquel®	50 to 300 mg per day
Olanzapine	Zyprexa®	8 to 20 mg per day
Ziprasidone	Geodon®	10 to 100 mg per day

Note: Dose ranges are approximate; other medications are available in this category.

One of the first drugs in this group, clozapine, has had some major side effects (including reducing the white blood count). Consequently, it is not used as frequently as the others and has not been as intensively studied in autism.

Another of these medicines, risperidone, has been very well studied and is now probably the most commonly used drug in the treatment of children with autism. A very large study on risperidone was recently completed in a large sample of children with autism as part of the Research Units on Pediatric Psychopharmacology Autism Network. In this study, children with autism and significant behavior problems were randomly assigned to an eight-week double-blind trial of either risperidone or placebo. The children in the risperidone group had a very large and significant reduction in irritability and were more likely to be rated as much or very much improved (all ratings were by clinicians who did not know whether the child was on the active medicine or placebo). There were some minor side effects of risperidone (fatigue, drooling, drowsiness), most of which passed quickly. The major side effect was weight gain (2.7 kg or almost 6 pounds).

In a second part of the study, children were followed over time in an open label study (that is, there was no longer any attempt to keep up the double blind part of the study). Children who responded well to risperidone continued to do so at a relatively low dose level (average dose of about 1.5 mg per day). After some months, children were then randomly assigned to a discontinuation trial (with some receiving the active medicine, others the placebo). Some children who had been on the active medicine were able to be tapered off the medicine successfully; others had the return of behavioral difficulties. The response to risperidone in this study was larger than the response to the first generation neuroleptics in older studies. Also, there were many fewer side effects, with weight gain emerging as one of the more common ones. It is worth noting that sometimes this weight gain can be substantial and it may not be easy or possible for a child to lose the extra weight even after the medicine is stopped.

There have been studies of other atypical neuroleptics as well, although they have not yet been quite as well studied as risperidone. In particular, olanzapine has showed some potential to reduce irritability, aggressiveness, overactivity, and obsessiveness in open drug trials. As was found in the RUPP study of risperidone, weight gain can be a significant problem. This weight gain is not always reversible. Some parents don't mind it (particularly if their child is on the thin side). However, substantial weight gain can be a problem for many children with autism who don't get enough exercise anyway.

First Generation Neuroleptics

Because these medicines have been around longer, they are sometimes called the first generation neuroleptics. These medicines are often used for treatment of severe behavioral difficulties such as aggression and self-injury, as well as agitation and stereotyped movements. Some of these medicines have been studied in controlled, double-blind trials in autism—usually over a period of several months. Improvements have been documented in such areas as agitation, withdrawal, and self-stimulatory movement. Many children respond well to these medicines.

In general, children should be prescribed the lowest possible dose of these medications, as some of the side effects occur more often at higher doses. (See the section on "Side Effects," below.) These medications are more likely to make the child feel drowsy or sleepy (with some causing more sedation than others). Sometimes sedation is mistakenly viewed as a positive response. That is, the child is no longer making much trouble. However, the child may also not be doing much learning!

There are a number of medicines in this group. Haloperidol (Haldol®) is one of the more potent members of this group and has been studied extensively in children with autism. It can be very effective in reducing high levels of activity, agitation, and stereotyped or self-injurious behavior. Studies of Haldol have demonstrated that it works quite well in children affected with moderate to severe autism. Significant behavioral improvement occurs at relatively low doses. Side effects are observed but are not usually common at such doses. It is usually started at a low dose and gradually increased. When effective, usually there are periodic attempts to lower the dose of medication. It is important that such drug "holidays" be planned to ensure that children receive only the lowest effective dose of medication. At very low doses, Haldol is not usually very sedating, but at higher doses, it can be.

Another medicine sometimes used in treating children with autism is Thorazine®. Thorazine is a lower potency major tranquilizer—that is, a higher dose needs to be taken to achieve the same effects as would be achieved with a higher potency medication such as Haldol. For example, about 100 mg of Thorazine equal about 1 mg of Haldol in terms of effectiveness. It's important to realize that the differences in potency in this and other groups of medications can make it difficult for anyone other than a professional to evaluate how high or low a dose of medication actually is. Thorazine is much more sedating than Haldol. This can be a benefit for some children. On the other hand, often sedation is a problem, but sometimes this can be avoided by giving a larger dose before bedtime when it may help the child get to sleep.

In between Haldol and Thorazine, there are a number of other medications. These tend to be intermediate in terms of potency and their side effect profile. Some of these medicines come as pills or tablets and some are available in liquid form (be sure to ask about this if your child has trouble taking pills).

Table 13-2 | Selected "First Generation" Neuroleptic Medications

Generic Name	Brand Name	Typical Range of Dose
Haloperidol	Haldol®	0.25 – 8 mg per day*
Thiothixene	Navane®	1 – 20 mg per day
Perphenazine	Trilafon®	2 – 16 mg per day
Trifluoperazine	Stelazine®	1 – 10 mg per day
Chlorpromazine	Thorazine®	25 – 400 mg per day**

Note: dose ranges are approximate, approval for specific ages varies, many other medicines are available in this category. Liquid forms (which may be easier to give and provide a range of dosing options) are also often available. Many similar drugs are available.

*least sedating and most potent but with the most motor side effects
**most sedating and less potent with fewer motor side effects

Side Effects. Side effects of the major tranquilizers include a group of unusual body movements that are made on an involuntary basis—that is, the child has no control over them. These are often referred to as "extra pyramidal symptoms" or EPS (a technical term that refers to the part of the brain that seems to be involved in causing them). These symptoms can include stiffness in arms or legs, shaking of the fingers or hands, restlessness (akathisia), stiffness of the neck, muscle stiffness, and unusual movements of the head and eyes. Often these problems appear in the first weeks or months of treatment. These dyskinesias (disordered movements) can sometimes also be seen when the medicine is discontinued or reduced (withdrawal dyskinesias).

The restlessness and some of the motor movements associated with these medications can be treated with other medications such as Cogentin® or Benadryl®, which can be given along with the major tranquilizer. Some doctors use these additional medicines almost routinely to try to prevent any of the acute movement problems.

Sometimes a movement problem called tardive dyskinesia occurs. This movement problem usually develops after months or even years of treatment, but sometimes more quickly. It takes the form of various involuntary movements of the body, extremities, or neck and may be associated with what appear to be grunts or tics. This condition can be confusing because at times it resembles the kinds of motor mannerisms frequently seen in autism. It is important to note that reducing the dose of medication may seem to make the tardive dyskinesia even worse.

Because tardive dyskinesia is sometimes irreversible, doctors should screen for it very carefully, both when they begin treatment with major tranquilizers and as they follow a child who is treated over time. That way if early signs suggesting tardive dyskinesia are present, the medicine can be stopped. There are specific rating scales that doctors and nurses can use to monitor the unusual movements sometimes associated with these medications.

Occasionally, when a medication is discontinued, withdrawal dyskinesias occur—that is, the child begins to exhibit some unusual movements. These usually persist for only a few weeks, but may be disturbing to parents and children. Adolescents and adults are more likely to have these than young children.

Other side effects sometimes observed in the first generation neuroleptics include true allergic reactions (not just motor side effects), which can cause serious medical problems. (It is important, by the way, for parents not to call other types of side effects "allergies." Sometimes you can inadvertently confuse a doctor by telling her your child had an "allergy" to a medicine when you really mean he had a side effect of some kind, and not a true allergic reaction.)

As a group, these medicines tend to have some of the same side effects as "cold pills" such as dry mouth, constipation, and so forth. Because these drugs are metabolized in the liver, sometimes they can cause problems and blood tests are periodically used to monitor liver, kidney, and other functions. In addition, all the medicines in this group have a slight tendency to increase the likelihood of seizures. Thus, their use should be considered carefully in a child with a seizure disorder. Furthermore, all the medications in this group often cause some degree of weight gain. Finally, individuals taking these medications (especially in high doses) need to be careful not to become too hot. A rare condition (malignant hyperthermia) can occur in children whose temperature increases dramatically. Children on these medications should be encouraged to drink a lot of fluids, particularly in the summer.

Again, it's important to keep in mind that often (but not always) side effects are dose related—that is, they are more likely with higher doses of medicine—but sometimes can be seen even on very low doses of medicine.

Stimulant Medications

Stimulant medications are very widely used in the United States for treatment of attention-deficit/hyperactivity disorder (AD/HD). It appears that these medicines work by increasing levels of a brain messenger chemical called dopamine. (Note that this is the opposite of the way the major tranquilizers work.) They work by helping the child focus, attend, and become less restless. These medicines are very effective in individuals with AD/HD; probably helping about 75 percent of those diagnosed with the disorder.

There are many different types of stimulant medications. They differ from each other in some ways. For instance, some are longer acting than others and some tend to be associated with different side effects. Side effects of these medicines in children with AD/HD include irritability, occasional worsening of attentional problems, sleep problems, and decreased appetite. Occasionally children have problems with dizziness and sometimes seem to become more moody or agitated. Children taking these medications sometimes develop tics (rapid, repetitive movements often involving the head and neck and upper body) or other habit problems (picking their skin), or, more rarely, hallucinations. There are a few side effects specific to some medicines in this group and not others. For instance, pemoline has been associated with liver problems.

Stimulant medications are sometimes used in children with autism spectrum disorders for the same reasons they are used in children with AD/HD—to help increase attention and help the child focus. Stimulant medications are not as frequently used in children with autistic disorder as they are used in children with Asperger's disorder and PDD-NOS.

The use of stimulants in autistic disorder is somewhat controversial at the moment. There are a handful of studies—not particularly strong ones, unfortunately—on both sides of this question. Sometimes children with pretty classic autism get *worse* on stimulants. Usually they become more agitated and engage in more stereotyped behaviors. A common report from parents is something like: "Doc, I thought the behavior was bad before but now it has taken off like a rocket!" However, the occasional child with autistic disorder does respond to stimulants. It is not clear why some children respond and others do not. We do know, though, that the way stimulants work, they sometimes produce stereotyped behaviors in typically developing children. We also know that the way the medicines work is the opposite of the way the major tranquilizers work (and they are the medicines most commonly given to treat just these behaviors in children with autism). On the other hand, the side effects of stimulants are relatively minimal and the medicine is cleared out of the child's system fairly rapidly. Accordingly, it may make sense to consider these medicines for a child who has major difficulties with attention.

In children with Asperger's syndrome and PDD-NOS, stimulants are frequently given and often well tolerated. For these children, the medications help the child focus and be more attentive in class, and teachers as well as parents may notice gains in the child's attention and on-task behavior. However, often there are other problems present that may not respond so well to the stimulant medications. For instance, the child may have difficulties with depression or compulsive routines or rigidities. Then the question of adding a second medicine to deal with those problems may come up (we'll return to this topic toward the end of this chapter).

When stimulant medications do work, they should be monitored over time. Given the medications' potential to decrease appetite, your pediatrician will want to monitor your child's height and weight every four to six months or so. If there are problems with growth and weight gain, you can try lowering the dose, using drug holidays, or switching to a different class of medicine. (Some of the antidepressants and antihypertensive medicines can also be used to treat attention problems.) As your child grows older (and if the medicine is still needed), the dose can be adjusted. It is also important to make sure your child still really needs the medication by occasionally having drug holidays—weekends, school breaks, or summer vacations where you stop or reduce the medicine, with the doctor's OK.

Table 13-3 | Selected Medications for Treatment of AD/HD

Generic Name	Brand Name	Typical Range of Dose
Methylphenidate	Ritalin®	Regular tablets –15-60 mg/day
	Metadate®	Extended release tablets
	Concerta®	Extended release tablets
Dextroamphetamine	Dexedrine®	10 to 40 mg/day
Atomoxetine	Strattera®	20 to 80 mg/day
Amphetamine mixture	Adderall®	10 to 40 mg/day
	Adderall XR®	Extended release tablets

Note that dose is adjusted based on child's size and clinical response. Except for Strattera®, the medications listed are stimulants and controlled substances.

Antidepressants and SRIs (Serotonin Reuptake Inhibitors) and Antidepressants

This group of medicines were originally developed for the treatment of depression and/or obsessive compulsive disorders. They seem to be particularly useful for children who either have many depressive symptoms, or, more commonly, for children who have problems with behavioral rigidity and rigid adherence to routines—similar to the problems seen in obsessive compulsive disorder.

The older medications in this group are the traditional antidepressants, which work on various brain chemical systems. The newer medications are the serotonin reuptake inhibiters (SRIs) and the *selective* serotonin reuptake inhibiters (SSRIs), which work by more specifically acting on the neurotransmitter serotonin. They prevent (inhibit) the re-absorption (reuptake) of serotonin after it is produced in the brain, thereby increasing the level of serotonin in the brain. The SSRIs are quite selective in how they act on serotonin—that is, they have little, if any, effect on other brain chemical systems such as norepineph-rine and dopamine. There is also one medicine in the group (clomipramine) that is less selective but still a potent reuptake inhibitor of serotonin (so is technically a SRI rather than an SSRI). Because the SSRIs are used more frequently, we'll discuss them first.

SSRIs

The SSRIs have attracted much interest for autism and autism spectrum conditions, because these medicines seem to be useful in treating the prominent behavioral rigidity, ritualistic behaviors, and rituals commonly seen. A number of studies, not always well con-trolled, have looked at how well the SSRIs work in autism. In general, these early studies have been encouraging, with many individuals responding positively, but research is still in the early phases. One complication is that, for reasons we don't understand, there seems to be a lot of variability in how individuals with autism respond. Some children respond well to a lower dose than a slightly higher dose; others to one of these medicines but not to another. It does seem that adolescents and children who are nearing adolescence respond better than younger children. However, these medicines can sometimes help younger children, too.

If your child is prescribed an SSRI, you will need to work fairly closely with a psychiatrist or other healthcare provider. First, because of the variable response in chil-dren with ASDs, the first SSRI you try may not be the most effective one. Second, it takes a relatively long time (weeks) to get the dose to a reasonable level and determine how effective the medication is for your child.

Side effects of these medicines are varied. They can include "activation" (increased irritability, restlessness, insomnia, and elation), which can be quite problematic. This acti-vation often is more likely with a bigger dose of the medication. One of these medicines, clomipramine, seems less likely to cause activation but unfortunately also seems to be less well tolerated by many children. There is also some potential for heart (cardiac) side ef-fects, so it is much less likely to be used than the other medications in this group. Other potential side effects of SSRIs include dry mouth, constipation, sedation, and weight gain.

Antidepressants

There is also an important role for the more traditional antidepressants in children and adolescents with autism who become clinically depressed. These medicines have been around for years. They are very effective in treating the clinical depression that often develops in adolescence for more able teenagers—who often have a growing sense of being different. Children with Asperger's disorder seem particularly vulnerable to this.

The antidepressants work on several brain transmitter systems, including seroto-nin, norepinephrine, and other brain systems. Because they affect multiple systems, they have the potential for causing various side effects. Some newer antidepressants, includ-ing Effexor® and Wellbutrin®, have different mechanisms of action, and therefore may have advantages in some instances.

Table 13-4 | Selected Antidepressants and SSRI Medications

Generic Name	Brand Name	Typical Range of Dose
Imipramine	Tofranil®	10-250 mg per day [1]
Desipramine	Norpramine®	10-250 mg per day [1]
Nortriptyline	Pamelor®	5-150 mg per day [1]
Clomipramine	Anafranil®	25-200 mg per day [1]
Fluoxetine	Prozac® Sarafem®	5-40 mg per day [2]
Citalopram	Celexa®	10-40 mg per day [3]
Fluvoxamine	Luvox®	12.5-200 per day [2]
Paroxetine	Paxil®	10-50 mg per day [2]
Sertraline	Zoloft®	12.5-200 mg per day [2]
Trazodone	Deseryl®	25-600 mg per day [2]
Venlafaxine	Effexor®	150-300 mg per day [3]
Bupropion	Wellbutrin®	150-400 mg per day [3]

Note: dose ranges are approximate, approval for specific ages varies, many other medicines are available in this category. Beneficial effects may take a period of time (weeks) to develop. Liquid forms (which may be easier to give and provide a range of dosing options) are available for some of these medications.

[1] Traditional antidepressants
[2] Selective serotonin reuptake inhibitors
[3] Newer antidepressant/SSRI with different chemical structure than the older medicines

Common side effects of antidepressants include dry mouth, constipation, and a tendency toward urinary retention. Other effects can include higher heart rate and blood pressure. Irritability and agitation can be a problem for some children, and sedation can be a problem for others. The drugs vary somewhat in their potential to cause sedation and agitation. If a bit of sedation is desirable (for a child who has difficulty falling asleep or is agitated), one of the medicines more likely to cause sedation might be used.

When stopping these medications, they should generally be gradually tapered off. This is because some children seem to have a kind of withdrawal reaction to discontinuing antidepressants and may experience nausea and vomiting, abdominal pain, headache, or other reactions to stopping too abruptly.

Because antidepressants can affect the heart rate and rhythm, overdoses of these medicines can be dangerous. Before starting either antidepressants or SSRIs, your child should have a good physical exam and medical history (with a special focus on any heart problems). A routine EKG should be done and your child's baseline heart rate and blood pressure should be determined. Blood levels can be monitored, if appropriate.

Mood Stabilizers

As you would expect from the name, the medications in this group all help to level out or stabilize mood disorders. The classic example of a mood disorder is something called manic-depressive illness or bipolar disorder. Individuals with bipolar disorder have major swings in mood. For instance, they may have periods (weeks to months) of serious depression followed by periods of having a normal mood and then by periods of elation and mania. The adult forms of the mood disorders are more straightforward to diagnose than the forms seen in children. In children, irritability, overactivity, and aggressive behaviors may characterize mood disorders. The up-and-down cycle of mood disorders can be a bit more difficult to see in children.

There has been some speculation that mood disorders may be increased in children and adolescents with PDD. These issues are somewhat controversial, given that, for example, irritability and overactivity are often seen in children with PDD.

In strictly diagnosed autism, the general response to mood stabilizers is not usually positive. However, these medications may be helpful if your child has symptoms suggesting that an additional diagnosis of bipolar disorder is justified—particularly if there is a family history of mood disorders. Children with cyclical patterns of mood problems and irritability, associated with insomnia and overactivity, may also be candidates for mood stabilizers. We have seen a few patients who have responded positively to mood stabilizers. These children had clear evidence of cyclicity in behaviors (swings from good weeks to weeks when the child's behavior was more out of control) and often there was a member of the immediate family who also had a mood disorder.

Medications used to treat mood disorders include lithium and some of the same medicines used to treat seizures (anticonvulsants). The precise way these medicines work is not known. Lithium is probably the best known of the mood stabilizers used with adults, although other anticonvulsants are more frequently used now and are more likely to be used in children.

There are some studies of anticonvulsants for mood problems in children with autism, but these are mostly reports of single or a few cases and tend not to be of the most rigorous quality. More research is clearly needed. Some of the medicines more frequently used to deal with cycles in mood association with overactivity and insomnia include carbamazepine and valproate (valproic acid), and also sometimes lamotrigine. In children with ASDs, problems that have reportedly improved on such mood stabilizers include mood problems, impulsivity, and aggression.

When anticonvulsants are used as mood stabilizers, levels of medicine are monitored through regular blood tests, both to be sure that an effective or therapeutic level of the medicine is reached and also to be sure that the level does not get too high. Typically, a child is put on a medicine for several days before the first blood level is taken. The blood level is usually taken about twelve hours after the last dose (usually first thing in the morning before the child takes the morning medication).

Various medical tests are usually done before starting treatment with mood stabilizers. Depending on the medication, these may include tests of the kidney and thyroid (particularly if lithium has been prescribed), as well as tests of the liver and blood counts for some of the other medicines.

Side effects of mood stabilizers can include sedation, changes in the blood count, and liver toxicity. Lithium can affect thyroid and kidney function, and also lead to a fair amount of weight gain, over time. (Because of concerns about lithium's side effects, it is used less often than some of the other mood stabilizers, but can still be used for children with major mood problems.) Your doctor should discuss all the potential side effects with you.

Table 13-5 | Selected Mood Stabilizers

Generic Name	Brand Name	Typical Range of Dose
Divalproex	Depakote®	Adjusted based on blood level
Valproic Acid	Depakene®	Adjusted based on blood level
Carbamazepine	Tegretol®	Adjusted based on blood level
Oxcarbamazepine	Trileptal®	Adjusted based on blood level
Lithium Compounds	Eskalith® Lithobid® Lithane®	Adjusted based on blood level

All these medicines require careful monitoring for side effects, including changes in the blood count, liver, thyroid, and kidneys.

Medicines to Reduce Anxiety

All of us have experienced anxiety. Anxiety can serve a useful function, such as reminding us of dangerous or risky situations. Sometimes, however, anxiety becomes a problem that needs treatment—for example, if someone is immobilized by chronic anxiety, or has panic attacks or specific fears that make it difficult to function in the day-to-day world.

As discussed in Chapter 12, children with ASDs also can have problems with anxiety. Sometimes this seems similar to the kinds of anxiety that others of us experience in confronting frightening or stressful situations. Other times the anxiety in autism is highly unusual and may be more related to difficulties in dealing with new situations or certain problem situations.

The medicines used in treating anxiety problems for typically developing children, adolescents, and adults can sometimes be successfully used in treating serious anxiety problems in children with autism spectrum conditions. However, as we'll discuss shortly, there has not been much research on using these medicines in autism. In addition, sometimes the same medicines that seem to help the rest of us relax can make children with autism worse—that is, more agitated and disorganized.

Several different groups of medicine can be used to reduce anxiety. Some of them may be familiar to you because you or someone else in your family has used them for anxiety (e.g., Ativan®). Others in this group may be less familiar. We'll discuss each group briefly.

Table 13-6 | Selected Anti-Anxiety Medications

Generic Name	Brand Name	Typical Range of Dose
Benzodiazepines:		
Lorazepam	Ativan®	0.5 to 2 mg per day
Clonazepam	Klonopin®	0.25 to 2 mg per day
Beta Blockers:		
Propranolol	Inderal®	10 to 120 mg per day
Nadolol	Corgard®	20 to 200 mg per day

Note: dose ranges are approximate, approval for specific ages varies, other medicines are also available.

Minor Tranquilizers

The minor tranquilizers are so called to make it clear that they work in a different way than the major tranquilizers (or neuroleptics). The minor tranquilizers have been widely used in adults and typically developing children to help deal with problems in anxiety—for example, before the person goes for dental work. These medicines have not been well studied in children with autism spectrum disorders, but they can be useful for the purposes for which they were intended. The minor tranquilizers include Valium® (diazepam) and Ativan® (lorazepam).

Occasionally children with developmental problems become somewhat more agitated on these medicines (this is called paradoxical agitation). If, for example, your dentist suggests you try one of these medications to help calm your child during a dental procedure, you may want to try a test dose at home first or in the doctor's office when you first arrive. There are some alternatives for sedation when these medicines don't work. For instance, occasional diphenhydramine (Benadryl®) works well. You can also discuss other alternatives with your healthcare provider.

Some individuals build up a tolerance to the minor tranquilizers. However, if these medicines do work for your child, they can be valuable when used on an occasional basis for situations you know will make your child very anxious. They should not be mixed with alcohol, since they each can make the effects of the other stronger. As when trying any new medicine, discuss with your doctor and/or pharmacist the other medicines your child is taking.

Beta Blockers

Another group of medicines called the beta blockers are sometimes used for children with autism and related conditions. These medicines were originally used as blood pressure medicines, but are now also used to deal with anxiety and irritability. There have been some open label studies and case reports of beta blockers in the treatment of anxiety, but good double-blind studies are not available.

These medicines have a number of potential side effects and it is important to weigh the pros and cons seriously before starting them. Side effects can include low blood pressure and problems with heart rate. These medicines can also make asthma worse.

You have to be careful to take the medicine as prescribed and taper it off when your child is through with it; the medicines have to be taken chronically (all the time) to work.

Alpha Adrenergic Agonists

Another group of medicines that were first used to lower blood pressure are sometimes used to treat behavioral problems. These medicines, called alpha adrenergic agonists, work through a different system than the beta blockers and can help in the treatment of tics (unusual, recurrent movements). For some children, they can also improve problems with over activity and inattention. They are sometimes recommended for children with autism, particularly for children who are irritable, hyperactive, and impulsive. Again, the data on using these drugs for autism spectrum disorders are unfortunately pretty limited.

Clonidine (Catapres®) has been used to treat tics as well as attentional problems; it can also be given as a patch and not just as a pill. A similar medicine is guanfacine (Tenex®). Typical doses for Clonidine are in the range of 0.1 to 0.3 mg per day, and for guanfacine they are slightly higher (0.5 to 2 mg per day). The medicines are given in divided doses by mouth (or by patch).

Because these medicines are also used to control blood pressure, side effects can include trouble with low blood pressure (hypotension) and the heart. As a result, your child will need an EKG before starting these medicines. Occasionally children may develop what is called orthostatic hypotension, or low blood pressure when standing up. This can cause dizziness when standing up. In addition, these medications can cause sedation, either at the start or over the long term. If sedation is a problem, the medication can be given mostly at night to help with sleep. It is particularly important that they be given as prescribed and tapered off slowly if they are discontinued. (Blood pressure can rapidly increase if these medicines are stopped too quickly.) Sometimes tolerance to the medicine seems to develop.

Opiate Blockers

There has been some speculation that some of the self-injurious behaviors in autism may be designed to induce the release of opiate-like compounds in the brain. The theory runs like this: Perhaps when individuals hit themselves or engage in other self-injurious behaviors, they generate a kind of natural "high" (similar to a "runner's high") because their bodies are producing a kind of internal opiate (like opium). If so, perhaps the same medicines that are used to block the effects of externally produced opiates (that is, opiate drugs such as heroin) might also serve to undercut this effect and thus eliminate, or reduce, the behavior. Another theory is that individuals with autism have a very high pain threshold and that self-injury is a form of self-stimulation. A small number of studies have raised the possibility that individuals with autism have higher natural levels of endorphins (the opiate-like compounds the body naturally produces). If so, it could be that self-injury is, paradoxically, an attempt by the child to make himself feel better.

Two different drugs that are ordinarily used to help people with opiate drug overdose problems have been used in children with autism spectrum disorders: naloxone

(Narcan®) and naltrexone (Trexan®). Since naloxone has to be given by IV, it is naltrexone which has been more extensively studied in autism. Studies were conducted starting in the late 1980s and continuing through the last ten years. Initial studies tended to be uncontrolled case reports, and, as often is the case early on, initial results were encouraging. Unfortunately, double-blind studies have not shown the same positive picture. Now most of the apparent benefit appears to be in reducing hyperactivity. (Again, this is a reminder of why it is so important to do double blind studies.) There is some suggestion that this group of medicines may cause worsened troubles in children with Rett's disorder. Side effects of these medicines include, notably, nausea and vomiting. At the moment, these medicines do not seem to have major usefulness in children with autism.

Combining Medications

Children with ASDs often end up being given more than one medicine for their emotional or behavioral problems. This practice, referred to as polypharmacy, is a complicated one. Sometimes two medicines are given because one is controlling side effects of the other. Sometimes a second medicine is added after a first one seems to work a bit but not as much as is wanted. Occasionally, taking two medicines together may mean that a lower dose of each can be used. Sometimes one medicine, which acts quicker, may be given while a longer-acting medicine is being introduced. Sometimes the doctor will feel that two conditions are really present and consider using two medications to treat them. (See the box on Co-morbidity on the next page.) These are just some of the possible reasons for giving more than one medicine at a time.

Unfortunately, there are a number of potential problems with taking multiple medicines. One is in sorting out which medicine is doing what, or, put in another way, how can you tell which medicine is being most helpful? In addition, there is always a tradeoff when using more than one medicine. For example, there may be more potential for side effects and more hassle in giving at least two medicines. Furthermore, the potential for drug interaction clearly increases, and it is important that your pharmacist and regular healthcare provider are aware of all the medicines your child is taking. Finally, some combinations of medicine clearly don't work and might be more risky than taking one medicine.

Occasionally, we have seen children with autism on many different medicines at the same time (the record is about ten) with the idea that each medicine is treating a different thing—anxiety, depression, attention, and so forth. In these situations, the child's behavior often deteriorates and it is impossible to figure out why and what to change. In general, with some important and sensible exceptions, it probably makes sense to start with one medicine. One exception, for example, is that many doctors feel that using a low dose of risperidone in addition to an SSRI may increase the effectiveness of both medications.

If your child's doctor discusses adding a second medicine, you should feel like you understand why she is recommending this. If things start to get very complicated and you are giving your child many different medicines, it may be time to step back and think about getting another opinion.

Autism and Co-morbidity

When one person has two or more diagnosed disorders, the disorders are said to be *co-morbid* (which merely means they occur together).

- In the past, many people thought that having a chronic condition such as autism (or any developmental disorder) almost seemed to "protect" the child from other disorders. The technical term for this is "diagnostic overshadowing."
- We now realize that having one disorder (like autism) makes the child more, not less, vulnerable to other troubles.
- There are many issues involved in disentangling the complicated effects of autism on behavior and emotional troubles—that is, in determining whether a difficulty is more part and parcel of having autism or truly a separate, co-morbid disorder.
- Particularly in the U.S., there is a tendency to equate symptoms and disorder. That is, if a child with autism has some troubles with attention, he will often be diagnosed as having AD/HD in addition to autism. However, many children with autism have difficulties with attention, but not necessarily of the type seen in textbook AD/HD.

Summary

Although many gaps remain, our knowledge of drug treatments in autism and related disorders has increased dramatically in recent years. While no medicine has, as yet, been shown to really improve the core difficulties of autism, medicines have been shown to help with some of the very problematic symptoms associated with autism. Medicines can be very effective in dealing with agitation, hyperactivity, anxiety, aggression, depression, and some aspects of obsessions and compulsions.

In thinking about medications for behavioral problems, always weigh the pros (potential benefits) and cons (potential side effects and problems). You should think about drug treatments if problems are quite severe, if they limit your child's opportunities to participate in his educational program or community activities, or if they negatively affect his quality of life (or the quality of your family's life). The medical professionals working with you should take a look at the "big picture" and help you get a good sense of the pros and cons involved. For some medicines, side effects are pretty minimal, and, depending on the situation, you might be more likely to think about using these medicines for a problem that is less severe or interfering. For medicines with more serious side effects, you may want to wait and see if the symptoms become more severe or interfering.

The doctor you work with should be in touch with your child's regular medical care provider, and, potentially, with school staff as well. It can be extremely helpful for school staff to collect data when a new drug (or any intervention) is tried to see whether there is a difference in behavior at school. The doctor you are working with may also want to use some rating scales or checklists as a way of monitoring the medicine (including potential side effects).

One of the exciting, but as yet unrealized possibilities is that in the future, as we discover more about what really causes autism, we may be able to develop much better treatments that target the core difficulties. In the meantime, we now have a number of medicines that can often be helpful.

Reference

Research Units in Pediatric Psychopharmacology (RUPP) (2002). Risperidone in children with autism and serious behavioral problems. *New England Journal of Medicine, 347:* 314-321.

Questions

Q. My three-year-old has just been diagnosed with autism. Does he need medications now to help with his behavior? Will he ever need medications?

In general, we try not to give medications to very young children because behavioral interventions have more potential payoffs and fewer side effects. By the time children are entering school (and sometimes sooner) medications can help deal with specific symptoms and problem behaviors—but they still don't substitute for a good behavioral and educational program. In terms of whether your son will *ever* need medications, it is hard to know. Many children do not, others do. The reasons why children would need medications vary a lot. Part of what you should consider as well is how disruptive the behavior is for you and your other children. Some parents are willing to try medications that may help with certain behaviors, whereas other parents feel that they or their child can learn to live with the behaviors.

Q. My twelve-year-old daughter has PDD-NOS and horrible problems dealing with new situations—to the point that she gets almost paralyzed. Are there any medications that might help?

There are several medicines that might help. Some of the SSRIs, and, for that matter, other antidepressant medications, have an effect on anxiety. These might be a bit more likely to help if the issues had to do with rigidity and a desire for order and compulsiveness. If the problem is a more general one with anxiety, there are other medicines that might help, including minor tranquilizers (Ativan®) and beta blockers (such as Inderal®).

Q. Our eight-year-old son has fragile X syndrome and autism. I've been told that children with fragile X syndrome always need stimulant medications to help them focus. Is this true?

Many, but not all, children with fragile X syndrome have attentional problems, so a decision on medication needs to be made relative to your child in particular. The problems which stimulants can help with include attentional problems and impulsivity. Occasionally stimulants make children a bit more irritable and may affect sleep. Also, stimulants sometimes decrease the appetite. This can be more of a problem for younger children who have not stopped growing, although the impact is usually very small. As with all medications, you need to balance the benefits and risk.

Q. Our eight-year-old son has had many behavioral difficulties over the years. He has had many different diagnostic labels and recently has been on a number of different medicines for his behavior. His behavior has deteriorated dramatically. He is now on five different medicines and it seems like we are juggling them all the time. We are at our wit's end. What can we do?

Think about admitting your child to a hospital (pediatric or child psychiatry service) where the diagnostic and medication issues can be carefully evaluated. One of the problems of using many different medicines is that it gets hard to figure out what medicine is doing what.

Q. We have a fifteen-year-old with Asperger's syndrome. He has done pretty well on an SSRI, but now our doctor wants to add a small dose of something he called an "atypical neuroleptic" because our son has gotten more irritable. Does this make sense?

Of all the various medication combinations that people use, this is one of the more common. Often children respond well to an SSRI initially, but as time goes on they seem to have a bit more trouble. Sometimes changing the dose of the medicine can help. Sometimes switching to a different SSRI may do the trick. Other times, particularly when new symptoms such as irritability arise, the doctor may think about adding one of the newer atypical neuroleptics such as risperidone. These seem to be safer than the older neuroleptics (such as Thorazine®) and have, in general, fewer side effects. They usually are used in a very *low* dose. It is possible that in addition to their effect on the behavior, they also may augment, or increase, the effect of the SSRI. That is, the SSRI may work even better.

Q. My son with Asperger's disorder has had a lot of trouble with anxiety. He was started on a new medicine that seemed to help but then he complained that his heart was racing. I talked to our doctor and we arranged for a visit with a local cardiologist. However, when we arrived for the appointment, it turned out the cardiologist was not participating with our insurance plan and I had to pay out of pocket. Is there a way to prevent this kind of thing?

It sounds like you and your doctor did many of the right things. The step that appears to have been left out was checking that the cardiologist was participating in your insurance plan. (Either you or your doctor's office could have asked—had they made the appointment—or the cardiologist's office could have asked.) It pays to investigate things ahead of time, and, probably even more importantly, it really pays to think about the kind of insurance policy you have. Often people don't have great choices of plans, but when you do, plans that allow you to pick specialists will give you the greatest range of choices. When you are looking at plans with selected panels of doctors, you should be sure that the list is up to date and also ask your doctor and your child's doctor about the reputations of the people listed. (See Appendix B for information about insurance.)

14 | Adolescence and Sexuality

Adolescence brings many changes for child and parent alike. Sexual maturation takes place as well as physical growth and many emotional and developmental changes. This can be a difficult time for both children and parents—even for children who are developing typically. It can be even more difficult for children who have sexual feelings but whose social and communication problems make it hard for them to talk about these feelings. For the highest functioning adolescents with autism or Asperger's disorder, relationships may be complicated by their difficulties making connections with peers or their feelings of rejection if others rebuff their attempts at friendship.

In this chapter, we discuss what you can expect during adolescence and how you may be able to make things go more smoothly. We start with a discussion of the facts about adolescence and puberty and then move on to talking about sexuality and coping with some problem behaviors. Keep in mind that, as always, we are talking about adolescence in general and that your primary healthcare provider as well as school staff and others can be good sources of information on your child's specific situation.

Adolescence: Basic Facts

Although most of us tend to think of adolescence as a time of turmoil, research has shown that this is not always so for typically developing children—indeed, it probably isn't even usually so. It is also true that some children with autism spectrum disorders go through adolescence fairly smoothly. Still, puberty (which marks the beginning of adolescence) involves a set of dramatic changes in a child's body, which can pose problems for any child. An increasingly adult body is also associated with a new set of societal expectations—which can be especially difficult for individuals with autism to grasp. What is acceptable and cute in a four-year-old may not be so easily accepted in a fourteen-year-old.

Puberty

Puberty is usually seen as marking the transition into adolescence. Children enter puberty when they begin the final process of sexual (reproductive) maturation. The overt physical changes of puberty are the result of complicated processes that really start before birth. Hormone systems, which previously had been relatively inactive, become much more active, resulting in dramatic changes in growth and in the body. In fact, the bodily changes of puberty are really only surpassed by those of infancy.

The bodily changes of puberty usually emerge over a period of about four years or so. Girls, on average, mature about two years earlier than boys. As levels of hormones start to increase, changes in both body size and what are called the "secondary sex characteristics" (increases in body and facial hair, in the voice, and in the breast and genital organs) become marked. In fact, the hormonal changes that trigger puberty start some years before the observable body changes. Various stages of puberty have been defined (see Table 14-1) in both boys and girls and serve as a rough guide to where in puberty an individual child is.

Table 14-1 | Stages of Puberty (Tanner)

Stage	Boys	Girls
Stage 1	preadolescent	preadolescent
Stage 2	slight amount of pubic hair, slight enlargement of penis and scrotum	sparse pubic hair, breasts begin to develop
Stage 3	increased pubic hair, penis longer, testes bigger	increased pubic hair, breasts enlarged
Stage 4	pubic hair pattern resembles adult pattern, but still sparser than in adult	abundant pubic hair (less than in adult), nipple becomes more prominent
Stage 5	adult male distribution of pubic hair, adult size testes and penis	adult female pattern of pubic hair, breasts of mature adult

Adapted from Tanner, J.M. *Growth at Adolescence*, 2nd ed, Oxford, England: Blackwell, 1962, and Daniel, W.A. *Adolescents in Health and Disease*, St. Louis: Mosby, 1977.

Sex Differences in Puberty

There are differences between boys and girls in how puberty develops. As mentioned, girls tend to mature before boys. For girls, signs of the beginning of puberty include breast development, with the onset of menses (menarche) happening fairly late in the process. For boys, growth of the penis and testicles and development of pubic hair will often be the first sign of puberty. Changes in hair (first in the underarms and then in the face) and voice happen a bit later. There are wide variations for both girls and boys related to when puberty starts and how long it takes to unfold. How long puberty lasts seems unrelated to whether it starts early or later. It does seem that with better nutrition and healthcare, puberty now occurs earlier than it used to.

With puberty come changes in body shape. Girls tend to develop broader hips and pelvic regions, while boys develop broader shoulders. Both boys and girls typically go through a "growth spurt," during which they may grow three or more inches a year. The growth spurt in boys is usually longer than it is in girls. Once the growth spurt of adolescence is over, boys tend, on average, to be both taller and heavier than girls. By the end of puberty, boys also generally have more muscles and are stronger than girls (although part of this may relate to cultural factors).

Perhaps the area of greatest concern during adolescence is that of growth and sexual development. Parents often worry when their children develop either very early or late. Your pediatrician can help assess how your child is doing in relation to other children of her age. He can also help you understand what changes to expect in your child over the following year. This can be especially helpful with regard to girls and when they might start to menstruate. Your doctor cannot tell you exactly which month your daughter will start, but he can usually tell you if he thinks it will be in the coming year.

Adolescence in Children with ASDs

Puberty is not typically delayed in children with autism and related disorders. However, the transitions and changes of puberty can be much more difficult for children with ASDs for many reasons. First and foremost, it is not always possible to totally prepare your child for the changes that she is about to experience. She may lack good communication skills or be unable to fully understand what you are trying to explain. In addition, the rapid mood changes that the parents of all adolescents try to cope with, and often find frustrating, can be magnified in children with disabilities. Aggressive behavior toward others and self-injurious behaviors can escalate. These behaviors can be harder to physically manage as your child becomes larger and stronger. (See the section on "Behavior Problems in Adolescence," on page 257.)

It is hard to know when behavior changes merely signify "normal adolescence" and when they are clues to new underlying problems such as the pain of an ear infection or a toothache. You may need to go to the doctor in order to rule out medical problems. In general, the start of adolescence is a good time for your child to have a scheduled physical—that is, at a time when your child is not sick and you can take longer with the doctor to talk about changes in adolescence. Bear in mind that now that your child is much bigger and stronger, it may be harder to manage her at the doctor's office. It may require more planning, extra hands, or special persuasion to be sure she gets all of the necessary tests or even all of the required immunizations.

Medical Problems

Adolescents with autism or PDD may develop any of the medical problems that other adolescents develop during this time of life. In addition, adolescents with ASDs have an increased risk of developing seizure disorders (see Chapter 9).

Nutritional Concerns. Adolescents need to eat more during growth spurts, so if your child is a very picky eater, it may require new efforts to get her to eat all that she needs. You may need to add extra calcium and iron during this period to ensure that she gets enough. You should discuss this with your healthcare provider. For some adolescents, obesity may be a concern, especially if your child doesn't have as many outside activities as a typical teenager.

Scoliosis. Adolescents need to be monitored for scoliosis (curvature of the spine) as they grow. Fortunately, most adolescents who have spinal curvature do not end up needing treatment. If the curve is severe, however, it may lead to problems with breathing. In that case the back will require treatment with bracing or surgery. Once your child has finished growing, the concern over scoliosis is over. The curve will not worsen significantly after that point.

Skin Problems. Another possible problem area for adolescents is their skin. Most will develop some acne during this time. If this is mild, you may not think that any treatment is necessary. If it is more severe, it may need to be treated so that it does not trigger scratching and picking of the skin, which could possible lead to more serious infections. Bad cystic acne can leave severe scars and you may feel treatment is worthwhile in order to try and avoid that. See Chapter 4 for more information on skin conditions.

Blood Pressure. Blood pressure problems will sometimes start during the adolescent years and your pediatrician will check for that each year at the annual check-up. Particularly if there is a history of high blood pressure in the family, it is important that the blood pressure be checked periodically.

Fatigue. Occasionally adolescents develop problems with their thyroid gland that requires evaluation and treatment. If left untreated, an underactive thyroid (hypothyroidism) can cause many problems, with fatigue being one of the most frequent symptoms. Infectious mononucleosis is another cause of fatigue among teenagers and others. Although people sometimes call this the "kissing disease," it is contagious and is not just passed through kissing (so teenagers who don't date can still get it). Your pediatrician will be able to diagnose this and give advice on its management. Particularly for girls who have heavy menstrual flows, anemia can be a problem and contribute to fatigue. A blood test can readily determine whether your child is anemic.

Sexuality

Developing sexuality poses a complicated set of issues for typically developing children, much less those with some developmental vulnerability. Some adolescents with autism will have strong sexual feelings; others won't. Some children, particularly higher functioning children, may be very motivated to have a girl friend or boy friend and sometimes this extra motivation helps the child make important gains. It is important to realize that sexual feelings are very much tied up with feelings about relationships—which means they are even more problematic for children with autism and related difficulties.

For typically developing children, sexual awareness comes early. Toddlers are aware of the differences between boys and girls by around age three and know their own gender. They also have a growing sense of their own bodies, and, through toilet training, an awareness of the distinction between public and private behaviors. As children become older, they want to understand more about their bodies and where babies come from. For the typically developing child, parents, teachers, and peers are all important sources of information. By adolescence there will be an interest in bodily changes such as menstruation and wet dreams and a strong awareness of appropriate and inappropriate sexual behaviors. Older adolescents cope with issues such as the distinction between love and sex, the importance of contraception and preventing sexually transmitted disease, and more adult-like notions of what long-term relationships mean.

For a child with an autism spectrum disorder, education about sexual issues is complicated by both language and communication difficulties and social problems. Sexual feelings can sometimes be quite intense—for lower and higher functioning children alike. Unfortunately, one of the prime sources of information available to typically developing children (i.e., their peers) is not so readily available to the child with an ASD. The child's learning difficulties and adults' anxiety may both pose further obstacles for learning.

Teaching Your Child about Sexuality

It is important to realize that helping prepare your child for adolescence and emerging sexuality really begins much earlier in life. You should try , whenever possible, to affirm the things that your child can do, and encourage an awareness of the importance of others and the many different kinds of relationships we can have. Early relationships with brothers and sisters and with parents will usually provide opportunities for learning about the differences between the sexes as well as about your child's own body. Because sexual issues are also very much relationship issues, it is important, early on, to encourage social skills. These can begin with very simple skills like greeting and leave-taking. Encouraging relationships both within and outside the home is important since these relationships will provide opportunities for learning and generalizing skills.

When you begin to teach your child more formally about sexuality, the first consideration is, of course, determining where your child is in understanding these issues. If your child is younger or more cognitively challenged, you may need to begin by helping her gain an understanding of privacy issues, a basic understanding of differences between the sexes, and so forth. As her understanding increases, you can begin to discuss issues that will be more important in adolescence, such as menarche and masturbation. It is also important to teach children about appropriate and inappropriate touching— that is, who can and can't touch the more private parts of their bodies (an issue that often will have come up already with their doctor).

Privacy and Modesty

Often the first difficulty parents face is teaching some ideas about privacy and modesty. This issue often arises early because you may need to spend a longer time teaching your child skills such as toileting and dressing.

Modesty is a difficult concept because it requires a *judgment* and an *appreciation of context*. You need to understand, for example, that it is all right to be naked in the shower or while changing clothes in a locker room but not "in public." Your child's difficulties with appreciating context and a tendency to rigidly over-generalize rules will usually make for some problems in teaching.

Problems in appreciating privacy and modesty rules cause endless troubles—starting at a fairly young age. A friend of ours, who once worked in a group home, tells a wonderful story of taking one of the clients in the home to a classical music concert. This rather large, nonverbal young man with autism loved classical music and seemed to enjoy the performance very much. The only problem arose when he went into the bathroom by himself. Shortly a torrent of men were pouring out the door. It turned out that the young man with autism had learned that when you go to the bathroom you take off all your clothes first and his doing this in the concert hall bathroom probably did not seem at all out of the ordinary to him!

In thinking about teaching modesty, there are several important considerations to keep in mind. First, what are the situations where privacy/modesty is needed? And second, who do you know who can help you do some teaching? For example, grandparents and siblings may be good resources, but casual acquaintances are not. Third, as with other tasks, you have to think about what you want to teach and the challenges for teaching. So, for example, given the difficulties children with autism have in generalization, you might want to teach your child to get dressed in her bedroom or bathroom and nowhere else (at least at first). Similarly, bathrooms are a good place to teach personal self-care and grooming. You can make a point of shutting the door to "have some privacy." You can also gradually teach the names of body parts and can point out differences between boys and girls and men and women. Some parents find it helpful to teach their child that the private parts of the body are the ones that are covered by a swimming suit. For additional guidance, you may want to refer to *Sexuality: Your Sons and Daughters with Intellectual Disabilities* by Karin Melberg Schwier and Dave Hingsburger (see Reading List).

Teaching Self-Care Skills

Often a lack of ability in self-care skills is a major, major problem for adults with autism spectrum disorders. Starting work on this area early really pays off in adolescence. If you have not started by adolescence, these skills can be very difficult to teach.

Modeling self-care skills for your child is one of the most useful (and least time-consuming) means you can use to help your child learn what she needs to do. For girls, the chance to watch Mom and sisters put on make-up and fix their hair can be important; for boys watching a father or older brother shave similarly can be helpful in the long run. You should also talk with your child and praise her for appropriate behavior; help her enjoy the experience of acting more "grown up." Although children with ASDs may overdo the interest in perfumes, aftershaves, or antiperspirants at first, it will be helpful for them in the long run.

Sometimes modeling and verbal guidance is simply not enough. In these situations, feel free to talk to classroom teachers and other care providers about strategies that may work for your child. For example, they may recommend using pictures and picture books to provide visual sequences of activities. You can laminate snapshots in a book or on a series of notecard-sized sheets (that you can then number and bind) to guide your child through the series of steps involved in, say, taking a bath. For example, you would take photos of:
- an empty bathtub
- turning on the water
- testing the water so it is the right temperature (depending on your bath set up, you can mark the faucet or water flow controller)
- getting undressed

- getting into the bath
- a systematic series of steps in washing
- getting out
- drying off
- cleaning out the bathtub
- getting dressed

At first your child will need more supervision, but as time goes on, you can let her have more independence and can praise her increased independence.

Masturbation

Most children with autism and related conditions will learn to masturbate. This can be a source of discomfort for parents. It is important to realize, however, that masturbation is very common in all children and adolescents and that the task for children with autism is to learn to do this in the privacy of their bedroom. Often masturbation will start in the preschool or early school years and you'll have the opportunity to explain (in as simple language as is needed) that we don't engage in that behavior in public. If you tell your child this, it is important that she indeed have access to some private places. You should try not to act upset. A matter-of-fact attitude is much better, since you may otherwise teach your child a very handy way of always getting your attention.

Some parents tell their child that bad things will happen to their bodies when they masturbate—this only adds to the child's confusion since it is untrue. Often much patience and work is needed. Visual supports and other learning aids can be helpful—for instance, learning to put out a sign that says "Do not disturb" (as in a hotel).

Sometimes masturbation during school can be a problem. Giving your child opportunities for frequent movement or objects to manipulate with her hands may be helpful. (An occupational therapist can recommend materials your child can fidget with, or you can check in a toy store.) Exercise, too, can help. The OT and special education teachers may help come up with some strategies for helping your child learn that masturbation in school is not appropriate.

Girls: Menstruation and Breast Development

As their breasts enlarge, girls with autism spectrum disorders need to understand that breasts are a private part of the body. They should know that other people should not be attempting to touch their breasts and that they should not show them to others. Higher functioning girls will want to know more about the functions of the breasts. As the breasts develop, the doctor will want to talk about breast exams (see the Reading List for some helpful books).

Like all girls, girls with autism spectrum disorders should be prepared in advance for the onset of their period. The Reading List gives some resources that may be helpful in educating girls about their bodies and the changes to expect. For children who are verbal, the chance to talk with their mothers or older sisters can be a big help. Do not overwhelm your daughter with information that she may not be interested in, but be prepared to answer her questions in a matter-of-fact way. For example, she may or may not want to know why women menstruate, but if she asks, provide truthful, factual information.

Some girls will be able to manage on their own with the help of their caregivers, but others may require more direct supervision or help during their periods. To teach basic skills like getting dressed independently, for example, you may want to use a waterproof marker to mark the front of underwear (or to mark where the front end of a pad should go). When your daughter is having her period, it may be helpful to teach her to change her pad at specific times, such as after math class and after lunch (particularly if she has trouble making this judgment herself). As with other self-help skills, photos or a visual outline of the steps involved may be helpful.

At least initially, someone may need to keep track of how often your daughter has a period and how long it lasts, and at times be sure that the pads are changed when necessary. Personal hygiene may require more intervention than before for some girls. Additional discussions about privacy may also be needed. For instance, more verbal and talkative girls will need to learn that one's periods are not a topic for general conversation. As parents you should also, of course, be mindful of the need to respect your daughter's privacy and sensitive to the situation and context where you discuss issues like this with her.

Some girls have cramps with their periods. These can start a day or so before the period or at the beginning of the period. Usually they only last a few days. For girls with poor communication skills, cramps may be a cause of behavior change at this time of the month. Menstrual cramps are often treated with nonsteroidal anti-inflammatory drugs (NSAIDs) such as ibuprofen. If the pain is severe and interfering with normal functioning, birth control pills may be used to prevent the cramps (see below).

Birth Control Pills

Birth control pills or other types of hormonal contraception can be very useful in helping teenaged girls and young women with autism manage their periods. First, they can help reduce heavy menstrual flow. Second, they make it easier to predict when a girl's period will start. That may be very helpful when a girl has major behavioral changes with her period or needs quite a bit of supervision when changing her pads and with general hygiene when she has her period.

If birth control pills are used, someone needs to be sure that they are taken every day as prescribed. An alternative is to use the patch form of hormonal birth control. A new patch is put on once a week for three weeks and then left off for one week so that the girl will get her period during that week. Hormone injections, given either monthly or every three months, have also been used for birth control or to control the periods and symptoms caused by them. For girls who have trouble remembering to take a pill every day, or for those who might take a patch off, the injections can be very helpful. In the future, we may see more hormonal contraception being used in such a way that some women will have a period only every few months. This may be particularly helpful in girls and young women with ASDs who have a very hard time coping with their periods and any associated symptoms.

There are many potential side effects to hormonal birth control, but in general it is very safe in teenage girls. The hormones can interact with some drugs, especially some antiseizure medications, so be sure that the doctor prescribing the birth control pills knows whether your daughter is on any other medications. Most teenagers placed on birth control pills are put on what are called "low dose" pills. That means that the amount of hormone in them is lower than in the past and there are many fewer side effects.

Some of the serious side effects that may occur with birth control hormones include increased risk of heart attack in women over the age of thirty-five who are smokers, increased risk of clotting problems such as stroke and thromboembolism, development of a nonmalignant liver tumor, and increased blood pressure.

Less serious but still problematic possible side effects include weight gain, nausea and vomiting, bloating, depression, and enlarged and sore breasts. In the past, higher dose pills often worsened acne. Now, with lower dose pills, many women find that their acne actually improves, and some physicians actually prescribe birth control pills just for that purpose.

As we have discussed concerning other medications, it is always important to discuss the potential benefits and risks of any birth control medication for your child with her physician (and with her, if appropriate) before deciding to put her on it.

PMS

It is important to realize that girls with autism may have premenstrual syndrome (PMS), but that it may be harder to diagnose in girls with severe communication problems. In such circumstances, it is important that parents are aware of the timing of what appear to be unusual, monthly "behavioral difficulties" which may actually represent a response to discomfort.

PMS symptoms can vary greatly between girls. Some will have few or no symptoms while others unfortunately can have many different symptoms. Both physical and emotional symptoms can be a part of PMS. Some of the most common physical symptoms include headaches, breast swelling and tenderness, change in appetite, weight gain, tiredness, and achy muscles and joints. Common emotional symptoms include irritability, depression, anxiety, poor concentration, and social withdrawal (which may be hard to separate from some girls' underlying behavior and social difficulties that are part of the ASD). Changes in sleep with either trouble sleeping or sleeping more than usual have also been described as a part of PMS.

The symptoms of PMS, as the name implies, usually appear in the second half of the menstrual cycle before the period starts. No one treatment has been found to work for all of the symptoms of PMS, or for everyone. For some girls, being aware that these symptoms can be expected at a certain time of the month can be helpful in dealing with them. Others have found that exercise is helpful in preventing or lessening the symptoms. Sometimes taking 1200 mg of calcium per day is recommended as a way to prevent PMS. This is the amount of calcium that is recommended anyway for children and adolescents during their years of rapid growth so that they will develop strong bones. Nonsteroidal anti inflammatory drugs (NSAIDs) such as ibuprofen and naproxen sodium, which are over-the-counter drugs, or prescription medicines of this type can be helpful for some of the physical symptoms of PMS.

For girls with severe symptoms of PMS, birth control pills have been used with very good results. Remember, you want to carefully weigh the potential risks with the hoped-for benefits before starting these. Antidepressants have also been used at times for severe PMS symptoms and have been very helpful for some people. Your daughter's doctor could discuss these options further with you.

Pelvic Exams

At some point, all girls need to start having an annual pelvic exam. If a girl is not having any problems with her periods or other aspects of her gynecological health and she is not sexually active, she can wait until sometime between eighteen and the early twenties before starting the annual exams. If there are problems sooner, she will need to be examined at that time.

Your daughter will require special care in preparing her for this exam. Your pediatrician may be able to do this exam or you may need to take her to a gynecologist. If possible, look for a gynecologist who is experienced in examining women with developmental disabilities. If you need to see a doctor that your child is not familiar with, it may take a few visits before your child will allow the exam. In any event, preparation with pictures and other aids will be helpful. Again, the Reading List has some resources you may want to use. Breaking the exam down into separate parts and explaining and demonstrating each part separately, using rewards for cooperation at each step can be helpful. Rarely, girls or women with autism are so resistant that they have to have some sedation or even anesthesia to be examined.

Boys: Wet Dreams and Sexual Maturation

Many changes also occur in the bodies of boys during puberty. As mentioned earlier, these include increased hair, growth of the body, change in voice, and development of the genitals. They also include wet dreams (emission of semen during sleep) and erections as sexual maturation moves along. These occurrences can be confusing. Boys who are higher functioning may be relieved to hear that this is a normal part of growing up. As with girls, advance preparation is helpful. (Often the father or a brother is the best person to do this.)

By this time in adolescence, it will be important that the doctor include examination of the genitals as part of the regular physical examination. This is also an opportunity for the doctor to teach the young man about self-examination of the testicles for lumps, if this is appropriate—that is, if the boy can understand the reason for doing it.

Teaching about Boundaries

The possibility of sexual or physical abuse is always a concern for parents. Parents of lower functioning children are often worried that they might not know about abuse if it occurs, and parents of higher functioning children worry that their child may easily be misled into inappropriate sexual activity. Fortunately, most children with autism spectrum disorders are closely supervised in their day-to-day activities and the opportunity for abuse does occur. Planning for activities and work should include consideration of who your child will be with and the safety of the situation. This may be a greater concern for more high functioning children because they may be allowed more independence and less supervision. They may not fully understand other people's intentions, however, and at times other people may not understand their behaviors.

Part of growing up is learning about boundaries and appropriate behavior on the part of others. Various programs and curriculums are available (see Reading List). These programs can help to teach about levels of intimacy in a very concrete way and help convey the idea that different adults have different relationships with the child. For example, for adult strangers hand shakes are appropriate; for closer friends and family members, other kinds of contact such as hugs may be appropriate. Clearly, teaching about strangers and being appropriately wary of strangers is important. For children who are verbal, the "No, Go, Tell" strategy may be useful. This method, described by Karin Schwier and David Hingsburger in *Sexuality: Your Sons and Daughters with Intellectual Disabilities* involves being able to say no to an activity, getting away from the situation, and telling others what has happened. (See the Reading List.)

Unfortunately, there will inevitably be some exceptions to the various rules you teach and sometimes these will come back to haunt you. For example, if you teach your child not to let strangers touch her, sooner or later she will see a new doctor who is a stranger to her, but who has a legitimate need to touch her.

Signs of Possible Abuse

Sexual or physical abuse can sometimes be easy to detect and sometimes more difficult. Among the many clues to possible abuse in typically developing children (which may also be seen in children with ASDs) are:

- unusual changes in behavior
- increased anxiety or depression
- avoidance of certain people or situations
- increased agitation or aggression
- withdrawal

Sometimes a marked increase in sexual activity (such as masturbation) may be the only sign. Physical symptoms or signs of sexual activity are obvious warning signs.

Discuss any suspicion of sexual abuse with your healthcare provider. And remember that, by law, the provider must contact child protective services if he or she thinks there is a possibility that your child has been abused.

Encouraging Healthy Sexual Relationships

People used to believe that the social problems of autism prevented sexual interest or relationships, but we now know that this isn't true. With earlier intervention and an emphasis on programs in communities, more people with ASDs are having meaningful relationships—sometimes including sexual relationships. Like many parents, you may have trouble viewing your child with autism as a sexual being and you may be concerned that she may be taken advantage of. However, it is important for her emotional health for you to allow her to explore her sexuality at the same time she is learning other positive ways to relate to others.

As you help your child learn to develop relationships, keep in mind that you want to:

a. make this a positive experience,
b. help your child learn about what *not* to do as well as what *to* do, and
c. remember that the overall goal is to help your adolescent develop a more positive view of herself.

As with other activities, experience is helpful. This experience may need to be carefully planned and monitored. For example, mixed (male - female) group activities present excellent opportunities for socializing. Explicit teaching can be helpful here, particularly for more verbal young people, and can emphasize important (but complicated) distinctions such as the difference between what we think and what we say. Understanding the distinction between public and private behavior is also important. Again, teaching your child when to say no, who can touch what and where, and when touching might be appropriate is also essential. For children who have not yet mastered them, there will be many chances to learn some of the appropriate social rules. Guided rehearsal and practice may also help—for example, in teaching your child how to act during a date. If your child has the chance to attend a social skills group with other teenagers, that may also be a big help.

Sometimes adolescents with Asperger's disorder or autism can be quite preoccupied with sex or with the issue of wanting a girl or boy friend. To some extent, these concerns are age appropriate and expected. They can, however, result in some very awkward moments if your child takes a rather literal, one-sided, approach to trying to obtain what she wants. For example, one teenager with Asperger's disorder would pick a girl and stare at her during lunch in the high school cafeteria. The girl would eventually come over to ask him what he wanted and he would then make a very explicit sexual request! This young man had to learn that while the girl had indeed asked him what he wanted, there is a rule against answering as frankly as he did.

In general, you should help your child deal with emerging sexuality by having open discussions with her with responses pitched to a level she can understand. These discussions should also make clear what the rules are for socially acceptable behaviors. It is important to keep in mind that sex is only part of what needs to be discussed. Your child also needs to understand the role that relationships play in sexuality and to understand the differences between having a friendship and a sexual relationship.

Occasionally, particularly for individuals with greater cognitive impairment, parents may need the help of a specialist in dealing with sex education issues. For example, you may want to consult a specialist if your child has real difficulty understanding basic issues such as masturbation and the need for privacy. Potential resources include your child's school, physician, or agencies such as your state department of developmental disability. Other parents can also be sources of good information.

Contraception

There are a variety of reasons that it might be appropriate to think about contraception for your son or daughter with autism. Some adolescents and young adults with autism spectrum disorders may be able to enter into a longer term relationship that involves a sexual relationship. For other young people, contraception might be an important safe-guard to consider when they move into a community living situation. Occasionally, birth control pills may be used to treat painful periods (dysmenorrhea) and sometimes for other medical reasons as well (see the section on "Birth Control Pills" on page 252).

Usually the issue of birth control looms larger in the mind of parents of girls, but even parents of boys with an ASD should realize that sexual activity brings potential risks of sexually transmitted diseases as well as of pregnancy. That is, if a young man is going to be sexually active he must understand the risks of unprotected sex. Some higher func-tioning young men may need help in understanding the use of condoms.

The issue of birth control and an awareness of the risks of unprotected sex (including pregnancy) should be discussed with the sexually active teenager and young adult. Your child's healthcare provider may be helpful to you in the process. As far as we know, individu-als with autism spectrum disorders are just as fertile as anyone else. In addition, if someone with autism conceives a child, there is some potential that she will pass along the risk for autism, if not the actual disorder, given that there seem to be strong genetic aspects of autism.

In the past, it was common for individuals (particularly women) with intellectual disabilities to be made infertile (sterilized) without their consent. Currently, laws about sterilization—as well as marriage and guardianship—vary significantly from state to state. In considering what is best for your own child, it is important to realize that sexu-ality does not have to lead to childbearing and that sterilization won't of itself make her less vulnerable to abuse. You should also remember that anyone who has the cognitive ability to make decisions about her own healthcare is entitled to do so, and decisions about your child's reproductive status very well may not be yours to make.

Behavior Problems in Adolescence

As he followed children over time, Leo Kanner, the man who first described autism, observed that some children made gains in adolescence and others had losses in their overall levels of functioning so that they didn't seem to live up to their earlier potential. We still see this pattern today and are not always sure why some children improve in adolescence and others have more trouble. Sometimes physical problems, such as the beginning of a seizure disorders, seem to be involved. We also know that there are many potential emotional and behavioral issues for children entering adolescence.

For children with autism spectrum disorders, the hormonal changes that precede the onset of puberty may exacerbate pre-existing behavioral difficulties such as aggres-siveness and self-injurious behaviors. For some children, the start of adolescence will bring on these types of behaviors for the first time. To complicate things further, the many changes in the body and an emerging sexuality may only add to life's confusions. Unfortunately, this is also a time when children are moving into more complex social and physical environments such as high school.

Behavior problems in adolescence often seem to start a year or so before the bodily changes which signal puberty. These may take the form of greater irritability, decreased attention, higher levels of activity, and stereotyped behaviors. Often these behaviors get better as the child enters puberty, but the increase in the child's physical size and the potential seriousness of the behaviors may be very problematic. As your child becomes older, you may need to add medications to help manage behavior problems, or, if she is already on medications, you may need to increase the dose or change to new medications. The strategies we discuss in Chapters 12 and 13 can be used effectively. Talk to your child's school staff as well about strategies that may help your child cope at school. An increase in physical activity may, for example, be helpful to some children.

Individuals who make major improvements in adolescence often have an emerging sense of being different and of wanting to "fit in." For these adolescents, it is important to support their desire and motivation to work toward more typical peer relationships. These individuals often receive the fewest services in school (because they indeed are doing well), but would greatly profit from explicit teaching about social relationships and real world skills.

Moving to Adulthood

As your adolescent becomes a young adult, you may need to find new healthcare providers. Some pediatricians may be willing to continue to care for your child into her twenties. As she reaches her thirties, or earlier with some doctors, you will need to find an internist or family physician to take care of her. The main reason you will eventually need to switch to an internist or family practice physician is that as your child grows older, she may develop the same kinds of medical problems that other older people get. That is, adults with autism are subject to all adult-related medical conditions, such as high blood pressure, high cholesterol, heart disease, etc. Your pediatrician may not feel comfortable treating these problems if they are not seen in children, and at times the pediatrician may not even recognize or think of problems that are only seen in adults.

Although autism has been recognized since the 1940s, relatively little has been written about adults with autism and their medical care. A particular challenge for parents of adults with autism and other pervasive developmental disorders is that many healthcare providers who typically work with adults are not knowledgeable about these disorders. Internists and general practitioners may have little or no training at all in the area of developmental diagnosis or developmental disability and may be hesitant to assume care for young adults with autism. Sometimes they are surprised or even shocked by the lack of cooperation on the part of an adult with autism. Other parents with older children with autism or PDD may be able to recommend doctors they have found who are willing to take on these young adults. Your pediatrician may be able to help in the transition by speaking directly with the new doctor about your child and her special needs.

Summary

In autism and related disorders, puberty is a time of growth and positive change for some children and a time of challenge for others. Helping your child cope with sexual feelings is an important part of helping her get through adolescence. We've emphasized that your child's adolescence will be easier if, earlier in childhood, you begin to help her understand societal norms about privacy and the importance of different kinds of relationships. Children with autism spectrum disorders may need help coping with emerging sexual feelings as well as their newly mature bodies. Teaching about boundaries and teaching about appropriate and inappropriate touching and behavior are all important. Some children have a worsening of behavioral difficulties in adolescence. Others begin having seizures during this time.

Keep in mind that no one goes through adolescence without at least an occasional problem. Your overall goals during adolescence are to help your child achieve as much personal independence and self-sufficiency as possible and also to help her deal with the reality of a new, changed body.

Questions

Q. My daughter is supposed to have her first GYN exam soon. Do we need to schedule this for the hospital where she can have anesthesia?

As for other developing young women, at some point your child's pediatrician or family doctor may recommend that you consult with a gynecologist. This may be routine—as your teenager approaches adulthood and needs regular care—or it may be because there is some problem. You should not assume that your child will absolutely have to have anesthesia. Probably it would be best to make an appointment for an initial visit with the gynecologist to let your child meet the doctor and have a discussion about what approach makes the most sense. When you schedule the visit, be clear about your child's special needs. Often mothers may decide to have their daughter use their own gynecologist, in which case you can discuss this issue with the doctor at your own check-up. See the Reading List for some resources (including picture books) that may help your daughter.

Q. My twelve-year-old son is just starting puberty and his skin has gotten to be a mess with acne. How can we help?

Unfortunately, acne is extremely common in adolescence as a result of hormonal changes in the body and changes in the skin. To minimize the problem, carefully wash twice a day (not excessively) and try some of the many over-the-counter products. For very severe acne, talk with your doctor or visit a dermatologist (skin doctor) about either topical (on-the-skin) or oral medicine. It usually takes at least four to six weeks before you can see the benefit of any new acne medicine, so you should wait that long before switching to a new medicine. See Chapter 4 for more information on skin problems.

Q. Our fourteen-year-old has made some nice gains in his cognitive and communication skills, but has a lot of trouble with self care. His father

still needs to get him into the shower. Is there some way we can work on his self-care skills?

Absolutely. You might want to talk with the school psychologist to get an assessment of current levels of self-care (adaptive) skills. There are several very good tests that can be used to do this, and, in conjunction with any cognitive or IQ testing already done, the psychologist may be able to generate for you a list of reasonable goals. The issue here is to pitch things at the right level for your child, keeping in mind that it is better to start a little slower and with things that are easier and then build on success as you move along. An experienced teacher or person who works with developmentally disabled children may also be a help. Sometimes it works well to have someone other than the parents involved. For example, one young man we know had pretty poor self-care skills but was really interested in fitting in at school. He took up swimming with the supervision of a college student who was able, fairly quickly, to get him up to speed. This activity helped him learn about getting dressed and undressed, as well as showering before and after swimming—one of the "rules of the pool."

Q. Our thirteen-year-old has autism and things were going pretty well until adolescence hit. He has had a lot more difficulty with attention and impulsive behavior. Our pediatrician tried stimulant medicines but these seemed to make things worse. What else can we try?

There are a number of different medications—depending on the specifics of your child's situation—that could be tried. Alternatives to stimulants include the antidepressants, some of the anti-high blood pressure medicines such as clonidine, and SSRIs. In some cases, neuroleptics (either the older or newer "second generation" medications) may be helpful. You should talk with your doctor about all these options. See Chapter 13 for more information about medications.

15 | Dealing with Developmental Deterioration

Most children with autism spectrum disorders do not lose developmental skills once they have acquired them. Unfortunately, however, developmental deterioration does sometimes occur in autism, as well as in two of the pervasive developmental disorders: Rett's disorder and childhood disintegrative disorder. In this chapter, we'll review what is known about regression and discuss some issues that are important to keep in mind if your child's behavior significantly deteriorates. This chapter won't be relevant for every reader. If it is not something you need to know about, skip it! On the other hand, if you have a child who has experienced a major loss in developmental skills, please read on.

Regression in Autism

When he first described autism, Leo Kanner mentioned that he thought autism was congenital—that is, that children were born with it. Subsequently, it has become clear that approximately 20 percent of children who are eventually diagnosed with an ASD seem to be relatively normal at birth but then lose skills and develop autism. These children fall into several distinct groups:

- Sometimes there is indeed a dramatic loss of skills and the development of what looks like autism. This occasionally occurs in children over age two who have had perfectly normal language, in which case a special diagnostic category (childhood disintegrative disorder or CDD) is used (and discussed in more detail later in this chapter).
- Sometimes regression happens in association with Rett's disorder (another topic later in the chapter).
- Sometimes regression seems to happen before the child has really acquired language (in which case, an autism diagnosis is made).
- In some cases, even though parents report a regression, careful discussion with them will uncover a previously unrecognized abnormality. For example, parents may report a regression in their child's behavior at eighteen months but then it turns out that their child hadn't ever used words and may have been lagging behind even before they started worrying about his development. Some researchers have studied home videotapes such as of first

birthday parties, and suggested that some differences in these children can be observed early on. This would suggest that these children probably had autism earlier, even though it wasn't recognized for awhile.

Sometimes when we talk with parents in some detail, we discover that what parents are really talking about when they use the word "regression" is not so much a regression as a "stagnation." That is, the issue really is that the child's development doesn't progress rather than that it regresses. For example, many infants (starting at five to six months) start to say "mama" or "dada," although they don't yet clearly associate this word with their parent. Occasionally, parents report that their child had a couple of possible words and then did not develop more. It is sometimes not clear, however, whether the child really had a good grasp of the words or was simply playing with making sounds as many babies do.

Other parents report a relative "late onset" of autism, and may not have become worried until their child was about twenty-four months old. Here the issue may be less one of regression and more the parents' growing awareness of their toddler's social difficulties and oddities. These children often have said first words on time and end up being higher functioning children with autism or PDD-NOS. Finally, sometimes it does appear that the child was developing reasonably normally and may have had several words but then did regress. These cases are probably a fraction of all cases where some concerns about regression are raised—perhaps a couple of percent of children with autism rather than 20 percent.

Although there has been great interest in regression in autism, the studies done have not usually shown much in the way of differences between these cases and other cases of autism. That is, there aren't many proven differences in symptoms or outcome in

Table 15-1 | Regression in Autism Spectrum Disorder—Subtypes

Type	Features
Childhood Disintegrative Disorder*	Normal development until at least age 2 years (usually 3 or 4 years), with dramatic loss of skills and development of autistic behaviors.
Rett's Disorder*	Normal development early on; then a decrease in the rate of head growth, loss of purposeful hand movements, other characteristic symptoms.
Subtypes of Autism: Developmental stagnation	Child seems to develop reasonably normally but then development slows down.
Late onset—higher functioning	Child talks on time but social and behavioral oddities more apparent after age 2 years
Regressive or "set back" autism	Child has several words and then loses them; behavior regresses

* Official diagnoses; note that although autism is a recognized diagnosis, the various subtypes of "regressive autism" are not.

children with autism who regress vs. those who don't—at least so far. (As you'll learn shortly, this turns out to be a complicated topic). This is particularly true when you take into account that children who are recognized earliest probably are the ones who have the greatest cognitive handicap. In addition, it is important to realize that all the various complexities in defining regression may complicate the research that has been done. For example, one researcher may take a parent's word that his child regressed, whereas another might seek corroboration from something like a videotape. Although it seems kind of arbitrary, these differences may make a major difference in how we understand the importance of regression.

At present, treatments for children with autism who have had a regression are no different than for other children with autism—unless a medical condition is found to explain the deterioration. With the exception of unrecognized seizure activity, the chances of finding an underlying condition are quite low, however. Still, the study of possible differences in these children remains an important area for research.

Childhood Disintegrative Disorder

As we discussed in Chapter 1, childhood disintegrative disorder (CDD) is a rare condition in which a child develops normally for several years (usually three to four years but sometimes even longer) and then has a very marked loss of skills and comes to look "classically" autistic. By definition, the child must have spoken on time and used language appropriately (speaking in sentences) before the regression, which, by definition, must be after age two years. It is probable that at least some children who apparently regressed at a very early age and are now diagnosed with autism may represent very early cases of CDD, but the current approach to diagnosis requires at least two years of normal development for a diagnosis of CDD.

Over the last century, slightly more than one hundred cases of CDD have been identified. You will see terms such as disintegrative psychosis or maybe Heller's syndrome used to refer to it in older papers. (Theodore Heller was the man who first described the condition back in 1908.) The psychosis idea was clearly a mistake; the term was used because people thought that almost every serious mental disorder was "psychosis." Today we use the term psychosis much more strictly for disorders which cause difficulties in distinguishing what is real from what is not, and it doesn't really apply to conditions on the autism spectrum.

CDD was added to the *Diagnostic and Statistical Manual of Mental Disorders* (DSM) in 1994. There was some controversy about including CDD in DSM for several reasons. One was that people thought that perhaps CDD always results from some medical condition—that it is essentially like a childhood onset of Alzheimer's disease. Interestingly, however, despite very careful medical evaluations (discussed below), usually no specific medical cause for CDD is identified. (This doesn't mean you shouldn't look, though.) Our current thinking is that probably CDD arises as a result of the operation of some factor or factors in development. For example, some gene or genes might turn off (or on) and disrupt development and lead to the development of CDD.

Another concern about adding CDD to the DSM was the concern that parents were perhaps mistaken about their children developing normally for the first several years. (That is, that these children had autism all along.) One of the advantages of home videotapes is that we can often now document the early normal development of children with CDD, showing that parents indeed are correct that their children certainly looked normal.

The data on outcome of CDD further support its inclusion as a separate diagnosis. See Figure 15-1 below.

Onset

As shown in Figure 15-1, the onset of CDD is much later than that for autism. The usual age of onset is between three and five years. Occasionally, the condition begins somewhat later in childhood, though always before age ten. The onset of this condition can be relatively sudden—over days to weeks—or it can be more drawn out—over weeks to months. Occasionally, the child becomes more anxious or agitated at the onset of CDD. He becomes less interested in the environment and starts to lose skills in multiple areas. Although he previously had talked normally, he loses the ability to speak entirely or can now say only an occasional single word. He loses interest in other people, including parents and siblings, and becomes socially withdrawn. Sometimes, if he had the ability to use the bathroom independently, he loses this skill and may again end up in diapers.

Not surprisingly, given the dramatic nature of this regression, parents are desperate. Usually they take their child for very extensive medical evaluations. Parents often presume (and until recently, so did most professionals) that some underlying medical condition is responsible for the child's regression. However, this seems not to be the case.

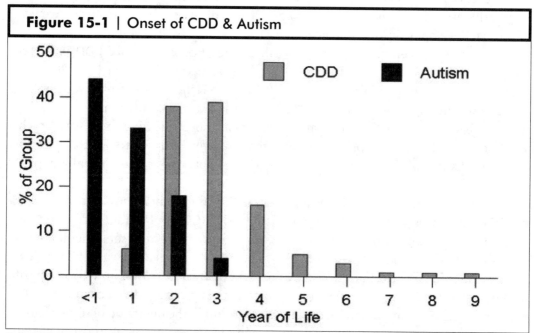

Figure 15-1 | Onset of CDD & Autism

Figure 15-1 Volkmar, Fred R., Ami Klin, Wendy Marans, and Donald J. Cohen (1997). "Childhood Disintegrative Disorder." See page 360 for complete citation.

Most children are given very extensive medical evaluations, and no specific cause for the condition can be pinpointed. This does not, of course, mean that one does not exist. However, it does suggest that we by no means understand the vast majority of cases of this rare and perplexing condition.

Clinical Features

The clinical features of CDD (the things a doctor can observe) are summarized in Table 15-2.

Table 15-2 | Childhood Disintegrative Disorder: Clinical Features

Clinical Feature	% of cases
Speech loss/deterioration	100
Social disturbance (loss of social interest)	99
Resistance to change/stereotyped behaviors	91
Overactivity	90
Deterioration in self-help skills	87
Anxiety, mood changes	74

Adapted, with permission, from "Childhood Disintegrative Disorder" in *Handbook of Autism and Pervasive Developmental Disorders*, 2nd edition (New York, NY: Wiley and Sons, 1997), p. 51. By definition, these features develop after 2 years of normal development.

Overall, more boys than girls appear to be affected. (It is likely that some girls with Rett's disorder were incorrectly thought to have CDD in the past.) Although CDD is clearly rare, it is unclear exactly how common the condition is since cases have probably often been incorrectly diagnosed. Probably the condition is about 100 times less common than autism.

Medical Evaluations

Usually parents become worried (and highly worried) very quickly once their child starts to lose skills. Often your child's primary doctor will be concerned. She may do some basic tests, such as tests of the thyroid and screening tests of blood and urine for disorders of metabolism. Looking for medical causes of regression is sufficiently specialized that your primary healthcare provider will want to get some outside help, and will send your child for more specialized evaluations. These might include consultation with a pediatric neurologist or specialist in genetics, since many of the medical conditions associated with loss of skills are the result of neurological illness (such as seizures) or genetic problems (such as tuberous sclerosis, discussed in Chapter 3). In coordination with your healthcare provider, the specialists will conduct a careful search for any genetic or neurological conditions that might explain the regression. These include a range of disorders, all of which are quite rare. A number of laboratory tests can be done to look for many of these conditions (see Table 15-3).

Sometimes development deteriorates following the onset of a recognized (or sometimes unrecognized) seizure disorder. Neurological examination and EEG should therefore definitely be performed. Rates of EEG abnormalities and seizure disorders in CDD are probably about the same as in autism. (See Chapter 9 for information about seizures in general and page 161 for information about the relatively rare syndrome of acquired aphasia (language loss) with epilepsy.) Some degree of loss of skills may also follow the onset of other medical conditions such as meningitis. In these instances, CDD would only be diagnosed if the characteristic symptoms that are so strongly suggestive of autism were present—that is, social and other abilities would need to be even more impaired than general development.

Most of the time, even after extensive testing, nothing specific is found. Even if a medical cause is found, the diagnosis of CDD is made. However, other aspects of treatment may change or there may be important information for the family (for example, about inherited conditions).

Table 15-3 | Tests for Medical Conditions When Development Deteriorates

Type of Test	What Is Being Looked For
EEG (Brain wave)	Seizure activity (see Chapter 9) may lead to loss of developmental skills; some types of seizures are associated with loss of language (see page 161 for a discussion of Landau Kleffner Syndrome).
Blood Tests	Blood tests are used to check for low (or high) levels of chemicals, for example, low thyroid (hypothyroidism) or for high levels of other chemicals such as amino acids.
Urine Tests	High levels of certain chemicals may be present in the urine in some disorders such as those that prevent the body from properly using amino acids.
Brain Scans (CT/MRI)	These are used to look for changes in the brain seen in some disorders; these may be general (throughout the brain) or localized to specific parts of the brain.
X-rays	Deformities in the bones are seen in some syndromes.
Other tests	In addition to standard physical or neurological examinations, other tests, including examination of the eyes, of hearing, of the skin, and other systems may be needed.

Outcome and Interventions

In about three-fourths of children with CDD, behavior and development deteriorate but then stabilize at some lower level. No additional deterioration then occurs, but gains are quite minimal. These children almost universally have some degree of intellectual disability (mental retardation). In other children (particularly when regression is associated with some other identifiable medical condition), deterioration is progressive—that is, it continues. Sometimes after the regression, some degree of recovery then occurs. For example, sometimes a child who had become mute regains the ability to say single words. In a handful of cases, children have made a major recovery after the deterioration. Unfortunately, the outlook for children with CDD is generally worse than for children with autism.

Except when deterioration is progressive, life expectancy apparently is normal. When deterioration is progressive, lifespan depends somewhat on what the underlying condition is.

As a practical matter, the behavioral and educational interventions for CDD are the same as for autism. These techniques include special education, behavioral treatments, and drug therapy. The goals are, as in autism, to select appropriate goals and services and then help the child benefit from services. Unfortunately, even when children with CDD receive the best possible services, they are more likely than children with autism to require residential programs. At present, no drug treatments are available to treat the underlying cause of CDD, but medications (see Chapters 12 and 13) can help deal with problem behaviors. When seizure disorders are present, drug treatments can also be helpful. (See Chapter 9.)

Rett's Disorder

As we discussed in Chapter 1, Rett's disorder is one of the more recently described autism spectrum conditions. Dr. Andreas Rett reported on this condition in 1966 after seeing two girls with the disorder in his waiting room; he then collected and reported on a series of cases.

Early on, there was much confusion about the possibility that Rett's disorder was a form of autism. As time went on, however, it became clear that, although some "autistic-like" features are present, they tend to diminish as the child grows older. In addition, the course of Rett's disorder is very different from that of autism. Rett's disorder was included in the PDD category of DSM primarily because there is some potential for confusion with autism (particularly early in life). It was also felt that Rett's disorder should be included somewhere, and PDD seemed the best fit.

At first, Dr. Rett thought that this condition could be due to high levels of ammonia in the blood. This turned out not to be true. Many years went by before a cause was found for at least some cases; in these cases an abnormality of a gene on the X chromosome seems to be involved. However, not every child with Rett's disorder seems to have this specific genetic abnormality. Research on the genetic basis of Rett's is continuing actively.

Originally, the condition was thought to be confined to girls. Since then, boys who have the disorder—or at least have the gene for Rett's disorder—have been seen, although not very frequently. Probably fetuses who are male and carry the gene are more likely to miscarry before birth.

Onset

In Rett's disorder, the mother's pregnancy, labor, and delivery are not typically unusual, and the child's very early development also seems to be fine. After some months or even a year or more of what seems to be normal development, progress starts to slow down. This has been termed "developmental stagnation." The child may also lose interest in the environment and the doctor may notice that head and body growth are slowing down. Often these changes are difficult to appreciate at first. Once development slows down, it may stabilize for a time before motor difficulties are observed (see next section).

Clinical Features

Rett's disorder usually begins much earlier in the child's life than CDD does and is associated with a decreasing rate of head growth and other unusual behaviors. Development may seem to be going reasonably well for the first twelve months or so (sometimes the onset is earlier or may be even a bit later). The slowed growth of the head leads to microcephaly—that is, small head circumference. The unusual behaviors and medical problems frequently associated with Rett's include:

- very unusual hand washing/wringing sterotypies (the child looks like he is constantly washing his hands)
- motor difficulties (ataxia), such as in walking (if the child has learned to walk he may become much more unstable on his feet)
- a loss of purposeful hand movements (the child has increasing difficulty using his hands for self-care, for drawing, and so forth)
- breathing problems may develop (breath holding spells and disorganized breathing patterns may be seen)
- seizures may develop (starting in the preschool years)

Children with Rett's disorder often seem less interested in other people, particularly during the preschool years, and there is some potential for a misdiagnosis of autism at this time. As time goes on, severe mental retardation develops. As we mentioned, seizures are also a common problem. Other problems such as breathing difficulties, bruxism (tooth grinding), motor problems, and scoliosis may be present. (See "Medical Treatment" below.) Sleep problems, including difficulties in getting to sleep and frequent awakenings during the night, are quite common. Social skills are, on balance, somewhat less severely affected than in autism, although the severe mental retardation contributes to problems in social interaction and communication. The motor difficulties also contribute to both, as well.

Medical Evaluations and Treatment

At present, the diagnosis of Rett's disorder is made based on clinical features and history. Not every child with Rett's disorder seems to have the same genetic abnormality. Once the genetics of Rett's get sorted out, it is possible that a blood test will always be used.

Children with Rett's disorder present some special challenges for medical care. They have multiple problems that involve treatment from a range of specialists. The problems can include difficulties with breathing, with tooth grinding, with diet and eating, with gross and fine motor movements, with seizures, and with posture and the skeletal system. For some children, difficulties with eating and lack of movement lead to constipa-tion, which can be quite severe. As a result, it becomes even more important that your child's primary physician be centrally involved in coordinating care.

Seizures

Epilepsy occurs in 75 to 80 percent of children with Rett's disorder. Most commonly, seizures are generalized tonic-clonic and partial complex, with other types less frequently observed. Often abnormalities on the EEG are seen before seizures develop. Treatment of seizures depends on the type of seizure (as discussed in Chapter 9). Some children with Rett's disorder are very sensitive to seizure medicines and may need careful monitoring. Sometimes seizures decrease in adolescence. Occasionally, children with Rett's have other behaviors (staring spells) that mimic seizures but do not represent actual seizures; if these are not seizures, they do not require drug treatment.

Breathing Problems

Difficulties with breathing can include:
- Hyperventilation (breathing rapidly) and apnea (stopping breathing)
- Breath holding and disorganized breathing (sometimes the child will actu-ally pass out; there is some potential for mistaking these for seizures)
- Swallowing air (aerophagia) and then regurgitating it (like burping)

The reasons for these behaviors are not known. They can present serious medical problems and even lead to death. These behaviors do *not* usually respond to behavioral interventions and should not be thought of as attention seeking! The efforts of respiratory therapists are sometimes needed, and special equipment such as apnea monitors may be useful.

Movement Problems

A number of different movement problems are often seen in children with Rett's dis-order, and usually the services of multiple specialists in both school and medical settings are needed. These may include occupational and physical therapists, as well as medical specialists in the muscular and skeletal system (orthopedists). Ongoing therapy has the potential to improve mobility. Given the up-and-down pattern of regression, it is important to continue this intervention over time—even when the child is having some loss of skills. As for other conditions, it is important that treatment be very individualized.

Children with Rett's disorder often have multiple movement problems. A general decease in muscle tone (hypotonia) along with ataxia (uncoordinated movements) and apraxia (unsteadiness) may be some of the earliest motor manifestations in the disorder. These problems lead to difficulties with walking and other problems in movement. The combination of difficulties with muscle tone, movement planning, and perception lead to an unusual, unsteady gait. As time goes on, difficulties with stability of the trunk further contribute to movement problems.

It is important to encourage (and maintain) the ability to walk independently and stay active as long as possible. Some children lose the ability to walk, and this can lead to other complications such as contractures (permanent tightening of muscle or tendon causing deformity) and bed sores. Various techniques can be used to help with walking.

Some of these are the same methods used with children with cerebral palsy or adults who have had a stroke. These might involve balancing activities or learning to shift weight. Some children also respond well to swinging and to vestibular stimulation (bouncing movement and so forth). Sometimes problems with the feet contribute to walking difficulties and need to be addressed as well. To complicate matters, children with Rett's disorder may be somewhat resistant to exercise or therapy activities and may also be slow to respond. Unfortunately, difficulties with hand movements and purposeful hand control can complicate the use of aids such as walkers.

The unusual hand movements in Rett's disorder can take various forms. Many children with Rett's make hand washing or hand wringing movements, but some children may make hand-to-mouth movements (e.g., pulling on the tongue). Often these movements change over time. Younger children may make quick, fairly simple hand movements. As children grow older, the movements may become more complex and then eventually less complicated. These movements often seem to increase when the child is stressed or upset; they may disappear (briefly) when the child is doing something. The movements do not seem to otherwise be particularly stimulated (in either direction) by the environment. Medications have not been particularly helpful in dealing with these movements. Occasionally, other techniques such as hand splints have been tried, but results are not always consistent. Assistive technology methods can be used to help increase functional movement of the hands.

As time goes on, children with Rett's may develop difficulty with spasticity (increased muscle tone). This can affect different muscle groups and varies in severity. Sometimes it causes very significant contractures. It may also contribute to some of the difficulties with deformities of the spinal column (scoliosis). Various activities (sometimes including pool-based hydrotherapy) may be helpful in preventing or delaying these problems. Scoliosis (curved spine) and kyphosis (hunch back) are fairly common in Rett's disorder. These problems further contribute to difficulties in walking and movement. Various exercises and physical therapy can be helpful. Special wheelchairs and other chairs that support the back and produce good posture may be needed.

Eating and Growth Problems

Difficulties with hand movements and lack of physical activity contribute to several interrelated problems, including poor growth and often constipation. Lack of good fluid and fiber intake contribute to the latter problem. As with other children, the first line of defense against constipation is changing the diet, such as by increasing fluids and high fiber-containing foods. Sometimes medical interventions such as those described in Chapter 4 are needed.

It is important to monitor growth of children with Rett's disorder and for parents to have the option of a consultation with a dietitian if weight is a problem. (See Chapter 4 for more detailed information about resolving constipation.)

Outcome and Interventions

Like other children with developmental disabilities, children with Rett's disorder should receive special education services individually tailored to their needs.

They will likely need the help of many professionals, including physical therapists, occupational therapists, speech-language pathologists, respiratory therapists, and orthopedic physicians.

Although some of the usual principles of behavior modification and special education can be used, it is important to realize that the hand movements that interfere with learning are involuntary behaviors not under the conscious control of the child. That is, you can't talk the child out of them and punishment won't work either. Behavioral methods can be used along with OT and PT procedures to help increase or maintain functional skills, such as in eating. Whenever possible, communication skills and basic self-care skills should be encouraged. Although medications for seizures are often needed, medications for behavior problems are usually not used.

Unfortunately, adults with Rett's disorder are quite disabled. Their ability to move, walk, and control hand movement independently is often limited. Although assessment can be difficult, many function in the severely impaired range on cognitive testing. It is worth remembering, however, that Rett's disorder is a fairly new diagnosis. As more researchers become interested in studying the disorder, there is hope that increased understanding will lead to more effective treatments. Animal models are being developed and new medications are being tried. For more information about Rett's disorder and new developments on the horizon, contact the International Rett Syndrome Association, listed in the Resource Guide.

Summary

In this chapter, we've briefly reviewed some of the autism spectrum disorders in which behavior and development deteriorates. This kind of regression most often occurs in children with childhood disintegrative disorder or Rett's disorder. A small number of children with "classic" autism also seem to have this pattern—most often before the age of two years. In general, regression is not expected in older children with autism, Asperger's disorder, or PDD-NOS.

Sometimes when children with autism are reported to have regressed, it really is more often a case of "developmental stagnation." That is, the child is not making as much progress as predicted, but he is not usually losing skills. Keep in mind that the behavior of some children with autism may deteriorate in adolescence, as discussed in Chapter 14. This change is *not* the same kind of regression we are talking about in this chapter.

Questions

Q. Can Rett's disorder co-exist with autism?

No. By definition, the two disorders are distinctive. There is a relatively brief "autistic-like" phase in Rett's disorder (usually in the preschool years) but after that, the conditions are quite different. Although children with

Rett's do have impaired social and communication skills, these are not of the same type seen in autism.

Q. What is the relationship between Rett's disorder and childhood disintegrative disorder?

The main, obvious relationship is that in both conditions there is some deterioration in the child's development and behavior. It is not at all clear that there is much of a relationship beyond this obvious one, though. Children with Rett's disorder are almost always girls. The regression often starts very early in life and has a characteristic course with slowing down of head growth, loss of purposeful hand movements, and development of unusual "hand washing" stereotypies. In CDD, the period of normal development is usually longer and the child has, by definition, progressed to the point of speech before the onset of a dramatic regression. Boys seem much more likely than girls to have CDD. The course of CDD seems much different than that in Rett's disorder as well. Usually children with CDD condition look like they have very severe "classic" autism and do not have the problems in movement or breathing that children with Rett's syndrome exhibit.

A gene has been discovered that seems to have some role in at least some cases of Rett's syndrome. Genes that might cause CDD have not yet been identified.

Q. Are there differences in treatment between autism and CDD?

Essentially, no—the treatments are the same. Educational, behavioral, and sometimes drug interventions are used in treating both conditions. The differences really lie in the initial evaluation. For CDD, there usually are much more extensive medical investigations to try to determine whether any other condition might account for the child's loss of skills.

16 | Complementary and Alternative Treatments

It is not surprising that many different treatments have been tried for a condition like autism—indeed, almost every kind of treatment you can think of has been tried over the years. Some treatments, such as Applied Behavior Analysis (ABA), have gone on to become widespread and scientifically accepted, while others, such as facilitated communication, have been discredited and faded from use. During the time between the emergence of a new treatment idea and the time when it is either adopted widely or disproved, parents are left to try their best to figure out whether the treatment or approach is worthy. The risks—in time, money, and wasted effort—are big, but so are the hoped-for benefits. This dilemma has led many families to search for and try different treatments.

This chapter focuses on some of the treatments that are often referred to as "alternative" treatments—undertaken *instead* of more conventional treatments—or, sometimes, as "complementary" treatments—undertaken in combination with more traditional treatments. Another way to refer to this group of treatments is as "nonestablished"—that is, the scientific research showing that the treatment actually works is either minimal or nonexistent. There can be a fine line between "established" and "nonestablished" treatments; sometimes, as research is done, treatments move between alternative and mainstream. At other times, as you will see, treatments that start out looking very promising don't pan out as hoped.

Because you will hear about many of these treatments, it is important that you have some information about them. We do not endorse any of these treatments, but want you to have information that can help you make informed decisions about your child. The lack of information does not mean that scientific support might not be available in the future—just that, at present, it is lacking, in our view. This prevents us from recommending these treatments to our patients.

The Life Cycle of Ideas

Some new ideas turn out to be right, while many others turn out to be wrong. Why then does it appear that new ideas in the autism field are regarded with great skepticism? Why do so many parents flock to embrace untried treatment ideas? The answer to these questions lies in the history of treatment of autism.

Treating children with autism has historically been hit-or-miss. Many different "treatments" have been tried, but only a few have yielded any significant benefits. In the past, when autism itself was poorly understood, there were virtually no effective treatments or approaches. Children with autism were considered schizophrenic and were often "hospitalized" in insane asylums. That approach, as well as a host of others, failed, leaving parents defeated and exhausted.

Given the challenges autism poses to families, it is natural that parents would search for treatment approaches that might benefit their child. During the past fifty years, many treatment ideas have been proposed, and many parents have been willing to try them on their children because no available treatments—even treatments that were scientifically endorsed at the time—seemed to work. The urgent need to help their child prompted parents to engage in their own trial-and-error investigation. When an approach seemed promising—based on the experience of one or more children—word would spread, and other parents would try the approach. Sometimes these ideas would come from parents; other times, from researchers or teachers. Sometimes, studies would be undertaken to test these approaches scientifically to determine if the success initially claimed could be verified objectively and duplicated with other children. Ideas that could make the leap from anecdotal success to general success remained, while ideas that couldn't, faded. That is the natural "life cycle" of ideas in autism, and, really, in all of science.

Two treatments illustrate this "life cycle" clearly. Behavioral treatments, particularly Applied Behavior Analysis (ABA), grew out of the awareness, in the 1960s and early 1970s, that the usual kind of psychotherapy didn't work for children with autism but that methods based on behavioral and educational interventions did help children with autism learn. A study by Ivar Lovaas in the late 1980s reported that intensive work using the ABA approach resulted in major improvements in both behavior and intelligence; subsequent studies have also shown gains for many children, although not as large as those seen in the first study. (You can find the exact references for these and related papers in the References.)

As word gradually spread in the autism community of the possible benefits of ABA, parents began to pioneer its use: They set up ABA-like programs for their child and advocated for its use in schools. At the same time, researchers, teachers, and clinicians began to use and study the method, which the original proponents enabled by sharing their data. They tried ABA on children with autism and methodically compared their behavioral and educational outcomes to those of other children with autism who did not receive therapy using ABA. As time has gone on and more research has been conducted, the uses, as well as some of the limitations, of the ABA approach have become clearer. For instance, it is clear now that early intervention programs that offer structured, intensive programming can be helpful, and many programs around the country now use aspects of these ABA methods in teaching children with autism.

Contrast ABA's history with that of facilitated communication (FC), which was introduced to the United States in the late 1980s. Interest in FC quickly spread because parents and teachers heard frequent reports about its success in enabling children with autism to communicate. FC's spread was fueled by high-profile media reports, parent and teacher testimonials, and the claims of its proponents. As explained later in this chapter, resistance was encountered by researchers who wanted to study the method to understand the critical question of how FC worked. This made collecting data to validate FC scientifically difficult. Nevertheless, the use of FC exploded, and, for a time, it seemed as if it would dominate autism treatment. Parents flocked to FC in the belief it would unlock their child's inner world, even forgoing other treatments. Later, when scientific research demonstrated that FC did not work, parents had to recover and regroup.

The failure of a treatment approach can cost children with autism and their families a great deal. Autism's history is rife with claimed cures that did not pan out. And when they don't, families are left to pick up the pieces and struggle on. Often, critical time has been lost, money spent, energy wasted, and hopes crushed. In our experience, we have seen this pattern over and over again. That is why we favor treatment methods that have been proven to work through careful, objective scientific studies that take the guesswork out of choosing treatment approaches. We want to make sure that the treatments we provide or recommend have proven benefits.

But progress in autism treatment is painfully slow and new ideas can appear to hold promise. So, what are parents to do between the time when they hear about the success of a treatment and the time when it is scientifically validated, especially when the clock is ticking with their child and the scientific process could take years to complete? We hope you can use the information in this chapter in conjunction with advice from your child's doctor, teachers, and therapists to steer your way through the maze of treatment approaches and make good choices for your child.

Understanding Research and Peer Review

One of the most important ways to determine whether a new or alternative treatment is worth trying is to review what has been published about the treatment. Seeing how treatments have been tested and analyzed can help in sorting through the many different treatment approaches available.

In reviewing information about treatments, you should give more consideration to treatments that are studied in carefully controlled ways and that are reported about in a reputable, scientific, reviewed journal. The best sources of information are peer-reviewed journals—publications in which other scientists and professionals evaluate each paper before it is published. The goal of review by a group of scientists other than the paper's author is to ensure some quality control and give the author the benefit of some independent opinion about the paper. Ultimately, this encourages the exchange of ideas and knowledge that has a better scientific basis. Thus, the goal of peer review is not to ban discussion, but rather to be sure that papers that do get published are of reasonably high quality. Even the best paper can be improved by peer review. Your child's physician may be a good source of information on how to evaluate information that appears in journals.

Even if a treatment is reported in a peer-reviewed journal, you should still evaluate the report carefully. It is important to look at the question being asked, the theory behind the research, the quality of the techniques used in the research study itself, the number of individuals being studied, and the claims made based on the findings. The issues involved in evaluating research vary to some extent depending on the kind of study being done, its methods, and its goals. For example, one element of a study—the size of the group studied—is critical to understanding the study's importance. For some purposes, even very small groups of children can be meaningfully studied. You can, for example, use information on just one child's behavior before and after an intervention to get useful information, if done in a careful, scientific way. However, most studies involve larger groups of children (rarely just an individual child). In general, the larger the group studied, the more confidence you can have in the results because it is harder to demonstrate what is called "statistical significance" with small groups.

It is also important to look carefully at exactly who is being studied and what measures the researcher has used to ensure that his or her research is as strong as possible. For example, in the best kinds of studies, there are attempts to measure and control for the important effects of just being in a study. This is called the placebo effect. The placebo effect refers to all the changes that tend to occur when people are involved in something new. Because of the novelty, participation in a study tends to make things better by itself. It is important to be sure that what is tested (a new drug or treatment) works even *better* than the placebo. The placebo effect has been vividly illustrated in recent work on secretin (discussed below), where, despite all the media hype, secretin has not been shown to be superior to a placebo.

Controlling for the placebo effect may involve using a control group, in which some of the children receive treatment A and others do not, or they receive treatment B instead. Likewise, to avoid the possibility that unintentional bias might distort the results, children can be randomly assigned to treatment groups. Careful attention to issues of diagnosis and assessment is also important. The best results may be achieved in children who don't have strictly diagnosed autism! All these precautions make good research challenging but very important to do.

The fact that a report about a treatment is published in a peer-reviewed journal does not necessarily mean that it is really true. Sometimes things happen by chance—whether in research or in the rest of life. Consequently, replication of research is always essential; that is, other research involving different groups must show the same results. Even if a study is published in a good journal and reports a positive result of treatment, the treatment must still work for other clinicians at other centers to be valid. Sometimes fluke results are observed which may mislead people into thinking a treatment works when it really doesn't. Put another way, the same treatment that works in one place should work in another.

Media and the Internet as Sources of Information

The Media and Autism

Mark Twain supposedly once said that there are three kinds of stories: Stories that are true, stories that are false, and stories you read in the newspapers! You should always keep this saying in mind when you hear reports on the television, radio, magazines, and newspapers. Most news people (including TV media people) try to be responsible. How-ever, given that the nature of the news business is to sell a product, you might expect that media professionals would be most interested in flamboyant and attention-getting sto-ries. It is less exciting, for example, to talk about how several years of patient behavioral work with groups of young children with autism makes a difference than it is to report that a new medicine or other intervention "cures" a single child (who may or may not have had autism in the first place). Rarely can media reports match the meticulous pre-cision of scientific research—the time constraints of media reports prevent in-depth prob-ing. You should also pay attention to what is not reported: Stories that "treatment X does not help autism" are also (usually) not of much interest. This is one reason for what scientists call a bias for only positive case reports to be published. Extravagant claims get attention. Truth and accuracy often do not.

Too often people's judgments go out the window when they read a sensationalized news account or see a TV story. We know parents who are stockbrokers, and, understand-ably, do a very careful job of researching any stock they are about to buy or recommend to their clients. Yet they seem perfectly happy to believe anything they hear about the latest untested treatments in autism and have indeed tried almost all of them.

The Internet and Autism

Evaluating claims for treatments posted on the Internet is even more challenging. The Internet presents some wonderful opportunities as well as many potential pitfalls. For parents, it can be a wonderful source of information. It can also help parents connect with each other and with professionals, as well as keep up with current research. One of the great beauties of the Internet is that it is a very free medium—people can say what they want. This is also one of its great dangers, since what people say may not always be true. The same considerations that apply to evaluating treatment claims apply to the Internet. There are some, and probably will eventually be more, sources on the Internet that rely on peer review or on another process of quality control, but at present it is usually very hard to know how to assess the validity of the various claims made. If you were to believe all the many reports of "cures" for autism, you'd think there wouldn't be

Evaluating Internet Resources

- Who is responsible for the information? What qualifications does this person or organization have? Who sponsors the site? Government agencies, universities and medical schools, public agencies, and peer-reviewed journals tend to have the most objective sites.
- Has there been some form of peer review or is what is presented a matter of opinion?
- Are there references or links to credible scientific organizations, papers, and books?
- Does what is said make sense? Who is the treatment supposed to work for and not work for? Is how the treatment is thought to work explained in ways you can understand?
- Does anyone make money on the treatment? Be very careful of sites that tell you to send money immediately. Give yourself time to check things out.

any more children with autism—unfortunately, this is not the case. Great care is required to avoid treatment whiplash.

There are several questions to ask yourself when you are trying to evaluate newspaper, television, or other media stories. First of all, is the story about a single case or a group of children? Is the story based on a scientific paper that has appeared in a reputable journal or is it reporting the claim of someone working more or less outside the usual scientific framework? What claim or claims are being made and do these make sense? If something sounds too good to be true, it probably is.

Thinking about Alternative Treatments

If you are exploring possible alternative or other less conventional treatments for your child, here are some questions to keep in mind.

1. Do the claims make sense?

What are the claims being made? Usually the more dramatic and flamboyant they are, the less likely they are to be true. Is there some attempt to provide a scientific explanation for the treatment? If so, does it make much sense? This can be one of the hardest things for nonprofessionals to figure out. You should use the same caution and good sense you would use in making a major investment—since you will be investing your and your child's time, and, often, your own money.

2. What is the evidence?

If advocates for the treatment claim they have evidence in favor of the treatment, ask to see copies of this evidence. Be very wary if:

- you are told that it is "going to be published,"
- you are simply given a list of individual testimonials supplied by the treatment advocate,
- you are told that the people doing the treatment are too busy curing autism (or don't have the time or money) to show that the treatment really works.

When you hear testimonials about successful treatments, ask exactly what was done and why. Often, you'll find that proponents of the treatment tried a variety of treatments simultaneously "rolled into" one; this makes it hard to understand which of the treatments, if any, was responsible for the change.

If the data supporting the treatment are based on reports of cases, be aware that case reports are sometimes the most difficult kind of evidence to interpret. This is so for any number of reasons. Perhaps the child did not have autism in the first place, or perhaps the researcher was not as methodical or objective as he or she should have been. Find out if there have been any attempts to have an independent assessment of the child or treatment.

3. Who was involved in the study?

Sometimes claims are made for treatments when it is not clear that the children studied really had autism in the first place. Other times the treatment proposed may be effective for only a very small subgroup of children with autism. Also keep in mind that a handful of children with ASDs do well—almost regardless of treatment. That is why controlled studies with groups of children are so important.

There are other problems as well. Autism is a chronic condition, and, as with any chronic problem, there will be ups and downs over time—periods when a child does better and periods when he does worse. Parents are more likely to seek out treatments when their child is having more trouble. Parents may attribute any improvement they see in their child to the treatment, when, in reality, it may have nothing to do with the treatment. Remember, too, that simply the wish and expectation that a child will "get better" may color objectivity (the placebo effect)—this is just as true for parents as it is for researchers!

4. How reputable is the publisher of the study?

In assessing treatment claims, it is also important to look at the publication—book, book chapter, newsletter, or pamphlet—in which the claim appears. The quality of these sources—the extent of peer reviewing—can vary tremendously. Chapters in books usually have been the subject of some editing, but only rarely are they peer reviewed. You can usually do some research on the authors of chapters or articles, however, and find out where they have been previously published and the universities, programs, or organizations with which they are affiliated. Evaluating newsletters, pamphlets, and similar publications can be more difficult. Consider the purpose of the publication. Is it intended as an advertisement or does it objectively present the treatment? Does it have a hidden or not-so-hidden agenda? Common sense in interpreting publications goes a long way. Your child's physician may be a good sounding board for assessing articles.

Even with papers published in well known, peer-reviewed journals, improvements can always be made. Science slowly accumulates knowledge based not only on what works, but also on what mistakes are made. As long as objectivity and careful scientific methods are maintained, reliable knowledge grows and evolves.

Warning Signs for Alternative Treatments

There are some important warning signs that suggest that a treatment should be avoided. If you were told that a new kitchen appliance slices, dices, balances your checkbook, mops the floor, and does the dishes, you would be skeptical. The same rule applies here—if the treatment is supposed to treat all aspects of autism or cure everyone, it is not very likely it works. Pay particular attention to the costs of the treatment—both the obvious cost in dollars, but also hidden costs such as your time and that of your child. Also be wary if treatment proponents explain that when it doesn't work it is because the parents or other people did not do it "quite right." Parents should never be blamed for the failure of a treatment they did not design. Legitimate treatments can be replicated so that success does not depend on procedures only the promoters know.

If you are a parent of a child with autism, you will hear a lot about alternative treatments. You also will see treatments come and go. We understand what motivates parents to want to try some of these treatments; however, we emphasize that in presenting them here we are not recommending them. In fact, sometimes we recommend against

Evaluating New Therapies

- What is the quality of the evidence? Word-of-mouth, case report, or a more controlled scientific study? Watch out for claims not based on solid, scientific information.
- Has a paper on the work been published in a peer-reviewed journal? If not, why not? If so, what is the quality of the science in the paper? Your doctor, school professionals, and consultants may be able to help judge quality.
- Has the finding been replicated? If not, be wary.
- Can the treatment be proven wrong? Be wary of treatments for which there are no objective, measurable methods to determine effectiveness. Treatments lacking a method to determine how and why they work rely on faith. Although faith is a powerful force, it cannot be tested objectively.
- What are the costs (financial and time) of the treatment? Be careful of treatments that require a lot of upfront costs. Also be very wary of treatments that consume a lot of your child's time (and often yours as well) when other treatments such as educational and behavioral intervention have already been shown to work.
- Who is the treatment designed to help? Treatments usually won't work for everyone. A claim that every single child is helped should arouse skepticism.
- What is the treatment supposed to do? Is there a theory behind the treatment? Has the theory been subjected to scientific testing? Again, your child's doctor and teachers can be helpful here.
- What is the evidence that it works and how was this measured?
- What are the side effects? All treatments have side effects. Are the potential side effects worth the potential benefits?

them. We encourage you to be an informed consumer for your child. Always find out what the potential risks as well as promised benefits are.

Even when treatments seem safe or innocuous, there may be some hidden dangers. For example, sometimes parents pursue a nonestablished treatment to such an extent that their child's education suffers. There is much evidence that educational interventions make a very big difference for children with ASDs. Often, the risk from alternative treatments is that they will deplete a family's resources—for example, when large amounts of time and money are involved. A greater risk is the lost opportunity to pursue educational approaches that have been shown to be effective.

Alternative Treatments for Children with Autism

This is, and remains, a free country, and we believe that parents are entitled (within reason) to make choices about the treatment of their child. By the same token, we feel that physicians and other professionals should be open to innovative treatments. However, we also believe that all of us should expect that treatments of any kind should be capable of validation—that is, that we ought to be able to show that they work. The sections that follow provide short summaries of some of the more widely discussed

Evaluating Promoters of Alternative Therapies

You can learn a lot about a treatment approach from assessing the organization, individual, or company promoting it. Here are some guidelines:

- Don't be fooled by a name. There have been many discredited treatments whose promoters attempted to lend legitimacy to themselves by calling their companies or organizations by prestigious-sounding names. Just remember, anyone can call their program by any name. It is nothing more than marketing and advertising.
- Follow the money. If payment is required for the treatment, find out where the money goes. Into the pockets of promoters? Into further research?
- Don't let the label "nonprofit" fool you. Just because an entity calls itself "nonprofit" does not mean that making lots of money is not its primary motivation. Anyone can create a nonprofit corporation and enrich themselves through it. Look behind labels.
- Don't be intimidated. You have a right to learn about possible treatments for your child. If promoters resist sharing information or do not allow methods to be studied, they may have something to hide. Avoid treatments whose promoters threaten those who challenge or question their treatment idea.

alternative treatments for children with autism, and presents what evidence there is about their effectiveness.

Facilitated Communication—A Treatment Proven Not To Work

At one time, facilitated communication was touted as a virtual cure for autism. It has now been clearly shown not to work. This is itself unusual: It is often much easier to show that a treatment might work than it is to show that it doesn't. Although parents of young children with autism spectrum disorders may not hear much about facilitated communication anymore, parents of older children may be familiar with it. In many ways it illustrates some of the dangers associated with what seem like relatively safe treatments. It also illustrates some of the basic questions to ask about alternative treatments.

Facilitated communication (also known as FC) got its start in Australia, where it was originally proposed to help children with significant motor problems to communicate. This intervention involved having a "facilitator" hold the hand of a child with the child's index finger pointed out, steadying the hand. With this support, the child allegedly was able to type out words or sentences on a computer keyboard or communicate by pointing to letters on a board or other communication device. It was claimed that children with autism who used this method communicated very effectively and at *much* higher levels.

This claim was a bit perplexing for several reasons. First, unlike children with cerebral palsy or serious motor problems, children with autism usually do not have difficulties using their hands. (Children with Rett's disorder are an exception.) Second, the kinds of communication that were claimed to come from the child were at an amazingly higher and more sophisticated level than ever seen before, far beyond what would be expected based on a child's tested speech and language abilities.

FC took a while to catch on in the United States, but was eventually popularized by a group of special educators who claimed that it could also be used for children with other kinds of problems, such as mental retardation. The idea behind FC was that children with autism were actually very highly intelligent but their motor problems made it difficult for them to show this. FC supposedly released them from difficulties they had in communication. With no apparent training, these children—including children who had never talked—were said to communicate in very sophisticated ways and demonstrate the ability to read and write (sometimes in several different languages— again with no formal training). Incredibly, many bright (and verbal) children with autism were said to be able to facilitate more effectively than they could talk—leading to the notion that you often had to ignore the words a child spoke and pay attention only to the FC. We once saw a child using FC who was, among other things, "asking" for changes in his medication based on what he had "read" in the *New England Journal of Medicine.*

Despite the attention, even hype, FC received—including in the *New York Times* and on ABC and CBS news programs—the hopes it raised were eventually crushed. FC was literally too good to be true. One of the first warning signs was the resistance of proponents to allow FC to be studied and validated. And skepticism was natural; the method defied logical explanation. For example, some children who allegedly communicated using FC did not even look at the keyboard. Sometimes facilitators claimed that attempting to "test" a child would ruin her trust in the facilitator. This also defied logic because the inability of children with autism to form relationships or attachments is one of the primary diagnostic features of the condition.

FC was not a difficult method to test once proponents could be persuaded to cooperate. One test arranged a child and her facilitator so that the child saw one thing and the facilitator another. The child was then asked to communicate what she saw. What the child typed was what the *facilitator* saw. Other studies looked at how well different facilitators performed with different children. Again, the kinds of "communications" produced had more to do with the facilitator than the child. Many, many studies quickly demonstrated that there was no validity to FC.

What difference does it makes anyway? What was the harm of giving FC a try? Unfortunately, FC, and the swarm of interest generated, led to a number of very real problems. First of all, educational programs for many children with autism were turned upside down, more or less overnight, as parents pulled their children out of special education and other intervention services to enroll them in classes where their "true" identities could be freed. Sometimes doctors were asked to prescribe medications on the basis of FC communication; some mental health workers even had group therapy sessions using FC. Most worrisome, however, was the potential for abuse of parents. Because many facilitators believed deeply in FC and were not conscious of what they were doing, sometimes very hurtful messages emerged from "facilitation." Often these messages disparaged parents—sometimes even claims of sexual or physical abuse were made, and some parents were reported to protective services on this basis alone. In the end, this "treatment" and the frenzy that surrounded it resembled the mass hysteria depicted in plays like "The Crucible."

There are many valid, effective methods for helping nonverbal children with autism and other developmental disabilities to communicate. Do not confuse these types of assistive technology or augmentative and alternative communication with facilitated communication.

Dietary Treatments

Chapter 6 discusses nutrition, which is as important for children with autism as it is for other children. Sometimes the diets of children with ASDs are complicated because of their extreme food preferences. Occasionally children with autism, like other children, have trouble with certain kinds of foods such as dairy products, and have to avoid them. Other children may need special diets to help control seizures. Children with autism may also be more likely to eat nonfood items such as dirt, clay, or paper. Obviously, addressing these nutritional issues can help children with autism lead healthier lives. Some parents, therapists, and researchers go further, however, and claim that various modifications in diet can lead to improvements in behavior, communication skills, or even cognitive functioning.

Although there is much interest in the effects of diet on autism, the quality of the scientific information available about dietary claims is, unfortunately, generally not very high. Careful, scientific studies are lacking, although some studies now in progress may give us better information in the future. Usually the claims for dietary treatments are based on unproven theories which try to account for the difficulties that children with autism spectrum disorders have. These may include supposed food sensitivities, such as to artificial food dyes or to products containing wheat or gluten, or allergies to some food or other substance. Occasionally very complex diets are prescribed—sometimes after a prolonged period of fasting, which can be dangerous.

At present, several dietary treatments focus on a presumed "gut-brain" or "bowel-brain" connection. That is, proponents theorize there must be some connection between diet and behavior because of what they claim are high rates of stomach/bowel problems in children with autism. However, one controlled study found no differences in terms of food intolerance, chronic gastrointestinal (GI) problems, and celiac disease when children with autism were compared to a matched group of children with autism (Black, 2002). Another line of thinking has focused on food allergy, and, particularly, on sensitivities to casein and gluten with the idea that abnormalities in the digestive system cause changes in the brain.

Most of the evidence supporting dietary claims is based on single case reports, or, at times, grouped case reports. Remember, in these types of reports, any number of factors—including the increased attention the child receives during the study—can explain the observed changes, rather than the diet itself. Controlled, scientific studies with groups of cases are not yet widely available. Without them, there is no reliable way to recommend any dietary treatment.

Many different types of dietary treatments have been proposed. The following sections discuss only some of them. All merit careful inquiry before trying them with your child.

Feingold Diet

About thirty years ago, Dr. Ben Feingold theorized that artificial additives (food colorings, preservatives, and artificial flavors and other ingredients) caused attention difficulties and hyperactivity. The original diet he developed involved eliminating all nonnatural ingredients. It was not particularly risky to a child's health and was quite popular for a time. A few parents of children with autism and related disorders still investigate this diet because their child also has difficulties with hyperactivity. There have been some attempts to combine the Feingold diet with the Gluten Free-Casein Free diet (see below). However, the Feingold diet has been evaluated in several carefully controlled scientific studies and has not been shown to work on the symptoms seen in children with autism.

Gluten Free-Casein Free Diet (GFCF)

Some children and adults (with and without autism) are sensitive to casein (a substance found in milk) or gluten (a protein found in wheat, rye, and barley) or both. These individuals need to be on special diets to prevent damage to their intestines and to avoid malnutrition and growth problems (see Chapter 6). Some people claim that many children with autism spectrum disorders have these sensitivities and that they lead to some of the behavioral and other problems seen in autism. At present, however, there is no solid evidence to suggest that sensitivities to casein or gluten are any more common in children with ASDs than in other children.

The GFCF diet requires eliminating milk products (the casein part of the diet) and substituting soy milk, tofu, and other foods that do not contain milk. Next, because gluten is found in wheat, other grains, and many food additives, they must be eliminated too. This can be quite hard to do. Usually, people use corn, rice, and other substitutes or buy commercially available gluten-free products. There are some special cookbooks that can help parents make GFCF food more appetizing for their children.

Advocates of this diet differ as to the length of time a child should try it to determine whether it helps (a couple of months seems to be the most frequent recommendation). Advocates for this diet also disagree as to whether a child needs to stay on the diet permanently.

Evidence supporting the use of the GFCF diet is made up largely of case reports and anecdotes. While a few studies have suggested some benefit for some children, these studies have not generally used control groups or other scientific controls. One small study by Knivsberg and colleagues (see reference list) suggested improvement in a group of ten children with autism treated with the GFCF diet for a year as compared to a matched control group (Knivsberg, Reichelt, et al., 2002). Studies with larger samples and good scientific methods are still needed, however. A further complication is that often this diet is tried in combination with other interventions, complicating the task of determining why changes might be observed.

If you want to try this diet, discuss it with your doctor and with a dietitian. Your doctor may suggest blood tests (or more specialized tests) to see if your child really is allergic to milk (see Chapter 6) or has a sensitivity to gluten. If you give the diet a reasonable period of time to work and it doesn't, then abandon it. There is possibly a slight risk of inadequate nutrition with this (and other specialized) diets. Be sure to discuss the issue with your healthcare provider and also find out whether he thinks your child may need vitamins to supplement her regular food intake.

Anti-Yeast Diets

Proponents of the anti-yeast diet claim that yeast causes an infection, which, in turn, causes autism. Children on this diet need to avoid foods that contain yeast (baked goods), as well as foods that are fermented (soy sauce) or aged in some way (cheeses). Sugar is also to be avoided. Because individuals on the diet do not eat baked goods, it is also a gluten-free diet.

Although claims have been made for dramatic cures using this diet, scientific support is lacking. As described below, the evidence supporting the idea of "yeast overgrowth" in children with autism is unproven. And there is no theory explaining just how this "yeast overgrowth" might cause autism or autistic behaviors.

Dietary Interventions—A Summary

At present, there really is not adequate scientific data to suggest that any of these diets actually work. Furthermore, these diets can be a real burden for parents, teachers, and the child. On the other hand, these diets are (generally speaking) relatively safe. In our work, we have not seen many children we were convinced were really helped through dietary interventions, but neither have we seen many children who were made worse, either. (Usually if a treatment works for some children, it won't work for all and may make some worse.) On very, very rare occasions, children have suffered as a result of these diets, sometimes because the family became so fixated on the diet that they failed to fully pursue interventions (such as educational intervention) that *do* work. Sometimes, the diet of a child with autism is so restricted that there are no food-based rewards that can be used in behavioral programs for them. Finally, research has found that some children develop nutritional problems as a result of severely restricted diets.

In summary, there is no good evidence favoring dietary treatments in autism other than the obvious ones. For example, if a child has lactose intolerance, eliminating milk from her diet may help her feel better, and, as a result, behave better. Our advice: Talk to your child's doctor and consult a dietician for information. Most of all, do not close your mind to proven interventions in your pursuit of dietary remedies.

Vitamins, Minerals, and Supplements

Vitamins are organic (carbon containing) chemicals which the body needs in small amounts for hundreds of important biological processes. For example, the body needs small amounts of Vitamin D to help build strong bones. Minerals are inorganic chemicals such as calcium, iron, and iodine that are also needed for some bodily functions. For example, iron helps the red blood cells function and iodine helps the thryoid gland function. Some other chemicals (such as lead and mercury) are either not needed by the body or are toxic. Dietary supplements are products which are meant to supplement the diet and may include vitamins, minerals, herbal products, or amino acids.

Over the last one to two hundred years, a number of diseases linked to vitamin or mineral deficiencies were identified and largely eliminated as a result of better attention to diet and vitamin supplementation. Using vitamins to prevent or treat specific vitamin deficiency diseases is extremely effective. Perhaps for this reason, a number of treatments involving using vitamins, often in large or "mega" doses, have been proposed for children with autism and other disorders—although it is very uncommon for children in the U.S., with or without ASDs, to have vitamin deficiencies. For instance, a recent television program touted the possible role of copper or zinc in autism—but based on very little evidence.

As with many treatments, there are reasons that, at least on the surface, vitamin therapies might seem like an attractive approach. It is clear that in children with vitamin deficiencies, learning (and many other aspects of life) can be severely affected. Seeming to bolster this connection, a number of studies—including studies of mega dose vitamin use in children with autism—have claimed to show that the treatment works. Unfortunately, these studies have a number of problems that make them hard to understand. Many are based on case reports, or, if large numbers of individuals are included, the studies do not include appropriate scientific controls of variables such as the placebo effect (explained above). One rigorous, double-blind, scientific study failed to find solid evidence for the use of megavitamins to treat autism or other developmental disorders (Findling and Maxwell, 1997). Two other similarly rigorous studies failed to show a benefit of the dietary supplement DMG (dimethylglycine). In sum, although less rigorous studies have sometimes suggested some benefit, more rigorous research has not.

The issue of exactly which vitamins to supplement has also been a source of disagreement. Because a variety of vitamins (typically including vitamin B6 and magnesium) are often mixed into a "a vitamin cocktail," tracking and analyzing results becomes extremely complicated. Although it is possible that a few children with autism *might* respond to vitamins, the data supporting this are very limited. One exception is that some experiments have found positive changes in a few children with fragile X syndrome (which is sometimes associated with autism) when given folic acid supplements.

At the usual doses, most megavitamins hold relatively little risk to children. However, higher vitamin doses can be associated with problems such as liver damage. Very high doses of vitamin B6 can cause nerve damage, as well as ulcers and seizures. High doses of folic acid can cause irritability.

Some homeopathic and naturopathic physicians recommend supplementing the diet with very small amounts of minerals in the belief that this may produce behavioral or developmental changes. Some years ago, a mother who devoutly believed in mineral supplementation told us that she was giving her child arsenic. We were horrified. Before calling the police, however, we learned that this was part of a "natural" treatment program and involved giving her child less arsenic than most of us are probably exposed to every day.

As with vitamin supplements, there is no good scientific evidence that people with autism who have adequate diets and do not have medical problems (such as anemia) need additional minerals. If your child eats a very restricted diet, however, you can consult a dietician to make sure she is getting enough of all the necessary nutrients. In addition, your doctor can do blood and other tests to check for vitamin deficiencies and anemia. Again, at usual doses, most of the proposed vitamin and mineral supplements probably won't do any harm. Still, it is important to discuss with your doctor all the medicines and dietary supplements your child receives since high levels of vitamins and minerals can sometimes cause health problems.

Chelation Therapies and Plasmapheresis

Although the body needs some kinds of minerals to grow and develop, there are a few compounds such as lead, mercury, and cadmium (what chemists call "heavy metals") that are not needed. In fact, these chemicals can cause serious problems when ingested. For example, the negative effects of high lead levels on children's development is well known. These effects can include attention and learning problems, as well as much more serious neurological problems if a child has very high lead levels. As a result, children are screened for high lead levels so that they (and maybe their environment) can be treated if this is found.

When children are objectively shown to have been exposed to minerals such as lead, chelation therapy might be medically necessary. This therapy involves administering medicine that is designed to bind with (stick to) the heavy metals and remove them from the body by way of the kidney. There is some risk of side effects (particularly on the blood count, liver, and kidney) and close medical supervision is important.

Advocates of chelation therapy for children with autism theorize that perhaps autism is caused by exposure to mercury or other substances—either before or after birth. Some people wonder whether the mercury that used to be in vaccines might cause autism. (Mercury is no longer in any vaccines except the influenza vaccine.)The scientific evidence for a mercury-autism connection is not strong. One of several studies on the older, mercury-containing vaccines showed that the very small amounts of mercury in vaccines were eliminated from the body very rapidly (Pichichero et al., 2002). In addition, chelation therapy has not seemed to help developmental functioning in children without autism who had high lead levels. In the absence of a demonstrated, documented problem, there is no reason to conduct chelation therapy in children with ASDs.

Another approach to removal of suspected toxic substances is plasmapheresis. In this medical procedure, plasma is separated from the rest of the blood. Then the plasma is discarded and the remaining blood is returned to the body along with a plasma replacement. There are legitimate medical uses for this approach in some conditions, but not in autism. For instance, it is used in some autoimmune disorders in adults, particularly when these have not responded to more conventional therapies. There is nothing about having autism that would be helped by plasmapheresis. In addition, this treatment carries the usual risks that are involved with IVs (infection), as well as the potential for serious (and potentially life-threatening) reactions.

Drug Treatments

As discussed in Chapter 13, a variety of medications are used by psychiatrists and other physicians to help improve some of the behaviors that often go along with ASDs, including anxiety, attention difficulties, behavioral rigidity, and other problems. Although not all parents and professionals agree with the use of these medications in children, they are not considered alternative or controversial treatments because scientific studies have shown that these medications are often effective in improving behavior. There are also many drug treatments for ASDs that *are* controversial or are considered alternative because there is no good data showing that they work. Some of the most commonly advocated alternative medications are described below.

Secretin

Secretin is a biological compound that serves as a hormone in the digestive tract and is used to help diagnose certain diseases of the digestive system. Interest in secretin started a few years ago, with news and television reports of a "dramatic cure" based on the report of three cases in a relatively obscure journal—the *Journal of the Association for Academic Minority Physicians*. A black market immediately sprang up for secretin, based on the theory that maybe there was something wrong with the digestive system in children with autism. Because secretin had to be administered via IV, it was somewhat more cumbersome to give than other medicines. Also, it was not clear how safe it was, much less how effective. However, the tremendous interest in this agent led to a series of much more rigorous scientific studies.

These more careful scientific studies have so far all failed to show significant improvement in autism following secretin treatment. The studies have included both single and multiple doses of secretin using different scientific control methods. Several hundred children have now been studied and secretin has not been shown to work in improving the symptoms of autism. (See the References and Reading List.)

Everyone would have celebrated if secretin had been shown to improve the functioning of children with autism. Sadly, it does not. The tremendous media hype over secretin, however, underscores the problems parents face in evaluating new treatments—particularly very new treatments where there is much excitement, but not much solid scientific data. As explained before, case studies of single subjects tend to be published only when the results appear to the researcher to be positive, and, because these studies are not controlled, it is essential to rely on studies that use more rigorous scientific methods.

The experience with secretin also highlights the problem of relying on the news media for medical information. The original and exciting story that secretin *might* have some benefit—blown horribly out of proportion by claims of cures and major improvement—got a lot more attention than the subsequent, much more painstaking, scientific studies that have *not* shown it to be effective. As one of us has said, "What makes an effective television program may not, of course, be the same as what makes good science" (Volkmar, 1999). Most of the time, important findings in medicine and science emerge in a painstakingly slow, step-by-step fashion as scientists build on each other's work, improving and refining it. Secretin is an example of a treatment where "too good to be true" unfortunately seems to apply.

Anticonvulsants and Steroids

During the past few years, claims have been made about the possible benefits of giving children with autism anticonvulsant drugs. These drugs play a proven role in treating children with diagnosed seizure disorders. However, there is much more controversy about using these medicines to treat children with autism spectrum disorders, some of whom may (or may not) have an abnormal brain wave test (EEG) but do *not* have seizures. Often these drugs are tried in children who have had some form of "regression" in the belief that seizures might be causing the regression. Scientific data to support the use of these medicines in children with autism who do not have seizures, however, are nonexistent. What's more, these medicines, like all medicines, can have serious side effects. Sometimes they "activate" the child—that is, they make her seem more "hyper" or energetic. This may give the impression that the child has suddenly made developmental gains—but these gains are lost over time as the child's system becomes used to the medication. This pattern is familiar to people who have been on steroids.

At present, scientific data does not support the use of anticonvulsants or steroids for an abnormal EEG in the absence of a clear seizure disorder. Talk with your child's neurologist about this in more detail.

Drug Treatments for Infections

One group of alternative therapies originates from the theory that autism somehow results from infections (either from bacteria, viruses, or yeast). According to this theory, treatment of the underlying infection should lead to improvement in the child's symptoms. Yeast infections have received the most attention. Many women have chronic, but very, very, mild yeast infections. It has been theorized that mothers of children with autism are more likely to have yeast infections that had never been recognized. This led a number of doctors to try medicines for yeast infections, such as Nystatin, to treat children with autism.

Somewhat surprisingly, many of the advocates of this treatment are not particularly concerned with determining whether mothers of children with autism can be shown to have had yeast infections. Also, they are not bothered that many women who have mild yeast infections have children without autism.

Potential side effects of treating children with medications for yeast infections include stomach upset, and, rarely, allergic reactions. Again, there is no reliable data suggesting that this treatment works in children with autism.

Another recent therapy has entailed the use of high potency antibiotics, based on the presumption that autism arises from some form of infection and the toxic by-products of infection. One small, open-label (uncontrolled) study used a powerful antibiotic in treating children with autism who had a history of regression, antibiotic use, and persistent diarrhea and reported some improvement in some of the children. The antibiotic used has its own set of side effects and the study needs to be repeated with better experimental measures. For now, there are not strong scientific data to support the use of antibiotics in treating autism, and you should bear in mind that antibiotics can have serious side effects.

IVIg Infusion

Some people have suggested that perhaps autism might represent an immune problem, particularly an autoimmune problem (where the body develops an adverse reaction to something within itself). Reliable blood tests are available to diagnose most autoimmune disorders (which in reality are quite rare). At least one of these disorders has been associated with the development of movement problems in children, but has not been shown to be more common in children with autism.

Some parents (and physicians) have explored ways to treat what are presumed to be autoimmune problems in children with autism. These include antibiotics (mentioned above), as well as intravenous (IV) immunoglobulin g. IVIg is a blood product that is isolated and transfused into a child. As with any IV procedure, there is some risk for infection, and also risks of kidney problems and neurological problems (including stroke). At the time we are writing this chapter, good scientific data to support the use of IVIg to treat children with autism are not available. In addition, one study has found that six months of IVIg treatment had no effect on a small group of children with autism.

Treatments Involving Sensory Input or Body Manipulation

As Chapter 11 discusses, children with autism frequently seem to have more trouble processing sensations. As a result, quite a few treatments aimed at improving how children deal with sensory input have been proposed. Some of these treatments are also advocated for children with other disorders, such as learning disabilities. This section addresses only the claims made about these kinds of treatments for children with autism.

Auditory Integration Training

Some people with autism have unusual sensitivities to some sounds and do not seem to pay enough attention to other sounds. Proponents of auditory training believe that these differences lead to distortions in perception and thus cause or contribute to a child's development and behavior. A program of therapy (costing hundreds, or, more typically, thousands, of dollars) is then devised to correct, at least in theory, these distortions. Based on the work of some French doctors, this treatment involves first identifying the sound frequencies that a children is overly sensitive (or not sensitive enough) to and then training her to better tolerate these sounds.

Most of the supporting evidence for auditory training is based on individual testimonials and case reports that are difficult to evaluate. Auditory integration training received a lot of publicity in the press some years ago. One early study reported positive outcomes from the treatment, but did not include a control group. In addition, the reported behavior changes were based on parent reports only (and the parents were very aware of their children's treatment). Better studies, which use more careful scientific controls, have not been able to show that this therapy is effective. Nonetheless, many practitioners are willing, for a fee, to use these methods. In the meantime, the American Speech Language Hearing Association (ASHA) has recently released a statement that this treatment does not meet scientific standards for effectiveness (see References).

Central Auditory Processing Treatments

Other treatments also emphasize listening. Some are designed to improve auditory processing—that is, how the brain interprets and makes sense of sounds. The idea is that communication problems stem from difficulties in processing auditory information somewhere along the pathway from the ear to the brain. Central auditory processing tests or special hearing tests are often used to identify the problem. Although many children with various disabilities, including children with autism, do poorly on these tests, the tests themselves require a lot of attention and self-control. Some children do poorly simply because it is hard for them to focus on the material. Some new tests try to deal with this problem by avoiding the need for a behavioral response, but it is not yet clear how well they work.

A significant problem with central auditory processing treatments is that, for children with language skills below about the level of a typical nine-year-old, the validity of central auditory processing testing is not at all clear. For many children with autism, this means that the testing is not valid. If the testing isn't valid, effective treatment programs can't be developed.

Treatment for central auditory processing disorders usually consists of behavioral treatments aimed at improving the auditory (listening) skills that are thought to be impaired. For example, the child might be asked to repeat strings of numbers to improve her auditory memory or to talk and draw at the same time to help her "integrate" activities in the brain. Although various practitioners (who can charge a hefty fee) provide treatment based on this theory, there is no solid scientific evidence that it works.

FastForWord®

Another program emphasizing improved listening and attending skills is FastForWord®, a computer-based program administered by professionals specifically trained by the program's producer. FastForWord® emphasizes exercises, games, and other activities intended to help children, including children with autism, understand spoken language or understand the relationship between spoken and written language. As with other "listening" programs, there is an important kernel of truth here: Many children with autism, in particular, have a much stronger interest in written letters and numbers than in spoken letters and numbers. The program's activities are designed to help children learn to listen "faster" to process the rapidly changing information provided in the sounds of speech. Other goals seem to include attempting to improve discrimination, auditory memory, and sequencing of material. Some of these techniques have been used for children with other kinds of learning problems.

Children can be enrolled over the Internet, for a significant fee, or receive training in the office of a therapist certified in the use of this method; software is also available and there are significant costs associated with this.

Several scientific papers have been published on FastForWord®. However, the data behind these studies have not been made widely available to other investigators, making it difficult to assess the method independently. This makes it hard to determine whether the method works for children with autism. Although it may help children with language problems, it is unclear whether it is superior to other methods used for the same amount of time.

Visual Therapies

There are at least two reasons why visual problems can further handicap a child who already has a disability. First, any loss of vision can be a serious obstacle to maximizing a child's potential through intervention. Second, providing information visually is often a particularly effective way to teach children with autism. Consequently, visual problems can interfere with your child's progress in several developmental and educational areas. What you hear in the way of human speech can be fleeting, but what you see (written signs, icons, or words) tends to be much more permanent. Indeed, many books have been written about using visual aids in teaching children with autism and in helping to deal with behavior problems (several of these are listed in the Reading List).

Fortunately, visual problems are not all that frequent in autism. There are, of course, some exceptions, but children with autism do not usually have obvious visual problems and they are often good visual learners. Nonetheless, various visual therapies—aimed at changing how your child sees or processes visual images—have been proposed for children with autism. More commonly these therapies are used for crossed eyes or other eye movement problems, but some practitioners, often optometrists, suggest them for children with learning problems. Sometimes these treatments and exercises are suggested as a way of reducing the need for prescription glasses, but occasionally they are suggested as a treatment for children with autism.

Typically your child is seen for an evaluation and then for follow-up, fee-based, therapy sessions. Often, special kinds of glasses—using colored filters or prisms—are recommended on the theory that they might filter out the frequencies in the light spectrum to which your child is sensitive. Many children with autism do not like to wear glasses and may be very resistant to them. Other kinds of vision therapies may involve rapid eye movement training with the goal of helping a child better process visual information.

Rigorous scientific evidence for visual therapies is lacking in autism. If your child needs glasses because she is farsighted or nearsighted or has some other eye problem, of course you should pursue treatment. There is no good evidence, however, that visual therapies are helpful to children with autism.

Body Manipulation Therapies

Over the years, a number of different therapies that involve some kind of manipulation of the body have come and gone. There have been claims for "nerve realignment," supposedly accomplished through manipulation of the back. Other therapies have involved working with a child to "relearn" skills correctly—for example, by teaching her to walk in the "proper" way. These therapies have no independent verification and it is a far stretch to believe that some of them could possibly work.

Recently, one of the more popular of these "body" therapies has involved holding. Holding therapy originates with the teachings of a famous ethologist (scientist who studies animal behavior) named Nikolaas Tinbergen. The idea of this treatment is that children with autism can learn to connect to others by holding onto them physically until they realize that they are connected with other people (the people doing the holding). This typically involves sessions in which a parent or therapist holds the child (who struggles initially at being held) until she stops fighting the holding. As you might imagine, many children with autism do *not* like to be held and so fights can ensue over the holding. Watching these sessions can be upsetting.

Like other physical treatment approaches, there is no good scientific evidence that suggests that holding therapy does anything for children with autism other than upset them, at least initially. And like other therapies, if the child does not get better, it is possible that the parents (who usually are doing the holding) may be blamed for doing it incorrectly.

Other body therapies have been proposed as well. For example, at least one study has shown some improvement in imitation and social skills in young children with autism who received massage several times a week as compared to children who were only held (see Reading List). There are also several studies that have shown that regular aerobic exercise for children with autism results in lower levels of some problem behaviors (see Reading List). These methods need further study.

You may hear about a range of other treatments, including cranial-sacral therapy, Feldenkrais, and similar treatments. These treatments often involve light pressure, massage, or modification of body movements. Although each of these has its own theory, there is no solid scientific data that these treatments help children with autism. In our work, we occasionally see parents who have spent a great deal of time and money pursuing them to no discernable benefit.

Options Method

The Options method grew out of the experience of two parents in dealing with their child with autism. In a series of books, Barry Kaufman describes how he and his wife spent long periods of time trying to follow their son's lead and reconnect with him. This method is expensive due to the training required and the amount of time expended. Some aspects of its philosophy are also controversial: for example, the assertion that a good part of the cause of autism is psychological. There is no solid scientific evidence to back it up, although the Kaufmans claim that their son recovered from his autism, and indeed he is listed as the co-author of one of their books.

Summary

This chapter reviewed some (but by no means all) of the more controversial therapies for children with autism and related disorders. Unfortunately, despite much interest, these therapies generally have very little, if any, solid scientific basis. The chapter has also presented the factors to consider when evaluating these therapies (and indeed all therapies) and those who promote them.

As a parent, you should be a well-informed consumer for your child. Seek out other parents, as well as professionals, to talk with. Make sure you think about the hidden, as well as the more obvious, costs. You should be particularly concerned about therapies that involve a direct, or even indirect, potential for harm to your child. In our work, we have seen some parents devote many months or years to the pursuit of "the cure" through an unconventional treatment program. This is a particular problem when this pursuit comes at the expense of their child's education.

Caution and common sense go a long way. Be appropriately skeptical of highly dramatic accounts of "cures" and "miracles" in television and newspaper stories. If you decide to undertake a treatment, you should know what the evidence is for the treatment, how long it will last, what it will cost, and what the potential good—and bad—effects of the treatment may be. It is important to realize that all children, including those with autism, change over time. Do not mistake the changes that occur naturally for those that might seem to result from treatments.

References

American Speech-Language-Hearing Association (1997-2003). ASHA adopts AIT policy. www.asha.org/about/publications/leader-online/archives/2003/q3/030805c.htm

Black, C., J. A. Kaye, et al. (2002). "Relation of childhood gastrointestinal disorders to autism: nested case-control study using data from the UK General Practice Research Database." *British Medical Journal* 325 (7361): 419-21.

Findling, R. L., K. Maxwell, et al. (1997). "High-dose pyridoxine and magnesium administration in children with autistic disorder: An absence of salutary effects in a double-blind, placebo-controlled study." *Journal of Autism and Developmental Disorders* 27 (4): 467-78.

Horvath, K., G. Stefanatos, et al. (1998). "Improved social and language skills after secretin administration in patients with autistic spectrum disorders." *Journal of the Association for Academic Minority Physicians* 9 (1): 9-15.

Knivsberg, A. M., K. L. Reichelt, et al. (2002). "A randomised, controlled study of dietary intervention in autistic syndromes." *Nutritional Neuroscience* 5 (4): 251-61.

Lovaas, O. I. and T. Smith (1988). "Intensive behavioral treatment for young autistic children." In *Advances in Clinical Child Psychology, Vol. 11*. B. B. Lahey and A. E. Kazdin, eds. New York: Plenum Press: 285-324.

Pichichero, M. E., E. Cernichiari, J. Lopreiato, and J. Treanor (2002). "Mercury concentrations and metabolism in infants receiving vaccines containing thiomersal: a descriptive study. *Lancet* 360 (9347): 1711-2.

Smith, T., A. D. Groen, et al. (2000). "Randomized trial of intensive early intervention for children with pervasive developmental disorder." *American Journal on Mental Retardation* 105(4): 269-285.

Volkmar, F.R. (1999). "Editorial - Lessons from Secretin." *New England Journal of Medicine, 341*:1842-1844.

AFTERWORD

Tremendous progress in understanding autism and related conditions has been made over the last sixty years. The pace of research over the past several years has increased considerably. We now know that autism is a brain-based disorder. We also have come to appreciate that autism is not as rare as people first thought, and may affect one in a thousand children. When you include all the conditions on the "autistic spectrum," one in several hundred children may be affected. We also know that educational and behavioral interventions can make a tremendous difference in the lives of children who have these conditions.

In this book, we have reviewed information on medical aspects of autism and other pervasive developmental disorders. While this information is not a substitute for having a good working relationship with a doctor who can give you *specific* information about *your* child, we do hope that it has given you some tips and points that are useful. In closing, we'd like to do some summing up. We'd also like to say a bit about ways parents can support each other and the brothers and sisters of affected children, about recovery in autism, and what the future holds for adults with these conditions.

Getting Quality Medical Care

Children with autism and related disorders have the entire spectrum of medical issues and problems that any typically developing child has. In addition, they face some special challenges for health care—sometimes as a result of associated medical problems and sometimes because the developmental challenges of autism pose further problems for them, and you, in working with healthcare providers.

Finding a Good Healthcare Provider

Some people seem to shop around for a doctor for their child like they shop around for a car—looking for the place with the best deal and lowest financing! Unfortunately, the crisis in our health insurance system has tended, if anything, to encourage this trend. We urge you to take the task of finding a primary medical care provider for your child very seriously. The healthcare provider may be a family doctor, a pediatrician, a nurse practitioner, or physician's assistant.

Above all, you should try to find someone who is easy for you to talk with and who is understanding of your child's special needs. Fortunately, more and more primary care doctors know something about autism, and, in contrast to the past, they are now more likely to have good information. One of the exciting things about medicine as a career is the opportunity to continue to learn, so even if you find a doctor who doesn't know much about autism but is willing to learn, that can be fine.

Sometimes you'll stay with the doctor who was seeing your child before you got a diagnosis. If you need to find a new doctor, other parents can be good sources of information, since they often will have done their homework on this and you can use their work effectively in your own search. School staff or early intervention providers may also be able to suggest doctors.

When searching for a new doctor, be sure you also check out the doctor's office and its staff as well. Ask yourself if you feel welcomed when you go for a visit; see if the staff seem to understand your child's difficulties. Take a look at other aspects of the doctor's practice as well. Does she have many partners (all of whom you might have to deal with in an emergency) or just a few? If your doctor has a solo (one person) practice, what are the arrangements for night call and "cross covering" (having other doctors share in taking phone calls and dealing with problems you may have at night and on weekends).

Working with Your Healthcare Provider

Because communication problems are part and parcel of having autism, your doctor will need to spend more time talking with you. As a result, you should always be a careful observer; you will know your child better than anyone. Get to know your child's doctor. Do *not* skip routine or well child checkups. If anything, children with autism spectrum disorders are better off having *more* well child checks than usual—to help them get acquainted and feel familiar with the doctor and office staff. Feel free to ask questions and get information. The doctor can provide you with valuable information, and you can do the same for the doctor. Finally, keep a record such as a notebook with reports of previous evaluations and past specialists; if your child receives medicines for behavior problems, a log or record book can be extremely helpful.

How Can You Be Involved?

As time goes on, you should make a point of getting to know other parents of children with disabilities—particularly those with autism spectrum disorders. These parents will sometimes have very helpful information or insights to share with you. Teachers and school staff, as well as early intervention providers and other professionals, are also potential sources of information. As with all information, you have to evaluate it and decide whether it is right for your child. There are a growing number of parent support groups around the country; some are at the local level, others at the state or national levels (see the Resource Guide for some well-established national support groups). Consider attending some of the local meetings. This may be easier for you as your child gets a bit older.

You will discover that many parents become active, at different levels, as advocates. This may be quite informal—for example, as another parent talks to you about the right your child has to educational services or about what healthcare providers to use or avoid in your area. Some parents become more active and may, for example, serve as parent advocates who will attend school meetings with you. Some parents and some parent groups are also active at the state and national level in advocating for laws and regulations and services as well as for research on autism. As children become older, many parents find that involvement in parent advocacy groups is a way for them to share and receive information and feel like they make a difference for their own and other children.

Taking Care of Your Family

Having a child with autism or any serious disability will have significant impact on family life. You have to cope not only with the special challenges of raising your child but also the needs of your other children and your marriage. Some of these challenges may crop up before you even know that something is "wrong" with your child, since sometimes a period of months or even years may go by before you get a diagnosis. At other times, and more and more frequently, you may get a diagnosis fairly quickly. For children with less familiar conditions, such as Asperger's disorder, it may take some time before you get the correct diagnosis. During this time, you and your spouse may have the persistent sense that something is wrong but not yet be able to put your finger on it. Once you have the correct diagnosis and have started an intervention program there will be new challenges.

For some parents, getting a diagnosis makes things feel better—you have a specific label, something you can talk to other people about, and you can begin planning for intervention. For other parents, learning that their child has a disability can bring out a sense of loss. You may grieve for the idealized child you wanted, and, perhaps briefly, seemed to have had. Or you may grieve for something very specific, such as the loss of your dreams that your child will be a soccer star or her class president.

In some ways, coping with a developmentally disabled child can be even more stressful than dealing with a child with a chronic physical disability. In large part this is because children with physical disabilities can have very good thinking skills. For parents of children with autism and related disorders, the stress of developmental disability is further compounded by the child's difficulty in relating socially. Concerns about the future and what it holds may understandably bother many parents. The Reading List has some potential resources for you.

Parents and Parenting

Parents have talked to us about many different problems they have had to face in dealing with their child's condition. Unlike a condition such as Down syndrome, the disability of autism is not overtly visible initially and you may find yourself explaining the condition to other people. If your child lacks a sense of fear or danger, you may always have to be "on guard" and aware of your child's location. Some parents see their child's lack of sense of danger as, at times, a further expression of their lack of attachment.

As children with autism get a bit older, parents—particularly those who have had other children—may find themselves adopting new parenting styles. The kind of laidback parents who did well with an older, typically developing child may discover that they have to adapt methods of teaching or behavior management that they would never have thought of before for their child with autism. One of the advantages of being involved with a parent support group is the discovery that you are not the only one who has to reinvent yourself as a parent. You'll also learn, as you see more children with autism spectrum disorders, what a tremendous range of conditions we are talking about! And it will be very obvious, as time goes on, that regardless of her disability, your child has her own personality.

Some parents discover that they become more and more focused on their child's disability and that they become more and more isolated. Although we can understand how this happens, it is not a good idea for many reasons. The more supports you have the better. These can include friends, extended family, members of your church and synagogue, neighbors, and others. Mothers may be more at risk for being stressed than fathers. This is probably in good part because, even with the increased role of fathers in caring for children in our society, mothers still often end up spending more time with the child. It may also be that fathers are a bit less likely to talk about their own feelings.

Some parents will discover that unexpected factors end up having a major impact on their parenting skills—for example, if a son is named for his father or another member of the family. Other things such as the sex of the child and individual differences in personality also influence the ways parents respond. For example, some parents respond to the news that their child has autism by moving into an action mode—they get busy looking for information, scouting out services and care providers, and generally keep themselves going. Other parents may be less active and involved in their child's educational and treatment program. Parents who are religious may discover that their faith is a major source of comfort and helps them cope more effectively. Or then again, they may begin questioning the beliefs they have had all their lives.

Lack of support may have implications for marital relationships. If, for example, parents are more isolated and stressed, they may give less support to each other. Although there is not good evidence of an increased risk for divorce in parents of children with disabilities, there is a high divorce rate in our society in general. Whether or not you and your spouse are divorced, it is vitally important for your children's sakes (and your own) that you—as parents—try to be supportive of each other. Parents need to be able to talk openly about their feelings with one another. Ocasionally a parent may discover that she could benefit from talking to a mental health professional about her feelings. This might come up, for example, if a parent blames herself (or her spouse) for the child's difficulties, or if a parent becomes isolated and feels depressed.

One of the good things about having two parents is that you can give each other good feedback when you make mistakes—you can also "spell" each other when either one of you is feeling very stressed out. If you are a single parent, it is important to find someone you can occasionally lean on to give you the kinds of feedback you would normally get from a spouse. For instance, you might want to cultivate a relationship with a fellow parent or a sibling of yours with whom you feel comfortable unloading your feelings from time to time.

When parents of children with autism make mistakes, they tend to be well intentioned. For example, sometimes a parent will be so overly involved and so busy coping that it is hard for her to step back a bit and get the big picture (is it really worth the hassle of visits to the orthodontist for your child's teeth to be perfectly straight?). Other times problems arise because a parent is spending less time attending to his or her spouse and other children and because the child with autism spectrum disorder is overly protected and not encouraged to be independent.

Siblings

Having a child with an autism spectrum disorder will definitely have an impact on brothers and sisters. You can expect that your other children will eventually notice problems and ask you about them. You can also expect that they will develop their own relationship with their brother or sister, however. Children handle these issues in many different ways. Your task as parents is to help them cope in ways that foster their development as well as that of their sibling with ASD.

Preschool is often an easier time for siblings, but things can begin to get a bit more complicated as they approach school age. Siblings may wonder what went wrong with their brother or sister, whether they can "catch" autism, why they don't have it, and so forth. Sometimes they may feel guilty that they were spared or that they have negative feelings about their sib. Again, open communication is important. School-aged siblings, like parents, will have many different styles of coping. Some come to act like little parents—taking on a care-taking role for their brother or sister. Others want to overcompensate by being the best possible student or athlete. Still others basically won't want to talk about it (or think about it). Sometimes siblings may become distressed or upset and may need help in talking about their feelings. Keep in mind that children may have complicated and changeable feelings; this is perfectly natural. You should be careful that your other children also feel that you care for them and that they also deserve your care and support.

Adolescence can be a difficult time for some sibs. Adolescents generally want to fit in and may be very conscious of even small differences from others, so you can imagine what it might mean to have a sibling who is very different. This may also be a time when the adolescent starts to think about the future and wonders what role she may have in the future in caring for her brother or sister.

In dealing with your typically developing children, try as much as possible to encourage honest and open communication. Encourage them to ask questions. You may be surprised at how young your child is when she starts asking questions about her sibling's disability, especially if your older child is the one with an ASD. Be a good listener. Give your typically developing children information that is appropriate to their age. On the other hand, don't overwhelm them with information! Realize that many of their worries won't be your worries—and you'll find this out only if they talk and you listen. Also keep in mind that it is not just what you say but what you do that is important. If you say one thing but act a different way, you are sending a powerful message to your child. An example might be if you minimize your child's disability and want your other children to also pretend that problems aren't there.

You can and should encourage your children to take an active role in their sibling's treatment program. Don't go overboard, however. You do not want the typically developing siblings to take on many of your jobs as a parent—as if they are being asked to be kids and parents too!

Take pleasure in the successes of *all* your children. They all need to feel as if you think they are special. Make sure that each of your children gets to spend some one-on-one time with you on a regular basis. Find ways to let them know that you care about them as individuals, and that that care is there even if you sometimes have to devote a large portion of your attention to one of their siblings.

What the Future Holds

We have talked already about some aspects of medical care for adults with autism. It would be typical for adolescents, as they become adults, to make a transition from a pediatrician to an internist or family practitioner. If your child is already seeing a family or general practitioner, this may not be an issue. Insurance coverage can be a complication and it would be good to start the process of planning for adult healthcare when your child is nearing the end of high school.

As your child moves through adolescence (or even before) you will undoubtedly begin to think about the future. Planning for adulthood should start many years before age twenty-one. You and your school should work very hard to help your child have as much independence as possible. The focus on adaptive skills that we mentioned in Chapter 3 is very important, since children with autism/PDD often learn things in isolation but then are not able to generalize skills into real-world settings. It is this generalization that is so important in terms of living independently as an adult.

There is good reason to think that with earlier detection and better and more intensive intervention, the overall outlook for children with ASDs is much better today than it was even ten years ago. At the same time, it is important to realize that some children with autism and related disorders don't make as much progress as we would like; as adults, these children often need some level of supervision and support. Other children make very significant progress over time.

Sometimes you will hear words like "cure" or "recovery." In general, it probably is best to think about major improvement rather than a cure. Sometimes "cure" or "recovery" becomes the goal and this can end up being the cause of trouble in a host of ways. For example, you may be dissatisfied with the progress your child does make, not give yourself credit for the gains you have helped foster, and so on.

Fortunately, a range of options in adulthood are now available for individuals with autism and related conditions. These include everything from living independently with a day job to living with more supports, such as in a supported apartment (where someone comes in periodically to check on things). Other individuals will move to a more supervised group home while others may stay with their parents. Employment options are also more extensive than they once were—ranging from a supervised workshop day job, to more supported employment in the community, to a fully independent job.

The goals for planning for adulthood vary considerably from child to child, depending on the child's needs and abilities, special challenges that may be present, and the child's motivations and interests. In general, your goal should be to strive for as "normal" a life experience as possible. Keep in mind that there will still be challenges and that it will be appropriate to think about treatment and education continuing even when formal schooling comes to an end. For higher functioning individuals, college and university attendance may be an option. Particularly for very bright individuals with Asperger's disorder, there may be a tendency to look at the most academically prestigious institutions. Keep in mind, however, that it often isn't the academics that are the challenge. Rather, it is the social and self-care skills which will limit the child's options. Often smaller liberal arts schools, particularly those which have developed programs for students with learning disabilities, may be your best bet if college is an option. For other students, vocational counseling can begin in high school with the aim of helping your child find a job that will be a good fit for her. The Reading List has some resources that may be helpful to you.

In closing, we hope that you feel that you've gotten some helpful information from this book. Please feel free to share it, or parts of it, with your healthcare provider. Note that in the Reading List we've specifically flagged some reading that may be most helpful for your child's doctor or other healthcare provider. We wish you, your child, and your family the best in pursuing a healthy and productive future!

Fred Volkmar, MD
Lisa Wiesner, MD

Diagnostic Criteria for Pervasive Developmental Disorders

DSM-IV Criteria for Autistic Disorder

A. A total of at least six items from (1), (2), and (3), with at least two from (1), and one each from (2) and (3):

  (1) Qualitative impairment in social interaction, as manifested by at least two of the following:

   (a) marked impairment in the use of multiple nonverbal behaviors such as eye-to-eye gaze, facial expression, body postures, and gestures to regulate social interaction

   (b) failure to develop peer relationships appropriate to developmental level

   (c) a lack of spontaneous seeking to share enjoyment, interests, or achievements with other people (e.g., by a lack of showing, bringing, or pointing out objects of interest to other people)

   (d) lack of social or emotional reciprocity

  (2) Qualitative impairments in communication as manifested by at least one of the following:

   (a) delay in, or total lack of, the development of spoken language (not accompanied by an attempt to compensate through alternative modes of communication, such as gestures or mime)

   (b) in individuals with adequate speech, marked impairment in the ability to initiate or sustain a conversation with others

   (c) stereotyped and repetitive use of language or idiosyncratic language

   (d) lack of varied spontaneous make-believe play or social imitative play appropriate to developmental level

  (3) Restricted repetitive and stereotyped patterns of behavior, interests, and activities, as manifested by at least one of the following:

   (a) encompassing preoccupation with one or more stereotyped and restricted patterns of interest that are abnormal either in intensity or focus

   (b) apparently compulsive adherence to specific, nonfunctional routines or rituals

   (c) stereotyped and repetitive motor mannerisms (e.g., hand or finger flapping or twisting, or complex whole body movements)

   (d) persistent preoccupation with parts of objects

B. Delays or abnormal functioning in at least one of the following areas, with onset prior to age three: (1) social interaction, (2) language as used in social communication, or (3) symbolic or imaginative play.

C. Not better accounted for by Rett's disorder or childhood disintegrative disorder.

DSM-IV Criteria for Childhood Disintegrative Disorder

A. Apparently normal development for at least the first two years, as manifested by the presence of age-appropriate verbal and nonverbal communication, social relationships, play, and adaptive behavior.

B. Clinically significant loss of previously acquired skills in at least two of the following areas:
    (1) expressive or receptive language
    (2) social skills or receptive language
    (3) bowel or bladder control
    (4) play
    (5) motor skills

C. Abnormalities of functioning in at least two of the following areas:
    (1) qualitative impairment in social interaction (e.g., impairment in nonverbal behaviors, failure to develop peer relationships, lack of social or emotional reciprocity);
    (2) qualitative impairments in communication (e.g., delay or lack of spoken language, inability to initiate or sustain a conversation, stereotyped and repetitive use of language, lack of varied make-believe play);
    (3) restricted repetitive and stereotyped patterns of behavior, interests and activities, including motor stereotypies and mannerisms.

D. Not better accounted for by another specific Pervasive Developmental Disorder or by Schizophrenia.

DSM-IV Criteria for Rett's Disorder

A. All of the following:
- (1) apparently normal prenatal and perinatal development
- (2) apparently normal psychomotor development through the first six months
- (3) normal head circumference at birth

B. Onset of all of the following between 5 and 48 months:
- (1) deceleration of head growth
- (2) loss of previously acquired purposeful hand movements, with the development of stereotyped hand movements (e.g., handwringing or handwashing)
- (3) loss of social engagement early in the course (although often social interaction develops later)
- (4) appearance of poorly coordinated gait or trunk movements
- (5) marked delays and impairment of expressive and receptive language with severe psychomotor retardation

Reprinted with permission from the *Diagnostic and Statistical Manual of Mental Disorders,* Text Revision, Copyright 2000 American Psychiatric Association.

DSM-IV Criteria for Asperger's Disorder

A. Qualitative impairment in social interaction of the type described for autism

B. Restricted, repetitive, and stereotyped patterns of behavior, interests, and activities of the type described for autism

C. Lack of any clinically significant general delay in language (e.g., single words used by age two, communicative phrases used by age three).

D. Lack of any clinically significant delay in cognitive development, as manifested by the development of age-appropriate self-help skills, adaptive behavior (other than in social interaction), and curiosity about the environment.

E. Does not meet criteria for another specific Pervasive Developmental Disorder.

Reprinted with permission from the *Diagnostic and Statistical Manual of Mental Disorders,* Text Revision, Copyright 2000 American Psychiatric Association.

Diagnosis of PDD-NOS

This category should be used when there is a severe and pervasive impairment in the development of reciprocal social interaction associated with impairment in either verbal and nonverbal communication skills, or with the presence of stereotyped behavior, interests, and activities, but the criteria are not met for a specific Pervasive Developmental Disorder, Schizophrenia, Schizotypal Personality Disorder, or Avoidant Personality Disorder. For example, this category includes "atypical autism"—presentations that do not meet the criteria for Autistic Disorder because of late age at onset, atypical symptomatology, or subthreshold symptomatology, or all of these.

B | Dealing with Insurance

The current crisis in the American health insurance system has had a negative impact on the quality, and, for that matter, on the quantity, of care provided to individuals with all kinds of disabilities. Unfortunately, despite the considerable hype in advertisements about various insurance and HMO programs (all of which seem to emphasize the word "care"), caring is often minimally available. Unless parents and others act as strong advocates for obtaining quality care, such care often is neither available nor provided.

In considering insurance plans, you should look at what the plan will provide in terms of continued care for developmental disorders, as well as for so-called "preexisting" conditions. Sometimes parents discover that insurance companies stop providing care when they switch insurance plans because the new insurance company claims their child was born with autism and had a "preexisting" condition. Another unfortunate tactic that insurance companies use is to try to avoid paying for ancillary but important services such as occupational or physical therapy or speech/language services; they may say these are provided only by the schools and not by the insurance company, which may attempt to limit access to more specialized care providers. This is unfortunate, because even when primary care providers are very interested in providing care, they often need the option of asking experienced specialists for help when problems arise.

As with anything else, if you do more homework in selecting an insurance plan you are much more likely to be satisfied with it. In the past, there were relatively few options available and most provided about the same kinds and levels of coverage. This is no longer the case. There are now many plans to choose from—in some ways, too many. Complexities with insurance arise because of understandable efforts on the part of both the government and the insurance industry to save money by making insurance plans efficient and cost-effective. Unfortunately, the effort to save money also means that insurance companies may not be as interested in covering individuals with chronic problems.

In selecting insurance, you can easily feel overwhelmed by the range of choices. Given that in most situations you are selecting a program that everyone in the family must use, you have to consider everyone's needs. Therefore you will have to keep in mind many factors. Relative to your child with ASD, it is very important to realize that often life is lived "in the fine print." That is, you should be very careful to read all the aspects of descriptions of the programs. You have to be educated as a responsible consumer for your child. Do not be afraid to ask questions. You have to remember the level of needs that your child has in terms of medical care, as well as the potential for additional needs in the future. Sometimes what seems like a great option in terms of low-cost medical care does not, in fact, seem so great in reality when you have to spend hours on the phone arguing with the insurance company over obtaining basic services.

Kinds of Insurance

Several different kinds of health insurance plans are now available. These include health maintenance organizations (HMOs), fee-for-service insurance plans, preferred provider plans (PPOs), government sponsored programs, and self-insurance.

Health Maintenance Organizations (HMOs)

The basic idea of an HMO is that you (and/or your employer) pay a certain amount (the premium) each month for a specified range of services. Essentially you are paying in advance for the services regardless of whether you use them or not. The idea of these "prepaid" programs is that the costs of all the various participants will average out over the month. One great advantage of these programs is that, in theory, you should not see another bill for medical services, having paid your monthly fee. Some plans, however, charge an out-of-pocket co-pay for certain services and/or for prescription medications.

An HMO offers several advantages. It is, at least in theory, comprehensive with a panel of possible caregivers, and it centralizes care and the finances. Having a centralized medical record can be a great help, as is having a primary healthcare provider who knows you and your child well. Another great advantage of the HMO is that preventive care such as regular check-ups is well covered. This offers many advantages for parents of children with autism, as it gives you and your child time to get to know the doctors and staff in situations where your child is not acutely ill. This will help your child be more comfortable in seeing the doctor at times when she is not feeling well. HMOs are often somewhat less expensive than other plans. The HMOs do, however, have some limitations.

Problems with HMOs arise due to the basic structure of this form of health insurance. Given that healthcare is centralized within a specific system, you usually can only see doctors and other healthcare providers who are part of the HMO. Sometimes this is not a problem, as there may be many doctors on the staff to choose from, including some who have experience in caring for children with autism and related conditions. However, in some plans there may not be any people who know much about the problems of children with ASD, or, for that matter, children with developmental difficulties. This can be a complication when you need additional services. For example, you may be perfectly satisfied with your pediatrician, but not like the choices available to you for a neurologist, ear doctor, or psychiatrist. In such cases, you may be able to ask if you can use "outside" care providers (providers who are not part of the HMO), but you may not be entitled to do this and might have to pay out of your own pocket if you decided to use such a physician. Another disadvantage is that you cannot go to see a specialist, even within the network, without first getting a referral from your primary care provider. This can be a real hassle if your child has chronic medical problems, such as seizures, and often needs specialist care, or if you want to deal with a psychiatrist of your own choosing about medications.

You may also encounter problems if you want the HMO to cover related services, such as speech-language therapy or occupational therapy. The HMO may tell you that these services should be offered by your child's school or that such services are not covered by your plan since this is not what it regards as part of routine, regular medical care. Because the HMO can be a relatively "closed" system, it may be hard for care providers to have access to the most advanced specialists who know about autism and similar conditions.

If you choose to use an HMO, it will be important for you to do some research in advance. You should find out:

- Exactly what services are covered.
- Whether any of the primary care staff (pediatricians and family care providers) know much about autism or are willing to learn. This is one of the most important things to find out. Sometimes, particularly in rural areas, the HMO may not give many choices for your primary care provider.
- Whether they have any of the doctors who have special expertise with children with autism.
- Whether you can use specialists who are not part of the HMO.
- How referrals to other doctors are made.
- Whether the program has any special exclusions that are relevant to your child. The HMO may decide not to let you enroll if it is aware that your child has a chronic disability.
- What the total cost to you will be. It is important that you look not only at the upfront cost (your monthly premium), but also the hidden costs (the money you may have to pay for services that are not covered by the HMO). For example, costs to you for outside specialists or prescription drugs or for a psychiatrist or child psychiatrist to talk with you about medications for behavioral problems.

You should also know that some programs, called combination programs, have features both of the HMO type plan and more traditional insurance programs; in some cases, these may be particularly good choices for your child. In addition, many HMOs have a point-of-service (POS) option. This costs a higher premium and, perhaps, a higher co-pay per visit, but allows you to see experts not on the HMO panel—a great advantage.

Fee-for-Service Insurance Plans

Fee-for-service insurance plans are the "traditional" kinds of health insurance. For many years only such plans were available. These plans usually, but not always, give you greater flexibility in deciding what doctors (or hospital) you wish to use. This, in turn, may give you the greatest flexibility in finding a physician who has the greatest compatibility with you and your child.

With these plans, you pay for the service and then you are reimbursed by the insurance company or sometimes the insurance company gets the bill directly from the doctor. In either case, the doctor gets paid for the services provided. In contrast to the HMO, you may more often have to pay some costs out of pocket over and above the cost of the premium; this can include things like co-pays, deductibles, and some bills for services the plan doesn't necessarily cover. It is important to realize that "out of pocket" may not mean small change and that the costs can sometimes add up quickly. The definition of what is medically necessary can vary; sometimes it may refer only to acute care, and important aspects of routine care such as check-ups or hearing aids may not be covered. For children with developmental difficulties, the lack of coverage of such basic services can be a problem.

As with the HMO, it is important in selecting a traditional fee-for-service plan that you know exactly what your policy will actually cover. Look especially under the section of the policy called Limitations or Exclusions. You should never just assume that all the services your child will need will automatically be covered.

Traditional fee-for-service programs are often provided by group plans to members or employees. The thought is that like with the HMO there is strength in numbers and group plans have some advantages in terms of lower costs, given the larger number of persons covered. Co-payments may also be lower with such plans. One of the problems with group plans is the enrollment period. Sometimes you can only sign up for the plans at a certain period in time. At those times, you may not necessarily have to fill out a health history so that the insurer may not necessarily know that your child has a disability.

Traditional fee-for-service plans can also be purchased on an individual basis, i.e., for a person or family. This approach is often much more expensive than coverage provided by group plans.

Preferred Provider Organizations (PPOs)

A PPO is a variation on the HMO and is the fastest growing type of coverage in the United States. In this program, your employer or insurance company essentially makes a contract with a group of doctors or hospitals to provide care for you and your child. Often, these may be the same doctors or hospitals who participate with HMO plans administered by the same company (e.g., Blue Cross/Blue Shield may offer several HMO and PPO options in your region, and many of the same providers may participate in both plans). Typically, the hospital or doctor agree to take a reduced fee in return for the PPO sending more patients, and patients pay a predetermined co-pay (such as $10 to $30) for each visit. The monthly cost for these plans is often somewhere in between the cost for HMOs (on the low end) and traditional fee-for-service plans (on the high end).

The PPOs have many of the same advantages/disadvantages as the HMOs. A significant advantage for families of children with autism, however, is that you can go outside of the network and always get at least some coverage (such as 60 to 80% of the "usual and customary" amount). This is very useful if you want to go out of state or out of network to see autism experts. Also, you can usually refer yourself or your child to any specialist within the network without having to get permission from a "gatekeeper" first—this can be very useful if you want to set up an appointment fairly quickly with a specialist.

One disadvantage can be that doctors you have been seeing may drop out of the plan if they decide, for example, that they're not being compensated enough. Also, especially in large urban areas, good doctors may have full case loads and not be accepting new patients (this also can be a problem with HMOs). Again, you have to be very careful to read the fine print to be sure that the particular plan is going to meet your needs.

Public Insurance Programs

Various public programs provide healthcare coverage for families who cannot afford other insurance. Such programs are funded by the federal government, the government of the individual state, a pool of funds, or some combination of state, federal, and private insurers. These include Medicaid or what sometimes is called medical assistance or Title 19.

Medicaid. Medicaid is a program funded both by the state and the federal government. It provides medical care for individuals with low incomes, as well as individuals who are eligible for Supplemental Security Income (SSI) or who receive what is now called Temporary Assistance to Needy Families (TANF). If you are enrolled in a Medicaid program, you receive a card which you must show every time you visit your doctor or receive medications or other medical supplies. Since the mid 1990s, most states have administered Medicaid through managed care organizations.

A range of services are provided under Medicaid including both in- and outpatient hospitalization services, laboratory services, services from physicians and laboratories, and X-rays. Although states generally must make some services available to individuals within certain groups, there is some variation from state to state. Usually, the primary care provider must ask for authorization for more specialized services; the range of choices of such services may be more limited than for other kinds of insurance.

Sometimes, even if your income is a bit higher than would typically be allowed, you can still qualify for support through these programs, particularly if you have a child with a disability. This can also happen, for example, if large medical bills reduce your family's income. There may also be income waivers available for parents of children who are considered to have significant disabilities. Eligibility for such programs varies from state to state and it is important that you check the requirements in your state.

Medicare. Medicare is a federal government program that covers a range of medical services. It applies to individuals who are senior citizens (over age 65) and to some people with certain disabilities. Although Medicare and Medicaid have similar names, they are in fact very different programs.

Self-insurance Plans

Sometimes an employer may be large enough to set up its own insurance plan. These so-called self-insured programs may seem, in many cases, very similar either to HMOs or to private, traditional insurance plans. However, the kinds of services provided may not be as extensive as those provided by other kinds of programs. Sometimes states mandate certain benefits, but individuals in self-insured plans may not be given all the mandates available. Another problem with self-insured plans has to do with denial of benefits. With the traditional programs, PPOs, or HMOs, you often can file a complaint.

The complaint is dealt with at the state level by the agencies that regulate these programs. Because self-insured plans are private, filing a complaint is more complicated and you have to be very careful to understand what is entailed in filing a complaint or using the so-called appeals process before you make a decision.

State Children's Health Insurance Program (SHIP or CHIP)

This is a federally sponsored, state administered program, created in 1997 to provide healthcare subsidies to children whose families earn too much for Medicaid, but who cannot afford other health insurance. The majority of states accept children of families who earn 200 percent or more over the federal poverty level. Services are usually the equivalent of those provided by company insurances. Information can be obtained from your State Department of Social Services.

The rules for this program vary from state to state and you must check with your state to see whether you qualify. Usually the family pays premiums as in traditional programs, and, as with the traditional programs, there may also be deductibles, other kinds of co-payments, and various healthcare options. You can find contact information and links to your state's SHIP program at www.cms.hhs.gov/schip.

Becoming an Informed Consumer

We realize that you may not have much, or indeed, any choice of insurance policies. This may be particularly true if you work for a small business that only offers one policy, or you risk running into preexisting condition exclusions if you switch, or there are few choices of providers in the town or area where you live. If you do have some choice, however, do as much work as you can before selecting an insurance policy. If you use benefits provided by your employer, see exactly what plans are available. If both parents are employed, you may have even greater access to a range of choices in insurance.

Unfortunately, reading the description of an insurance plan, much less the policy itself, can be very confusing. Feel free to ask for help. For example, your employer may have an insurance office that can help answer your questions. If you are using a private insurance agent, this person can also answer many questions. Your current healthcare provider may be able to give you good information; parents of other special needs children, particularly if they also are employed by your company, can be good sources of information as well.

It is very important to educate yourself about what is covered so you will not have an unexpected surprise in discovering that the plan won't cover services your child needs. Be sure to understand exactly what is covered, what your deductibles and co-pays are, what the exclusions are. Be careful not to be misled by what appear to be lower deductibles. Sometime it will cost you more to have a plan that has a lower deductible than a higher one. This can be confusing because you think that in fact you are "getting a deal." In fact, the policy with the high deductible cost may be the least expensive in the long term.

Particularly if you are using a group insurance plan, you may not have easy access to the actual insurance policy or agreement between your employer and the insurance company. In this situation, what you often see is a fancy-looking brochure. Although this may be beautifully done and seem very reassuring, please remember that this brochure is not the policy and is not what is legally binding. Always ask to examine the actual insurance policy or contract and feel free to ask your employer's benefits office for help in understanding it.

In looking at the insurance policy, be careful to look at what is *not* covered (excluded services). These exclusions often include medications or certain medications and specific services, such as mental health services, and occupational or speech-language therapy. Check to see whether "preexisting conditions" are excluded. (Autism and related disorders are always going to be "preexisting," since you already know your child has a problem.) Sometimes there is a waiting period for so-called preexisting conditions. You might have to wait six months or sometimes even as much as a couple of years before you can receive reimbursement for some services.

Remember that insurance companies also must abide by the laws, which vary from state to state in terms of kinds of benefits that must be made available. Some states mandate certain services that must be available for children with autism. Look into other questions such as whether there is a cancellation provision to the policy. That is, can the insurance company decide to cancel your plan either for you as a group or for your individual child—for example, if you have too many expensive claims. Look to see whether there are rights of so-called conversion (meaning you can take a group policy and change it to an individual policy). This is important when your employer decides to change the group policy. It may be very difficult for your child to be enrolled in a new program, but it would then be important that you can continue the old policy as an individual policy.

There are some other things to check as well. Look to see what the maximum liability of the policy is. Sometimes insurance policies have a clause that states the total amount of money that the insurer will pay over the life of the child. This would be more of an issue if you are not able to switch easily to another policy once you use up the lifetime maximum on the first policy. Policies may also include a certain maximum amount for a year's coverage. Check to see whether there is so-called coordination of benefits. This applies when both a mother and a father receive different insurance programs through their occupations—sometimes you can get caught in the "cross fire" between the various insurance companies.

Dealing with Disputes

Sometimes, even when you have done all your homework, problems will arise. For example, you may discover that the doctor you have used for years does not participate in the plan you have just joined. Or you may discover that a private insurance program has changed its policy so that a previously approved service is no longer covered, or that the care provider you really wanted is no longer participating with the insurance plan. Sometimes you may want services that the insurance plan says are not covered but that you feel should be, either because you have read the policy or because you know that in your state such services are mandated, by law, to be covered.

When problems arise, keep in mind that a basic motivation of the insurance company is to make money and avoid spending it. You'll be in a stronger position to convince them that they have to spend the money if you have done your homework—both on the specific insurance policy and what is legally mandated in your state. Make sure you know the name of the office in your state which regulates insurance programs; this office can also help you know your rights and sometimes may be helpful in resolving problems with the insurance company. You can find links to state insurance departments on the website of the National Association of Insurance Commissioners at www.naic.org or you can contact the Help Desk at 816-783-8500 for help locating contact information for your state office.

Some insurance plans have specific ways for dealing with disputes that you can use. You may be able to call a patient representative or counselor or benefits coordinator—often, particularly if you are dealing with a large company or HMO, this will be the one person you can expect to be able to call on over time and who can help you deal with problems from within the system. Keep in mind, however, that a large insurance company may have a large staff with a fair amount of turnover. Always try to talk to the same person if you can, and, in any case, always keep a record of who you talked to.

The following are some of the principles that can guide you in resolving problems.

Be an effective advocate for your child: Always remember that you are your child's best advocate. You will know what your child needs and should not be shy in asking for it. While you should be assertive, try not to be angry or confrontational. Being assertive means you should be knowledgeable but also willing to listen. You should not be content to have a problem or complaint swallowed up in red tape.

Keep a record: Always keep a record of who you talked to and when, as well as what you were told. Keep in mind, however, that while you are keeping a record, the HMO or insurance company may as well—including a computer record each time you talk with someone at the company. Keep copies of any letters or other materials that support your request. Also keep copies of any information or correspondence from the insurance company. After you have a phone conversation, make a note to yourself or write a short letter that summarizes your discussion and send it to the insurance company or HMO (but keep a copy for yourself). It may be easiest if you keep a notebook and then put things in chronological order so you can easily find them.

Be prepared: You should know, in advance of talking with the company, exactly what you want and what the problem is. Be prepared ahead of this call with all the basic information such as policy number, the claim number, and so on. If you have any additional information that supports your request, be prepared to share it. For example, you might have additional supporting letters from doctors or copies of articles that support the use of the treatment you request.

Make good use of others: Particularly if you are using a group insurance plan, the insurance office in your company may be helpful in dealing with the insurance company. Your healthcare provider may also be very helpful. Sometimes the support of other parents or other individuals who have had experience within your organization with the same insurance program can also be helpful. Use parent advocacy groups at the local, state, and national levels as sources of information as well (see Resource Guide for some national resources).

Know the system and try to work with it: Know what your rights are within your state and within the insurance company. Try to move your dispute through the system as quickly as you can. Sometimes you will discover that the person you are talking to at the insurance company is not the person who will actually make the decision about your request—if this is so, ask to speak with the person really in charge. Also think about asking your child's doctor to write a letter or to offer to speak with the person in charge. If things seem to have stopped dead in their tracks, call or write again; sometimes the insurance company may hope that your complaint will "go away" if it takes its time responding to you.

What to do when the system doesn't work: Too many parents do not realize that they do have the right to file a complaint with the state. Usually, however, you will not want to file a complaint with the state insurance agency until you have used all your options in dealing with the insurance company or HMO. Similarly, you usually should not immediately think about a lawsuit. This is very expensive and there is no guarantee that you'll win in the end. However, for some parents there may be legal advocacy groups who could help you on a reduced fee basis.

Parents should carefully consider insurance plans and the special needs of their child when they consider relocating or changing jobs. Until the time that we have universal health care coverage in this country, such concerns should, unfortunately, be central in the minds of parents of children with autism spectrum disorders.

GLOSSARY

AAC: *See* Augmentative and Alternative Communication.

ABA: *See* Applied Behavior Analysis.

Abscess: An accumulation of pus, usually caused by an infection.

Absence Seizure: Once called a petit mal seizure, this type of *seizure* is characterized by blank staring and eye blinking.

Accommodation: An adaptation of the environment, format, or situation made to suit the needs of those participating.

Adaptive Behavior (Functioning): The ability to adjust to new environments, tasks, objects, and people, and to apply new skills to those situations; the capacity to meet the demands of daily life for personal self-sufficiency and independence.

Adenoids: Soft tissue in the upper part of the throat, behind the nose, that may become enlarged and contribute to problems with breathing or ear infections.

AD/HD: *See* Attention-Deficit/Hyperactivity Disorder.

Age Equivalent Score: The age (in years and months) that the child's performance would be typical of in the "normal" population. For example if the child's ability to understand words was an age equivalent of 2-10 this would mean it is the kind of score that an average 2-year 10-month-old child would achieve. This is not the same as *standard score*.

Allergy: A hypersensitivity to a specific substance which results in the immune system trying to defend the body against the substance, triggering adverse symptoms such as runny nose or itchy eyes and skin.

Amblyopia: Loss of vision in one eye due to the child's failure to use both eyes equally during the developmental period.

Anemia: A condition in which there are insufficient red blood cells in the bloodstream.

Anesthesia: A substance administered to reduce pain or consciousness and make a medical procedure more comfortable; local anesthesia reduces sensation in one part of the body, while general anestheisa produces complete loss of consciousness.

Anesthesiologist: A medical doctor who administers anesthesia.

Anticonvulsant: Medication used to control *seizures*.

Antihistamine: The type of drug most often used for treating allergies.

Anxiety: A feeling of unease, dread, fear, or "nervousness," which can be accompanied by physical symptoms such as increased heart rate or sweating. Some degree of anxiety may be normal (for example, in new situations), but when anxiety is irrational, excessive, or causes distress or impairment, it can be part of an *anxiety disorder.*

Anxiety Disorders: Psychiatric illnesses characterized by high levels of anxiety that cause distress or impairment to the individual. Types of anxiety disorders include phobias (fear of some specific thing), generalized anxiety disorder, panic disorder, and post traumatic stress disorder, among others.

Applied Behavior Analysis (ABA): A behavioral approach that uses researched-based, highly structured teaching procedures to develop skills in individuals. An emphasis is placed on modifying behavior in a precisely measurable manner using repeated trials. *See also* Discrete Trial Teaching; Behavior Management Plan.

Apraxia: A disorder that makes it difficult or impossible for an individual to plan and sequence movements needed to accomplish a task.

Asperger's Disorder: A *pervasive developmental disorder* characterized by early language and cognitive skills that seem relatively normal, but significant difficulties with social skills.

Aspiration: Breathing a substance (such as food or bacteria) into the lungs.

Assessment: The process used to determine a child's strengths and weaknesses. Includes testing and observations performed by a variety of professionals, including special educators, psychiatrists, psychologists, speech-language pathologists, etc. Also called evaluation.

Assistive Technology: A tool or device that increases, maintains, or improves the abilities of a child with disabilities to function. Examples include communication devices, computers, adapted pencil grips.

Asthma: A condition in which the airways in the lungs become inflamed and narrow often due to oversensitivity to a trigger (such as pollen, exercise, or smoke) that does not affect normal lungs.

"At Risk of Experiencing Developmental Delay": The term applied to children under the age of three who have not been formally diagnosed with a specific condition. This label may render them eligible for *special education* services.

Ataxia: Difficulty coordinating movements of the body, as in walking.

Atonic Seizure: A type of *seizure* causing sudden loss of muscle tone.

Attention: The ability to focus on and sustain concentration on a task. *See also* Attention Span.

Attention Deficit Disorder (ADD): A term sometimes used for a condition that does not include the *hyperactivity* found in *AD/HD*.

Attention-Deficit/Hyperactive Disorder (AD/HD): A condition characterized by distractibility, restlessness, short *attention span*, impulsivity, and *hyperactivity*.

Attention Span: The amount of time one is able to concentrate on a task.

Audiologist: A healthcare professional who evaluates hearing and prescribes assistive listening devices (such as hearing aids).

Auditory: Relating to the ability to hear.

Augmentative and Alternative Communication: Any method that assists or supplements speech and language (augmentative communication) or replaces speech as the primary communication system (alternative communication). Examples include sign language, picture cards, or electronic communication devices.

Aura: A sensation (such as a strange feeling or vague fear) that precedes some types of *seizures*.

Autism: A form of *pervasive developmental disorder* characterized by difficulties in social interaction and communication acquisition and use, as well as odd or unusual mannerisms, behaviors, and habits. *Mental retardation* is frequently present.

Autism Spectrum Disorder: Another term sometimes used for *Pervasive Developmental Disorders*.

Autistic Disorder: The "official" term for *autism* used in the *Diagnostic and Statistical Manual of Mental Disorders*.

Autistic-Like Behaviors: Behaviors that include verbal and physical *perseveration* and rituals, poor eye contact, and limited *social awareness*; sometimes seen in individuals with *developmental disorders* who do not have autism.

Avoidant Personality Disorder: A disorder characterized by long-standing feelings of social inhibition, oversensitivity, and feelings of social inadequacy. This condition is typically diagnosed in adults; as children, these individuals often are shy and become more so during adolescence.

Barium: A chemical used in tests of the digestive tract; typically the patient swallows a barium liquid or a piece of food coated in barium and X-rays are used to track the progress of the barium, which shows up as white on X-ray.

Behavior Management Plan: A plan designed to modify or reshape the behavior of an individual with *disabilities* that addresses existing behavior, *interventions*, support, and goals.

Bilirubin: A pigment formed by breakdown of hemoglobin and found in bile. High levels may indicate liver disease.

Biofeedback: A method used in teaching relaxation through which the individual learns to control heart rate or some other observable measure of anxiety.

Bipolar Disorder: The condition, formerly known as manic-depression, in which an individual experiences periods of *depression* and/or periods of more elated (even abnormally positive and excited) mood.

Birth to Three Program. A program that provides *early intervention*.

Bruxism: Grinding the teeth.

Cardiac: Related to the heart.

Case Manager: A person who coordinates services for individuals with *disabilities*. *See also* Service Coordinator.

Case Reports: Accounts of individual patients' responses to treatment; sometimes used as proof that a treatment works, but more properly regarded as an indication that the treatment may merit more formal research.

Casein: A substance found in milk and in products derived from milk.

CDD: *See* Childhood Disintegrative Disorder.

Celiac Disease: A disorder that results in sensitivity to *gluten* in food, and which results in damage to the lining of the small intestine if a gluten-free diet is not followed.

Cerebral Cortex: The outer layer of the brain, which is involved in sensory and motor functioning, as well as complex cognitive tasks.

Childhood Autism. *See* Autistic Disorder.

Childhood Disintegrative Disorder (CDD): A rare form of *pervasive developmental disorder* in which a child, who has developed typically in early childhood, begins to display *autistic-like* characteristics. His or her abilities are said to "deteriorate" from earlier, more capable behavior.

Childhood Schizophrenia: A psychiatric disorder with symptoms that include disturbances in form and content of thought, perception, emotions, sense of self, relationship to the external world, and other behaviors. Childhood schizophrenia is very rare.

Chromosomes: The microscopic rod-shaped bodies in the nucleus of cells which contain the *genes*. Unless they have a chromosomal disorder such as Down syndrome, people have twenty-three pairs of chromosomes in their cells.

Chronic: Long-lasting or permanent.

Cognition: The ability to know and understand the environment and to solve problems.

Comorbid: Related to two or more disorders occurring in the same individual.

Complex Partial Seizure: A type of seizure confined to one area of the brain which causes jerking or unusual movement in one part of the body and may eventually result in loss of consciousness.

Compulsions: Either repetitive behaviors (such as repeatedly checking that a door is closed) or thoughts (such as repeating words silently to oneself) which have the apparent goal of preventing or reducing anxiety; the person may feel that something bad will happen if they do not engage in the activity.

Computerized Tomography (CT) Scan: A diagnostic procedure in which a computerized picture of cross sections of the body is created by passing X-rays through the area that is being studied at various angles.

Conductive Hearing Loss: Hearing loss that results from a blockage in the middle ear or external ear canal (such as from fluid) which prevents or reduces transmission of sound to the inner ear.

Congenital: Present at birth.

Constipation: Infrequent or hard stools.

Controlled Substance: A medication specially regulated by the government because of its potential for abuse.

Convulsion: A *seizure*.

CPR: Cardio-pulmonary resuscitation; the process of attempting to restart someone's heart or breathing in an emergency by delivering a specific sequence of breaths to the mouth and compressions to the chest.

Decibel (dB): A unit of loudness used in assessing hearing; people with normal hearing can hear sounds that are 15-20 dB or softer.

Dehydration: The loss of excess amounts of body water.

Dementia Infantilis: An old term for *childhood disintegrative disorder.*

Development: The process of growth and learning during which a child acquires skills and abilities.

Developmental Delay: In children birth to eighteen, *development* that is significantly slower than average.

Developmental Disability: A condition originating before the age of eighteen that may be expected to continue indefinitely and that impairs or delays *development.* Such conditions include *autism, pervasive developmental disorders,* and *mental retardation.*

Developmental Evaluation: *See* Assessment.

Developmental Milestone: A goal that functions as a measurement of progress in development over time; for example, rolling over from back to front or speaking in two-word phrases.

Developmental Test: A test, usually given to preschool children, which assesses developmental skills in multiple areas—for example, gross and fine motor, language, and cognitive abilities.

Diabetes: A chronic disorder of carbohydrate metabolism that results in abnormally high sugar levels in the blood and sugar in the urine, excessive urination and thirst, and sometimes other symptoms. Type 1 diabetes results when the body produces little or no insulin (a hormone that regulates the metabolism of blood sugar) and must be treated with injections of insulin. Type 2 diabetes may develop due to obesity and can often be controlled through diet and medication.

Diagnostic and Statistical Manual of Mental Disorders (DSM IV): A manual published by the American Psychiatric Association that defines and describes the diagnostic criteria for mental disorders, and provides systematic descriptions of them.

Diarrhea: Abnormally watery or frequent bowel movements.

Dietitian: A professional with expertise in food and nutrition; registered dietitians have completed an internship and passed a national exam. (This is in contrast to a nutritionist, who does not have to meet any particular qualifications to use that title.)

Disability: A term used to describe a delay in physical or cognitive *development*. The older term, "handicap," is also sometimes used.

Discrete Trial Teaching: An instructional technique that is part of *Applied Behavior Analysis*. This technique involves four steps: 1) presenting a *cue* or *stimulus* to the learner; 2) obtaining the learner's response; 3) providing a positive consequence (reinforcer) or correction; and 4) a brief 3-5 second break until the next teaching trial is provided. *See* Applied Behavior Analysis.

Disintegrative Psychosis: Another term for *childhood disintegrative disorder.*

Dopamine: One of the *neurotransmitters* in the brain; it is presumed to play a major role in regulating movement.

Down Syndrome: A congenital disorder caused by the presence of an extra copy of the twenty-first chromosome; it is usually associated with some degree of mental retardation, low muscle tone, speech and language delay, and sometimes, *autistic-like behaviors.*

DSM IV: *See* Diagnostic and Statistical Manual of Mental Disorders (DSM IV).

Early Intervention: A specialized way of interacting with infants to minimize the effects of conditions that can delay early development. Early intervention may include services from an infant educator, a physical therapist, an occupational therapist, a speech-language pathologist, and/or other professionals with expertise in teaching developmental skills to very young children.

ECG: *See* Electrocardiogram.

Echolalia: A parrot-like repetition of phrases or words just heard (immediate echolalia), or heard hours, days, weeks, or even months before (delayed echolalia).

Eczema: Inflammation of the outer layer of skin, resulting in an itchy, scaly rash.

EEG: *See* Electroencephalogram.

EKG: *See* Electrocardiogram.

Electrocardiogram (ECG or EKG): A recording of the heart's electrical impulses. A painless procedure, it involves attaching electrodes to the individual's chest and other body parts and connecting them by wires to an electrocardiograph machine.

Electroencephalogram (EEG): The test used to determine levels of electrical discharge from nerve cells; used in diagnosing *seizures*.

Engagement: The ability to remain focused and interactive with (or responsive to) a person or object.

ENT: A physician who specializes in disorders of the ear, nose, and throat; also known as an otolaryngologist.

Epidemiology: The study of the incidence and distribution of diseases and other factors related to health.

Epilepsy: A recurrent condition in which abnormal electrical discharges in the brain cause *seizures*.

Epinephrine: Adrenaline—A hormone that is important to the body's metabolism and in helping the heart work and in relaxing muscles in the lungs.

Etiology: The study of the cause of disease.

Eustachian Tubes: Small tubes leading from the middle ears to the passageway behind the nose and throat area (the nasopharynx); these tubes regulate air pressure in the ears.

Evaluation: *See* Assessment.

Expressive Language: The use of gestures, words, and written symbols to communicate.

Family Physician: A physician who sees both adult and child patients.

Fever: An abnormal elevation of body temperature.

Fiber: The indigestible part of carbohydrates, essential to the digestive process.

Fine Motor: Relating to the use of the small muscles of the body, such as those in the hands, feet, fingers, and toes.

Folic Acid: A vitamin found naturally in leafy green vegetables, nuts, and organ meats that is important in the formation of red blood cells and in the production of DNA. Also called folate.

Fragile X Syndrome: A condition caused by a *mutation* in the *genetic* information on the X *chromosome*. (The X chromosome is one of the two so-called sex chromosomes; children with two X chromosomes are girls, and those with an X and a Y chromosome are boys.) Fragile X often causes *mental retardation* or learning disabilities, language difficulties, distinctive physical characteristics, and sometimes *autistic-like behaviors* or autism.

Free Appropriate Education: An education that is provided to a child without cost to the parents, and that is expected to provide some educational benefit to him.

Frequency: In audiology, a unit used to measure pitch (how high or low a sound is).

Functional Behavior Analysis: Observing a child's behavior and evaluating its purpose.

Generalization: Transferring a skill taught in one place or with one person to other places and people.

Genes: The microscopic sequences of protein and DNA found on the *chromosomes* which determine which traits an individual inherits from his parents.

Genetic: Inherited; relating to the genes.

Geneticist: A professional who evaluates people for genetic disorders and may provide counseling and information about these disorders.

GERD: Gastroesophageal reflux disease: a condition in which stomach acid and other stomach contents flow up into the esophagus and sometimes the mouth, damaging tissue and causing pain, vomiting, or other symptoms.

Gluten: A protein found in wheat, rye, barley, and other grains.

Grandiosity: A feeling that one is more powerful or important than one really is; sometimes a symptom of *bipolar disorder.*

Grand Mal Seizure. *See* Tonic Clonic Seizure.

Gross Motor: Related to the use of the large muscles of the body, such as those of the back, legs, and arms.

Guardian: A person appointed by law to manage the legal, medical, and/or financial affairs of someone else.

Hand Flapping/Hand Biting: *Perseverative* behaviors often seen in people with *developmental disorders.* These behaviors may be motivated by a *sensory* need, or a desire to focus and calm oneself or to escape from a demand.

Heimlich Maneuver: A procedure used to help someone who is choking by delivering a hard, upward thrust beneath their breast bone until the object that is causing the choking is dislodged.

Heller's Syndrome: An alternate (older) name for *Childhood Disintegrative Disorder.*

Hepatitis: An inflammation of the liver.

Hives: An itchy rash, usually caused by an allergic reaction.

Homeopathic: Related to homeopathy—the theory that diseases can be cured by giving very small doses of drugs that cause symptoms of the disease you are trying to cure.

Hormone: A chemical produced by an organ or gland in the body that is released into the bloodstream and affects activity elsewhere in the body.

Hyperactivity: A nervous-system-based difficulty that makes it hard for a person to control *motor* (muscle) behavior. It is characterized by frequent movement, rapidly switching from one activity to another, or having difficulty remaining seated or controlling restless movements.

Hypotonia: Low (reduced) muscle tone; muscles feel "floppier" than usual, and it takes more effort to initiate movement and maintain posture.

ICD: The *International Classification of Diseases*; the manual used in place of the DSM in countries other than the U.S. for diagnosing medical disorders.

IDEA: *See* Individuals with Disabilities Education Act.

Identification: The determination that a child should be evaluated as a possible candidate for *special education* services.

IEP: *See* Individualized Education Program.

IFSP: *See* Individualized Family Service Plan.

Imitation: The ability to observe the actions of others and to copy them in one's own actions. Also known as modeling.

Immunization: The process of inducing protection against an infectious disease by administering a *vaccine*.

Impetigo: A contagious, bacterial skin infection characterized by reddened skin that can blister and fill with pus.

Impulsivity: Behavior that is characterized by acting without thinking through the consequences of one's actions.

Inclusion: Placing children with *disabilities* in the same schools and classrooms with children who are developing typically. The environment includes the special supports and services necessary for educational success.

Individualized Education Program (IEP): The written plan that specifies the special education and other services (such as occupational or speech therapy) the school has agreed to provide a child with *disabilities* who is eligible under *IDEA*; for children ages three to twenty-one.

Individualized Family Service Plan (IFSP): The written plan that specifies the education and *related services* to be provided to children eligible for *early intervention* under *IDEA* and their families; for children birth to age three.

Individuals with Disabilities Education Act (IDEA): A federal law originally passed in 1975 and subsequently amended that requires states to provide a *"free appropriate public education* in the *least restrictive environment"* to children with *disabilities*. This is the major special education law in the U.S.

Infantile Autism: *See* Autistic Disorder.

Input: Information that a person receives through any of the senses (sight, hearing, touch, feeling, smell).

Insistence on Sameness: A tendency in many people with *autism* to become upset when familiar routines or environments are changed.

Instrument: A set of questions or activities administered to evaluate functioning; a test.

Intellectual Disability: An alternate term for *mental retardation.*

Intelligence: The ability to learn, think, and use knowledge to deal with problems.

Intelligence Test: A tests that examines various aspects of intelligence; commonly verbal (language related) and nonverbal (non-language related) tasks are examined. The score from an intelligence test is typically expressed as an *IQ.*

Intelligence Quotient (IQ): A numerical measurement of intellectual capacity that compares a person's chronological age to his or her "mental age," as shown on *standardized tests.* These scores are distributed on a bell-shaped curve, often with 100 being average. IQ scores below 70 are in the mentally retarded range; above 130 in the gifted range.

Internist: A physician who specializes in internal medicine, or the diagnosis and non-surgical treatment of illnesses, particularly in adults.

Intervention: Action taken to improve a child's potential for success in compensating for a delay or deficit in their physical, emotional, or mental functioning.

In Utero: within the uterus or womb.

IQ: *See* Intelligence Quotient.

IV: This abbreviation for intravenous (in the vein) is often used as shorthand for "intra-venous catheter"—a means of delivering medication or nutrition straight into the blood-stream by inserting a thin tube into one of the patient's veins.

Ketogenic Diet: A diet that is high in fat and very low in protein and carbohydrates that is sometimes helpful in controlling *seizures.*

Landau-Kleffner Syndrome (LKS): A disorder that has some similarities to *childhood disintegrative disorder.* The child loses the ability to understand and use spoken language (after previously having normal abilities) and usually experiences seizures. Children with LKS may regain all or some of their language skills over time and become seizure free.

Language: A system of symbols (spoken, written, signed) used to communicate. *See* Expressive Language; Receptive Language.

Learning Disability: Learning difficulties in one or more specific areas of study (such as reading, spelling, or math) that are greater than would be expected based on the individual's overall *intelligence;* this contrasts with *mental retardation,* where abilities are significantly below average in all areas. (To make matters confusing, in some coun-tries such as England, the preferred term for mental retardation is learning disability.)

Least Restrictive Environment (LRE): The educational setting that enables a child with disabilities to have the maximum contact with typically developing children while allowing him to make appropriate progress in the curriuculum.

Magnetic Resonance Imaging (MRI): A computerized diagnostic procedure that involves creating cross-sectional images of the body or its organs by exposing the patient to a magnetic field. No radiation is used.

Malnutrition: Nutritional intake that is insufficient to promote or maintain growth and *development*.

Malocclusion: An abnormal relationship between the upper and lower jaw, resulting in a faulty bite (e.g., underbite, overbite).

Mannerisms: Repetitive, seemingly purposeless movements or sounds; *stereotyped behavior*.

Medicaid: A joint state and federal program that offers medical assistance to people who are financially needy and are therefore entitled to receive *SSI*.

Medicare: A federal program, not based on financial need, that provides payments for medical care to people who are receiving Social Security payments.

Megadose Vitamin Therapy: Using vitamins in dosages that are at least ten times the recommended daily allowance.

Mental Age: *See* Age Equivalent Score.

Mental Retardation (MR): The term used in the U.S. to describe people who score in the lowest three percentiles on cognitive assessment tests (generally 70 or below) and who also have significant difficulties with *adaptive behavior*. May also be referred to as intellectual disability.

Mercury: A heavy, silver metal that is liquid at room temperature; in the past, used in some preservatives for *vaccines*.

Mixed Hearing Loss: Hearing loss resulting from both *conductive hearing loss* and *sensorineural hearing loss*.

MMR: The abbreviation for the measles, mumps, and rubella *vaccine*.

Modeling: *See* Imitation.

Motor: Relating to the ability to use muscles to move one's body parts.

Muscle Tone: The degree of stretch or relaxation in a resting muscle. *See also* Hypotonia.

Mutation: A change or alteration in *genetic* information.

Myoclonic Seizure: A *seizure* that produces brief, involuntary jerking of muscles.

Naturopathic: Referring to "natural" treatment with sunshine, water, exercise, or other naturally occurring agents; without drugs.

Nebulizer: A device used in the treatment of asthma that produces a medicated mist to be inhaled.

Negative Reinforcement: Any situation or stimulus whose removal or avoidance increases a specific response. For example, typically developing children display good behaviors in the classroom so as to avoid the teacher's disapproval.

Neuroleptic: A group of medicines (sometimes referred to as major tranquilizers) that act on various chemical systems in the brain—particularly those involving the *neurotransmitter dopamine*.

Neurologist: A physician specializing in medical problems associated with the brain and nervous system.

Neurotransmitter: A chemical substance in the brain that allows the transmission of impulses from one nerve cell to another. Abnormal levels of neurotransmitters may result in difficulties with mood, attention, impulse control, etc. *See* Dopamine; Norepinephrine; Serotonin.

Nonverbal Learning Disability: A pattern of strengths and weaknesses that includes relatively better verbal abilities than nonverbal abilities (which can be quite impaired), as well as difficulties with social skills and motor skills. NVLD appears to be common in individuals with Asperger's disorder, but is not synonymous with Asperger's disorder.

Norepinephrine: A *neurotransmitter* that plays a role in maintaining blood pressure and also in regulating various behaviors. Also known as noradrenaline.

Nurse Practitioner: A registered nurse who has additional training in medical practices and therapies.

Obesity: Weight that is 120 percent or more of the desired body weight for height. For example, if the desired body weight for height is 100 pounds and a child weighs 120 pounds or more, he is obese.

Obsessive Compulsive Disorder (OCD): A disorder that causes *anxiety* due to abnormal recurring thoughts or images (e.g., fear that the door is unlocked) which the individual can only dispel by performing a specific act (e.g., repeatedly checking to make sure the door is locked).

Occupational Therapist (OT): A therapist who specializes in improving the *development* of *fine motor* and adaptive skills.

Ophthalmologist: A physician who specializes in diagnosing and treating eye and vision problems; ophthalmologists can perform surgery and prescribe medications, as well as prescribe corrective lenses.

Opiate Antagonist: A medicine the reverses the effects of opiate drugs.

Optometrist: A specialist in diagnosing and nonmedical treatment (e.g., with prescription lenses) of vision problems.

Oral Motor Skills: Skills involving muscles in and around the mouth, including chewing, swallowing, and forming speech sounds.

Orthodontist: A dentist who specializes in diagnosing, preventing, and treating irregularities of the teeth and jaw.

OT: *See* Occupational Therapist.

Otitis Media: An inflammation or infection of the middle ear.

Otolaryngologist: A physician specializing in the ear, nose, and throat; also known as an ENT.

Otoscope: A lighted instrument that is inserted in the outer ear to examine the ear canal and eardrum.

Paradoxical Reaction: The opposite reaction than would typically be expected.

PDD: *See* Pervasive Developmental Disorder.

PDD-NOS: *See* Pervasive Developmental Disorder-Not Otherwise Specified.

Pediatrician: A physician who specializes in the care of infants, children, and adolescents.

Perineum: In females, the area between the anus and the vagina, and in males, the area between the anus and the scrotum.

Perseveration: Seemingly purposeless, repetitive movement or speech that is thought to be motivated by a person's inner preoccupations.

Pervasive Developmental Disorder (PDD): An umbrella category in the *DSM* for a range of conditions that can include symptoms such as difficulties with communication and social skills, unusual interests or habits, and *insistence on sameness*. The PDDs are: *autistic disorder, Asperger's disorder, PDD-NOS, Rett's disorder,* and *childhood disintegrative disorder.* The term may be used synonymously with a*utism spectrum disorder.*

Pervasive Developmental Disorder-Not Otherwise Specified (PDD-NOS): A *pervasive developmental disorder* that includes most characteristics of a*utistic disorder* but not enough to meet the specific diagnostic criteria for a*utistic* d*isorder.*

Pervasive Lack of Relatedness: A condition characterized by an individual's extreme difficulty relating to objects or people in a typical or appropriate fashion.

Petit Mal Seizure: *See* Absence seizure.

Physical Therapist (PT): A therapist who specializes in improving the development of *gross motor* skills.

Pica: The eating of nonfood substances.

Placebo: A "dummy" medication or treatment used as a control in testing another medication or treatment in order to see whether the "real" treatment is more effective than no treatment.

Placebo Effect: The tendency of patients who are receiving a *placebo* to feel better or to be perceived as doing better when they are participating in a new treatment or study.

Play Therapy: A diagnostic and treatment method sometimes used by child psychologists in which the child is encouraged to play or draw as a means of expressing his thoughts or feelings.

Positive Reinforcement: Providing a pleasant consequence after a behavior in order to maintain or increase the frequency of that behavior.

Potency: Strength, as of a medication.

Pragmatics: The use of language for social communication. Includes requesting, protesting, commenting, sharing information, and the knowledge of the "rules" governing conversation.

Pressure Equalizing Tubes: Tiny tubes inserted into the eardrums to allow fluid to drain from the middle ear; sometimes referred to as grommets.

Prompt: Input such as physical guidance or a verbal or visual reminder that encourages an individual to perform a movement or activity.

Prompt Dependence: When an individual requires a *prompt* in order to perform a taught task or behavior.

Proprioception: The body's innate sense of its position in space.

Psychiatrist: A medical doctor who diagnoses and treats mental illness; in contrast to a psychologist, he or she may prescribe medications in treatment.

Psychological Assessment: An assessment of various abilities, often including intelligence, adaptive skills, visual-motor skills, attentional skills, and other skills.

Psychologist: A professional who specializes in the study of human behavior and treatment of behavioral disorders and administers tests (e.g., of intelligence).

Psychosis: A mental disorder that alters an individual's understanding of reality, and may include delusions, hallucinations, or disturbed thought processes.

Psychotherapy: Treatment of mental disorders such as anxiety through psychological means (such as counseling and talking).

Psychotropic Medications: Medications that alter brain function. Psychotropic drugs are often used in the treatment of mental illness and sometimes for certain autistic behaviors.

PT: *See* Physical Therapist.

Puberty: The stage of physical development at which sexual reproduction first becomes possible.

Reactive Attachment Disorder: A disorder that develops in infants and young children as the result of emotional or physical neglect or abuse; children with the disorder have social skills delays and difficulty bonding with others.

Receptive Language: The ability to understand spoken and written communication as well as gestures.

Reflex: An involuntary, unlearned response to a stimulus.

Refractive Error: An inability of the eye to sharply focus images due to problems with the length of the eyeball, the shape of the cornea, or the power of the lens; nearsightedness and farsightedness are examples of refractive errors.

Regression: The loss of skill or ability.

Reinforcement: Any consequence that increases the likelihood of the future occurrence of a behavior. A consequence is either presented or withheld in an effort to prompt the desired response. *See* Positive Reinforcement; Negative Reinforcement.

Related Services: Services that enable a child to benefit from *special education*. Related services include speech-language, occupational, and physical therapies, as well as transportation.

Reliability: In psychological testing, the degree to which a test produces about the same results each time a particular individual is administered that test.

Repetitive Speech: Also called *echolalia*. *See also* Perseveration.

Rett's Disorder: A rare *pervasive developmental disorder* that affects mostly females, is characterized by typical early development, and later, a pervasive loss of social, cognitive, and physical skills. Some improvement in these areas may take place in late childhood. Many children with Rett's disorder develop *seizure* disorders.

Rigidity: Inflexibility of behavior; needing things to happen in a very specific way in order for them to "feel right" to the child.

Ritualistic Behavior: Seemingly purposeless behavior that a child always engages in when in a particular situation. For example, on entering a room, a child may always have to turn the lights off and on twice.

Rubella: German measles; a disease that causes a mild rash in adults but that can lead to birth defects if a woman contracts it while pregnant.

Rumination: Regurgitating food and chewing on it again.
Schizophrenia. *See* Childhood Schizophrenia.

Schizotypal Personality Disorder: A personality disorder (usually seen in adults) in which there is discomfort with close personal relationships and often eccentric behavior. Odd beliefs and thinking may be present. This is sometimes confused with *Asperger's disorder.*

Scoliosis: Abnormal curvature of the spine.

Screening Test: A test given to groups of children intended to determine which children need further *assessment.*

Secretin: A naturally occurring hormone that aids in digestion; some people have theorized that a deficiency of secretin plays a role in causing symptoms of autism.

Sedation: The process of reducing anxiety, nervousness, or wakefulness with medication; it may or may not involve loss of consciousness.

Seizure: A change in consciousness or behavior or involuntary movement produced by abnormal electrical discharges in nerve cells in the brain.

Selective Mutism: A disorder characterized by failure to speak in specific situations despite speaking in other situations.

Selective Serotonin Reuptake Inhibitor (SSRI): A medication used for treating depression or anxiety that works by preventing *serotonin* produced in the brain from being reabsorbed quickly, thus increasing the amount of serotonin available in the brain.

Self-Regulation: The capacity to remain organized in the face of external or internal stimulation.

Self-Stimulation: The act of providing physical, visual, or auditory stimulation for oneself; rocking back and forth and *hand flapping* are examples.

Sensorineural Hearing Loss: Hearing loss caused by damage to the inner ear or to the auditory nerve, which transmits sounds to the brain.

Sensory: Relating to the senses.

Sensory Integration: The ability to receive *input* from the senses, to organize it into a meaningful message, and to act on it.

Serotonin: A neurotransmitter that is believed to play a role in mood regulation and sleep; levels of serotonin may be deficient in children who have depression or anxiety.

Service Coordinator: The individual designated to oversee the education and *related services* for a child with *disabilities* and the services provided to his or her family. *See also* Case Manager.

Side Effect: An effect which results unintentionally from the administration of medication; manifestations of side effects from medication vary from person to person.

Simple Partial Seizure: A type of *seizure* causing involuntary jerking of muscles that does not result in the loss of consciousness.

SLP: *See* Speech-Language Pathologist.

Social Security Administration (SSA): The federal agency that administers both *SSI* and *SSDI*.

Social Security Disability Insurance (SSDI): Money that has been funneled into the Social Security system through payroll deductions on earnings. Workers who are disabled are entitled to these benefits. People who are born or become disabled before the age of twenty-two may collect SSDI under a parent's account if the parent is retired, disabled, or deceased.

Social Skills: Learned abilities such as sharing, turn-taking, asserting one's independence, and forming attachments, that allow people to effectively interact with others.

Social Worker: A professional who aids and counsels others to function within society; he or she may help to secure services such as counseling, financial assistance, or respite care.

Special Education: Specialized instruction to address a student's unique educational *disabilities* as determined by an *assessment* and as specified in a child's *IEP.* Instruction must be precisely matched to the child's educational needs and adapted to his or her learning style.

Speech/Language Pathologist: A therapist who works to evaluate and improve speech and *language* skills, as well as to improve *oral motor* abilities.

SSA: *See* Social Security Administration.

SSDI: *See* Social Security Disability Insurance.

SSI: *See* Supplemental Security Income.

SSRI: *See* Selective Serotonin Reuptake Inhibitor.

Standard Deviation: A measurement of the degree to which a given test score differs from the mean (average) score. On many IQ tests, for example, the mean or average score is 100 and the standard deviation is 15 (so a child who scored one standard deviation below the mean would have an IQ of 85). The majority of children (94 percent) score within two standard deviations (30 points) above or below the mean of 100 (between 70 and130).

Standard Score: A test score based on the normal distribution curve (the "bell curve"). In tests scored with standard scores, 100 usually is considered exactly average, with scores from 85 to 115 considered to be in the average range.

Standardized Test: A test that is administered in exactly the same way each time and that is designed so that results can be compared with the performance of other individuals who have taken the test.

Statistical Significance: An estimate of the likelihood that an observed result is not simply due to chance; the usual level of statistical significance (probability of or less than 5%) means that there is 1 chance in 20 that the event would have happened as a result of chance alone.

Status Epilepticus: A life-threatening condition in which *seizures* continue without a break for many minutes and the child remains unconscious.

Stereotypic Behavior: Purposeless, repetitive movements or behaviors such as hand flapping.

Stereotypy: *See* Stereotypic Behavior.

Stimulant: A *psychotropic* drug often used to control *hyperactivity* in children.

Stimulus: A physical object or environmental event that may trigger a response or have an effect upon the behavior of a person. Some stimuli are internal (earache pain), while others are external (a smile from a loved one).

Strabismus: A condition in which the two eyes do not work together; one or both eyes may turn inward or turn outward, or the gaze of one eye may be higher than the other.

Stridor: A crowing sound made when inhaling due to a narrowed upper airway.

Subthreshold: Not meeting full criteria (guidelines) for a diagnosis.

Supplemental Security Income (SSI): A program of payments available for eligible people who are disabled, blind, or elderly. SSI is based on financial need, not on past earnings.

Sustained Release: A long-lasting form of medication in which small amounts of the medication are released over time rather than releasing all of the medication immediately upon ingestion.

Swimmer's Ear: A painful infection of the outer ear; common in children who often go swimming.

Syndrome: A group of symptoms or traits that, occurring together, are characteristic of a particular disorder.

Tactile: Relating to touch.

Tactile Defensiveness: Oversensitivity or aversion to touch.

Tardive Dyskinesia: A condition characterized by involuntary jerky movements of the mouth, tongue, lips, and trunk. Some medications prescribed for behavior control may contribute to the development of this condition.

Thimerisol: A mercury-based substance formerly used to preserve some vaccines such as the *MMR*.

Tics: Involuntary, purposeless movements or sounds that occur, for example, in *Tourette syndrome*. Tics are usually distressing to a child who has them, in contrast to *stereotypic behavior,* which children with autism find pleasurable or neutral.

Tolerance: A diminished ability to benefit from some drug due to repeated or prolonged administration.

Tonic-Clonic Seizure: A type of seizure with two phases: a tonic phase, in which the body stiffens and the child loses consciousness; and a clonic phase, in which the muscles alternatingly jerk and relax.

Tonsils: The two masses of tissue on either side at the back of the throat that help defend the body from infection.

Tourette Syndrome: A *disability* characterized by vocal and movement *tics* that change in severity and nature over time.

Transition: The period between the end of one activity and the start of another.

Transitional Object: An object such as a blanket or stuffed animal that a young child habitually uses to comfort himself.

Tuberous Sclerosis: A congenital disorder in which benign tubers develop in the skin, organs, and brain, and which sometimes includes *seizures, autism,* and/or *mental retardation.*

Tympanometry: A test performed to measure the amount of pressure in the middle ear; abnormal pressure may indicate middle ear fluid or difficulties with Eustachian tube function.

Vaccine: A solution that is administered orally or as an injection in order to help the body create defenses against a specific disease. Vaccines contain bacteria or viruses (or parts of them) that ordinarily cause disease, but have been altered so that they won't cause an infection.

Vestibular: Pertaining to the *sensory* system located in the inner ear that allows the body to maintain balance and enjoyably participate in movement such as swinging and roughhousing.

Visual Imagery: Using recalled scenes or visual images in an attempt to relax or to tolerate more stressful situations.

Visual Motor: Related to the use of the eyes to discriminate and track objects and to perceive environmental *cues*. Visual *motor* skills are required to carry out tasks such as putting a puzzle piece into a puzzle or a key into a keyhole.

RESOURCE GUIDE

This section includes a small sampling of the many organizations and websites that can be helpful to families of children with autism spectrum disorders. The resources listed here were chosen because they can be especially useful in understanding healthcare issues related to autism. Bear in mind that there are also many other wonderful resources that we were not able to include due to space constraints. The authors do not necessarily endorse the views and services of these organizations.

Autism Spectrum Disorders

Asperger Syndrome Coalition of the United States
P.O. Box 351268
Jacksonville, FL 32235-1268
866-4-ASPRGR
www.asperger.org
A national nonprofit organization committed to providing up-to-date and comprehensive information on Asperger syndrome and related conditions. Offers articles as well as contact information for support groups that serve people with AS and related conditions and their families.

Asperger Syndrome Education Network (ASPEN®)
www.aspennj.org
info@AspenNJ.org
A regional nonprofit organization that provides general information to families and individuals whose lives are affected by Asperger's and related disabilities, and advocates for improved programs and services. Website includes many useful articles on AS, information on ongoing research, and a list of local support organizations across the U.S.

Autism Society of America
7910 Woodmont Ave., Ste. 300
Bethesda, MD 20814
301-657-0881; 800-328-8476
www.autism-society.org

A national organization of parents and professionals that promotes a better understanding of autism, encourages the development of services, supports autism-related research, and advocates on behalf of people with autism and their families. Has a national network of local chapters and acts as an information clearinghouse.

Autism Society Canada
P.O. Box 635
Fredericton, New Brunswick
Canada E3B 5B4
506-363-8815
www.autismsocietycanada.ca
A national nonprofit organization committed to advocacy, public education, information and referral and advocacy. Has links to provincial autism societies and information related to Canadians with autism.

Cure Autism Now (CAN)
5455 Wilshire Blvd., Ste. 715
Los Angeles, CA 90036
888-8AUTISM; 323-549-0500
www.canfoundation.org
A nonprofit organization dedicated to funding and promoting research with direct clinical implications for the treatment and cure of autism. Website includes links to information on ongoing clinical studies, research abstracts, news related to autism, and books and products.

International Rett Syndrome Association
9121 Piscataway Rd.
Clinton, MD 20735
800-888-RETT; 301-856-3334
www.rettsyndrome.org
The national organization for families affected by Rett syndrome. Provides information, referrals, encourages public awareness of the condition, and supports research.

National Alliance for Autism Research
99 Wall St., Research Park
Princeton, NJ 08540
888-777-NAAR (6227)
An alliance of families and researchers working to fund and accelerate autism research.

National Autistic Society (England)
393 City Rd.
London EC1V 1NG
United Kingdom

+44 (0)20 7833 2299

www.nas.org.uk

   The UK's foremost organization for people with autism and those who care about them. Organization can provide information on support groups for parents and siblings and "holiday facilities" specifically for young people with autism, and website offers information geared specifically to siblings as well as to parents. The affiliated Centre for Social and Communication Disorders can provide complete diagnostic and assessment services for individuals with ASDs.

Online Asperger Syndrome Information and Support

www.aspergersyndrome.org

   This website contains articles about specific issues (social skills, education, diagnosis, etc.) related to Asperger's disorder; links to products or other resources; message boards for parents, people with AS, and professionals; lists of private schools and camps, etc.

Yale Developmental Disabilities Clinic

http://info.med.yale.edu/chldstdy/autism

   Has information about PDDs and assessment, clinical and research programs, references, and many links to national and local autism resources.

Associated Disorders

The Arc

1010 Wayne Ave., Ste. 650

Silver Spring, MD 20910

301-565-3842

www.thearc.org

   A grassroots organization (formerly known as the Association for Retarded Citizens) that works to include all children and adults with cognitive and developmental disabilities in every community. Sponsors local chapters that provide support and offers a wide variety of publications on its web site.

Epilepsy Foundation of America

3231 Garden City Dr.

Landover, MD 20785

800-EFA-1000; 301-459-3700

www.efa.org

   The national organization for individuals with seizure disorders and their families. Provides information and referrals, supports research, and promotes awareness.

FRAXA Research Foundation

45 Pleasant St.

Newburyport, MA 01950
978-462-1866
www.fraxa.org
This organization funds research into finding a treatment or cure for fragile X syndrome. Website has helpful information and links.

LD OnLine
www.ldonline.org
A very comprehensive website that focuses on providing in-depth information about learning disabilities and AD/HD, but also has information of use to parents of children with any disability. Topics covered include assessment issues, special education, speech and language delays, social skills, processing disorders, nonverbal learning disabilities, and more.

National Fragile X Foundation
P.O. Box 190488
San Francisco, CA 94119
800-688-8765; 925-938-9300
www.nfxf.org
Provides information and support to families of children with fragile X, promotes awareness of fragile X syndrome, and encourages research. Website includes a great deal of useful information.

NLDline
www.nldline.com
An online source of information about nonverbal learning disorders; the site offers many articles on educating, raising, and recognizing children with NLD, as well as other topics of interest such as bullying, executive function, and Asperger's disorder.

NLD on the Web
www.nldontheweb.org
A comprehensive source of online information on nonverbal learning disabilities; articles cover the basics, assessment, educational issues, etc., with links to other sites of interest.

Nonverbal Learning Disorders Association
2446 Albany Ave.
West Hartford, CT 06117
860-570-0217
www.nlda.org
An international nonprofit organization that facilitates education, research, and advocacy for individuals with NLD. Hosts conferences, has a network of support groups, and a website with information and many useful links.

Tuberous Sclerosis Alliance
801 Roeder Rd., Ste. 750
Silver Spring, MD 20910
800-225-6872; 301-562-9890
www.tsalliance.org

The national organization for tuberous sclerosis; it funds research, promotes public awareness, operates a network of support groups, and produces on-line and print publications about tuberous sclerosis.

Tuberous Sclerosis Information Page
National Institute of Neurological Disorders and Stroke
www.ninds.nih.gov/health_and_medical/disorders/tuberous_sclerosis.htm

A web page about tuberous sclerosis that is periodically updated with new information and links.

General Healthcare Issues

American Academy of Child and Adolescent Psychiatry
3615 Wisconsin Ave. NW
Washington, DC
202-966-7300
www.aacap.org

This professional organization for child and adolescent psychiatrist offers a series of publications on mental health issues called "Facts for Families," which are available online or in print format. Website has a Referral Directory that allows you to search for a child psychiatrist by locality and specialty.

American Academy of Family Physicians
P.O. Box 11210
Shawnee Mission, KS 66207-1210
800-274-2237
www.aafp.org

The website of the American Academy of Family Physicians (a professional organization for family doctors) offers many helpful fact sheets on health topics, drugs, self-care, and healthy living, many of them available in Spanish as well as English. You can also search for a family doctor on the website.

American Academy of Ophthalmology
www.aao.org

The website of the American Academy of Ophthalmology has links to a number of patient education materials on eye problems and eye care, as well as an online database of ophthalmologists.

American Academy of Pediatrics

141 NW Point Blvd.
Elk Grove Village, IL 60007
847-434-4000
www.aap.org

The website of the American Academy of Pediatrics (a professional organization for pediatricians) allows you to search for pediatricians by location, and also offers a number of fact sheets on healthcare of children and adolescents. The AAP also publishes a number of books for parents.

American Dental Association

www.ada.org

The website of the ADA (a professional organization for dentists) allows you to search for dentists who belong to the ADA by specialty (such as pediatrics) and location.

MedicAlert® Foundation International

2323 Colorado Ave.
Turlock, CA 95382
800-432-5378
www.medicalert.org

Sells IDs (bracelets or medallions) engraved with an individual's medical condition and a toll-free number that healthcare professionals can call for information about the individual's health condition, medications, and allergies before emergency treatment; as part of the service, parents are notified if anyone calls the number on behalf of their child. Charges a fee to join and an annual membership fee.

MEDLINEplus

www.MedlinePlus.gov

A searchable database, geared to nonmedical professionals, of healthcare topics and news. From this site, you can click on "Other Resources" to link to MEDLINE, which includes many more articles, but is geared to healthcare professionals. Both MEDLINEplus and MEDLINE are services of the U.S. National Library of Medicine and the National Institutes of Health.

(To access MEDLINE directly, go to www.ncbi.nlm.nih.gov/pubmed.)

Medscape

www.medscape.com

A searchable database of articles that have appeared in professional medical journals and newsletters. On the Medscape website, you can also sign up to receive free weekly email newsletters on key medical news and clinical advances in pediatrics, psychiatry, or other areas (you designate the areas you are interested in).

National Association of Insurance Commissioners

816-783-8500

www.naic.org

The national organization for state insurance commissioners, the NAIC has resources for consumers such as tips on purchasing all types of insurance and avoiding fraud; the website has a link to state insurance department websites.

State Children's Health Insurance Program (SHIP)

Centers for Medicare and Medicaid Services
7500 Security Blvd.
Baltimore, MD 21244
877-267-2323; 410-786-2000
www.cms.hhs.gov/schip

SHIP is a health insurance program for children whose families cannot afford health insurance but earn too much to qualify for Medicare. Individual states have different criteria for qualifying. See website or contact the office for state contact information.

Dietary Concerns

American Dietetic Association

120 S. Riverside Plaza, Suite 2000
Chicago, IL 60606
800-877-1600
www.eatright.org

The largest national organization for food and nutrition professionals, the ADA offers a "Find a Nutrition Professional" link on its website, as well as many pages of nutrition information geared to consumers.

Celiac Disease Foundation

13251 Ventura Blvd., Ste. 1
Studio City, CA 91604
818-990-2354
www.celiac.org

Provides information and support for people with celiac disease and their families, supports research, publishes a newsletter.

Food Allergy and Anaphylaxis Network

10400 Eaton Place, Ste. 107
Fairfax, VA 22030
800-929-4040
www.foodallergy.org

Promotes public awareness and research into food allergies and offers online and print publications; will also send "allergy alerts" via email about products that are being recalled due to mislabeling or contamination.

Gluten Intolerance Group of North America
15110 10th Ave. SW, Ste. A
Seattle, WA 98166
206-246-6652
www.gluten.net

A nonprofit organization that offers information, support, and educational materials, sponsors a children's camp, and advocates for changes in legislation affecting people with gluten intolerance. Its "Quick Start Diet Guide for Celiac Disease" can be downloaded from the website.

Safety

Child Passenger Safety Website
www.nhtsa.dot.gov/people/injury/childps

This website, run by the National Highway Traffic Safety Administration, offers tips on properly installing car seats and booster seats, and rates many different models of car seats.

National Safe Kids Campaign
1301 Pennsylvania Ave. NW
Washington, DC 20004
202-662-0600
www.safekids.org

A national nonprofit organization dedicated to prevention of unintentional childhood injury. They offer tips on keeping kids safe around the home and in the community and information on products recalled because of safety hazards.

Other Useful Resources

American Occupational Therapy Association
4720 Montgomery Lane
P.O. Box 31220
Bethesda, MD 20824-1220
301-652-2682
www.aota.org

AOTA, the professional association for occupational therapists, has publications about OT and can refer you to an OT in your area.

American Speech-Language-Hearing Association (ASHA)
10801 Rockville Pike
Rockville, MD 20852
800-498-2071

www.asha.org

ASHA, the professional organization for speech-language pathologists, has information on therapy and speech and language issues and can refer you to an SLP or audiologist in your area.

Behavior Analyst Certification Board

519 E. Park Ave.
Tallahassee, FL 32301
www.bacb.com

Website provides details about credentials necessary to be certified as a behavior analyst and the organization can assist in locating a behavioral consultant.

Disability Resources, Inc.

www.disabilityresources.org

An extensive collection of links to information on many disabilities, including autism spectrum disorders, and to resources and support available in each state.

Family Village: A Global Community of Disability-Related Resources

www.familyvillage.wisc.edu

This website has a great deal of information about disability and the family, autism, and other disabilities, as well as links to other sites, online support groups, listservs, etc.

Sensory Integration International

P.O. Box 5339
Torrance, CA 90510
310-787-8805
www.sensoryint.com

This organization conducts research into sensory integration dysfunction, provides training for therapists, and offers information and publications as well as referrals to therapists.

Sensory Integration Network

www.sinetwork.org

This website posts resources about sensory integration, including links to research studies, frequently asked questions, equipment and treatment suggestions, and information about publications. It also allows you to search for an OT with expertise in working on SI problems.

TEACCH

www.teacch.com

Provides information on the TEAACH program (Treatment and Education of Autistic and Related Communication Handicapped Children), including excellent sources of information, reading lists, organizations and support groups, and an introduction to autism.

Computer-Based Assisted Learning Resources

Attainment Company
P.O. Box 930160
Verona, WI 53593-0160
800-327-4269
www.attainment-inc.com
> Life skills materials (board games, software).

Closing the Gap
526 Main St.
Henderson, MN 56044
507-248-3294
www.closingthegap.com
> Clearinghouse for information on computer-related technology for children with disabilities.

Inspiration Software, Inc.
www.inspiration.com
> Organizational software (including Kidspiration®) particularly helpful for children with organizational difficulties.

Intelli Tools®
1720 Corporate Circle
Petaluma, CA 94954
800-899-6687
www.intellitools.com
> Software and technology adaptations.

Don Johnston, Inc.
26799 W. Commerce Dr.
Volo, IL 60073
800-999-4660
www.donjohnston.com
> Reading and writing solutions (equipment and software) for children with disabilities.

Laureate Software
110 E. Spring St.
Winooski, VT 05404
800-562-6801
www.laureatelearning.com
> Educational software for children with disabilities.

This is a *selective* list of materials that parents and professionals may find helpful in learning more about the healthcare needs of individuals with autism spectrum disorders. It includes publications of a more technical nature that we referred to in writing this book, as well as publications written expressly for parents. An asterisk indicates materials that are highly recommended for parents; MD indicates works of greatest interest to healthcare providers.

General References

MDBatshaw, Mark, M.D. *Children with Disabilities*, 5th ed. Baltimore: Paul H. Brookes, 2002.
    This is a very well done medical book focused on developmental disabilities.

Bondy, Andy and Frost, Lori. *A Picture's Worth: PECS and Other Visual Communication Strategies in Autism.* Bethesda, MD: Woodbine House, 2001.
    An introduction to the steps involved in teaching a nonverbal child to use PECS to initiate communication with others.

*Cohen, D.J. and Volkmar, Fred R., M.D., Eds. *Handbook of Autism and Pervasive Developmental Disorders,* 2nd ed. New York, NY: John Wiley & Sons, 1997.
    This is a very comprehensive book (one of us is an editor) which may give you more information than you want (but some people prefer that rather than the reverse). This is being redone as a 3rd edition. Sections cover aspects of diagnosis, assessment, and treatment.

Dillon, Kathleen. *Living With Autism: The Parents' Stories.* Boone, NC: Parkway Publishing, 1995.
    After an introduction to autism, this book presents the family and parenting stories of several families with a child with autism.

Gray, Carol. *The New Social Story Book.* Arlington, TX: Future Horizons, 2000. (www.futurehorizons-autism.com)
    As we discuss, social stories can be very useful in helping to prepare a child with ASD for a medical procedure or to teach behavioral expectations. This book explains the rationale for using social stories and gives many examples.

*Harris, Sandra L. and Weiss, Mary Jane. *Right From the Start: Behavioral Intervention for Young Children with Autism.* Bethesda, MD: Woodbine House, 1998.
   An introductory guide, written for parents, to Applied Behavior Analysis and early intervention programs for young children. Clear explanations in easy-to-understand language.

Hyatt-Foley, D. and Foley, M. *Getting Services for Your Child on the Autism Spectrum.* London: Jessica Kingsley, 2002. (www.jkp.com).
   The book provides honest and practical advice, invaluable to anyone whose child is diagnosed with an ASD.

Kephart, Beth. *A Slant of Sun: One Child's Courage.* New York: Quill, 1999.
   A beautifully written account of a mother and her young son with autism. National Book Award Finalist.

McClannahan, Lynne E. and Krantz, Patricia J. *Activity Schedules for Children with Autism: Teaching Independent Behavior.* Bethesda, MD: Woodbine House, 1999.
   A concise guide to using activity schedules to help children with ASDs master sequences of behavior, such as brushing teeth or washing hands.

Naseef, Robert A. *Special Children, Challenged Parents: The Struggles and Rewards of Raising a Child with a Disability.* Baltimore, MD: Paul H. Brookes, 2001.
   Written by a psychologist, who is also the father of a child with autism, this book discusses the struggles and rewards for parents with a child with autism.

[MD]Ozonoff, Sally, Rogers, Sally J., and Hendren, Robert O. *Autism Spectrum Disorders: A Research Review for Practitioners.* Washington, DC: American Psychiatric Assn. Press, 2003.
   An excellent general introduction to autism of particular interest to general practitioners and pediatricians. Many outstanding chapters.

Park, Clara Claiborne. *The Siege: The First Eight Years of an Autistic Child with an Epilogue, Fifteen Years Later.* New York: Little, Brown, 1990.
   This is a classic account of a family's experiences raising a daughter with autism.

Volkmar, F. R., Ed. *Autism and Pervasive Developmental Disorders.* New York, NY: Cambridge University Press, 1998.
   Written for college students, this book provides a more detailed summary of work on diagnosis, genetics, treatment, and so forth.

Wheeler, Maria. *Toilet Training for Individuals with Autism and Related Disorders: A Comprehensive Guide for Parents and Teachers.* Arlington, TX: Future Horizons, 1998.
   Offers many suggestions in toilet training children with autism. Lots of advice and examples.

*Wing, Lorna. *The Autistic Spectrum: A Parent's Guide to Understanding and Helping Your Child*. Berkeley, CA: Ulysses Press, 2001.
> *An excellent introduction to autism and related conditions written by a professional who also is the parent of a child with autism. A really outstanding book.*

Chapter 1: Autism and Related Conditions: An Overview

Brill, M.T. *Keys to Parenting the Child with Autism*. 2nd ed., Hauppauge, NY: Barrons, 2001.
> *A concise but helpful summary with valuable information for parents.*

*Powers, Michael D., Ed. *Children with Autism: A Parent's Guide*, 2nd ed., Bethesda, MD: Woodbine House, 2000.
> *An excellent resource for parents. Highly readable and full of useful information on a range of issues.*

[MD]Rutter, Michael, Bailey, Anthony, Simonoff, Emily, and Pickes, Andrew. "Genetic Influences in Autism." In *Handbook for Autism and Pervasive Developmental Disorders*, 2nd ed. D.J. Cohen and F.R. Volkmar, M.D., Eds. New York: John Wiley & Sons, 1997.
> *Excellent summary of genetic research.*

*Siegel, Byrna. *The World of the Autistic Child: Understanding and Treating Autism Spectrum Disorders*. New York: Oxford University Press, 1998.
> *An excellent and helpful guidebook for parents with sections on understanding the causes of autism. A new edition is due out soon.*

Sigman, Marian and Capps, Lisa. *Children with Autism: A Developmental Perspective*. Boston: Harvard University Press, 1997.
> *An excellent summary of work on autism from two outstanding psychologists.*

Weber, Jayne Dixon. *Children with Fragile X Syndrome: A Parents' Guide*. Bethesda, MD: Woodbine House, 2000.
> *A well-written introduction to fragile X syndrome, written for parents and families.*

Chapter 2: Getting a Diagnosis

[MD]American Psychiatric Association. *Diagnostic and Statistical Manual of Mental Disorders (DSM-IV)*, 4th ed. Washington, DC: American Psychiatric Association, 1994.
> *This is the manual used for the diagnosis of all pervasive developmental disorders, including autism.*

Atwood, Tony. *Asperger's Syndrome: A Guide for Parents and Professionals*. London: Jessica Kingsley Publishers, 1997. (www.jkp.com).
This is an excellent book on Asperger's disorder. It addresses a number of issues including dealing with problem behaviors.

Bashe, Patricia Romanowski and Kirby, Barbara L. *The Oasis Guide to Asperger Syndrome*. New York: Crown Publishers, 2001.
Very good overview of Asperger's disorder.

MDFilipek, P. A., Accardo, P. J., Ashwal, S., Baranek, G. T., Cook, E. H., Jr., Dawson, G., et al. (2000). Practice Parameter: Screening and Diagnosis of Autism: Report of the Quality Standards Subcommittee of the American Academy of Neurology and the Child Neurology Society. *Neurology, 55*(4), 468-79.
A summary of current recommendations for physicians in screening for autism.

Howlin, Patricia. *Children with Autism and Asperger Syndrome: A Guide for Practitioners and Careers*. New York: John Wiley & Sons, 1998.
Excellent summary book.

Klin, Ami, Sparrow, Sara, and Volkmar, Fred. *Asperger's Disorder*. New York: Guilford Press, 2000.
Written primarily for teachers and professionals, there are good chapters on diagnosis and intervention.

Lord, Catherine. "Diagnostic Instruments in Autism Spectrum Disorders." In *Handbook of Autism and Pervasive Developmental Disorders*, 2nd ed., D.J. Cohen and F.R. Volkmar, M.D., Eds. New York: John Wiley & Sons, 1997, pp. 460-83.
Excellent review of checklists and rating scales designed to aid the diagnosis of autism.

*Powers, M.D. and Poland, J. *Asperger Syndrome and Your Child: A Parent's Guide*. New York: Harper Collins, 2003.
An excellent book for parents.

Sparrow, S. (1997). "Developmentally Based Assessments." In *Handbook of Autism and Pervasive Developmental Disorders,* 2nd ed., D. J. Cohen & F. R. Volkmar, Eds. New York: Wiley, pp. 411-47.
A helpful review of various assessments/tests.

Towbin, Kenneth. "Pervasive Developmental Disorder Not Otherwise Specified." In *Handbook of Autism and Pervasive Developmental Disorders*, 2nd ed., D.J. Cohen and F.R. Volkmar, M.D., Eds. New York: John Wiley & Sons, 1997, pp. 123-47.
Summary of work on PDD-NOS; one of the best resources for parents of a child with PDD-NOS.

Volkmar, Fred R., Klin, Ami, and Cohen, Donald J. "Diagnosis and Classification of Autism and Related Conditions." In *Handbook of Autism and Pervasive Developmental Disorders,* 2nd ed., D.J. Cohen and F.R. Volkmar, M.D., Eds., New York: John Wiley & Sons, 1997, pp. 5-40.
   Summary of current definitions of autism and related conditions.

MDVolkmar, Fred, Klin, Ami, and Pauls, David. (1998). Nosological and Genetic Aspects of Asperger's Syndrome. *Journal of Autism and Developmental Disorders, 28,* 457-63.
   Discusses genetics of Asperger's disorder as well as definition.

Chapter 3: Raising a Healthy Child with an Autism Spectrum Disorder

Baldwin, Ben. *The Complete Book of Insurance: The Consumer's Guide to Insuring Your Life, Health, Property, and Income.* Chicago: Irwin Professional Publishing, 1996.
   Written to help parents make informed decisions about buying insurance; covers all of the types of insurance and selecting an agent.

DeWilde, S., I. M. Carey, et al. (2001). Do Children Who Become Autistic Consult More Often after MMR Vaccination? *British Journal of General Practice* 51(464), 226-7.
   A study suggesting no effect of MMR on rates of autism.

Fombonne, E. and J. E. H. Cook. (2003). MMR and Autistic Entereocolitis: Consistent Epidemiological Failure to Find an Association. *Molecular Psychiatry 8,* 133-134.
   An excellent review of the scientific literature on MMR and autism.

Hollins, Sheila, Bernal, Jane, and Gregory, Matthew. *Going to the Doctor.* London: St. George's Mental Health Library, 1996.
   An excellent picture book on going to the doctor. (There are also other helpful books in the series, including about getting a blood test and going to the hospital.) Can be obtained from the Royal College of Psychiatrists (www.rcpsych.ac.uk/publications/bbw).

Kranowitz, Carol Stock. *101 Activities for Kids in Tight Spaces.* New York, NY: St. Martin's, 1995.
   Very nice book with a range of activities to use in keeping your child occupied.

Stratton, K., et al., Eds. *Immunization Safety Review: Measles, Mumps-Rubella Vaccine and Autism.* Immunization Safety Review Committee - Institute of Medicine. Washington, DC: National Academy Press, 2001 (can be ordered online at www.nap.edu).
   Reviews the evidence on measles vaccine and autism.

Stratton, K. et al., Eds. *Immunization Safety Review: Thimerosal Containing Vaccines and Neurodevelopmental Disorders.* Immunization Safety Review Committee - Institute of Medicine. Washington, DC: National Academy Press, 20001 (can be ordered online at www.nap.edu).

Taylor, B., E. Miller, et al. (1999). Autism and Measles, Mumps, and Rubella Vaccine: No Epidemiological Evidence for a Causal Association [see comments]. *Lancet 353* (9169), 2026-9.
  A study of a large group of children (nearly 500) with autism. This study looked at immunization data and found no changes with the introduction of MMR vaccination.

Taylor, B., E. Miller, et al. (2002). Measles, Mumps, and Rubella Vaccination and Bowel Problems or Developmental Regression in Children with Autism: Population Study. *British Medical Journal 324* (7334), 393-6.
  In this study, the proportion of children with autism who had regression or bowel symptoms did not change over a twenty-year period.

Volkmar, F. R., Cook, E., Pomeroy, J., Realmuto, G., and Tanguay, P. (1999). Practice Parameters for the Assessment and Treatment of Children and Adolescents with Autism and Pervasive Developmental Disorders. *Journal of the American Academy of Child and Adolescent Psychiatry*, 38(12), 32S-54S.
  Guidelines for assessment and treatment of autism spectrum disorders.

Chapter 4: Coping with Common Medical Problems

[MD]Dykens, Elisabeth and Volkmar, Fred. "Medical Conditions Associated with Autism." In *Handbook of Autism and Pervasive Developmental Disorders*, 2nd ed., D.J. Cohen and F.R. Volkmar, M.D., Eds. New York: John Wiley & Sons, 1997.
  Discusses common medical conditions associated with autism.

[MD]Lacamera, Robert and Lacamera, Ann Cobb. "Routine Health Care." In *Handbook of Autism and Pervasive Developmental Disorders*, 2nd ed., D.J. Cohen and F.R. Volkmar, M.D., Eds. New York: John Wiley & Sons, 1997.
  Good summary of needs for healthcare in autism.

Pace, Betty. *Chris Gets Ear Tubes.* Washington, DC: Gallaudet University Press, 2002.
  A step-by-step description of what your child can expect before, during, and after surgery if he needs to get ear tubes.

Royston, Angela. *Why Do My Eyes Itch: And Other Questions about Allergies.* Oxford, England: Heinemann Library, 2003.
  Questions and answers about all sorts of allergies for children in late elementary school or middle school.

Chapter 5: Handling Visits to the Emergency Room or Hospital

Civardi, Anne and Bates, M., Eds. *Going to the Hospital*. Tulsa: EDC Publishing, 2001.
A children's book with well done illustrations; could easily be used in helping many children prepare for a visit to the hospital.

Hollins, Sheila, Avis, Angie, and Cheverton, Samantha. *Going into Hospital*. London: Gaskell and St. George's Hospital Medical School, 1998.
An excellent picture book - provides a good introduction to what's involved in going to the hospital. Can be obtained from the Royal College of Psychiatrists (www.rcpsych.ac.uk/publications/bbw).

Rogers, Fred. *Going to the Hospital*. Tulsa: EDC Publishing, 2002.
A children's book by Mr. Rogers on going to the hospital. The photographs are excellent and this would be a good book to use in preparing a child for a hospitalization.

Chapter 6. Growth and Nutritional Issues

[MD]Ahearn, W.H., Castine, T., Nault, K., and Gina, G. (2001). An Assessment of Food Acceptance in Children with Autism or Pervasive Developmenal Disorder Not Otherwise Specified. *Journal of Autism and Developmental Disorders, 31,* 505-11.

Cornish, E. (2002). Gluten and Casein Free Diets in Autism: A Study of the Effects on Food Choice and Nutrition. *Journal of Human Nutrition and Dietetics, 15,* 261-69

Duyfee, Roberta Larson. *American Dietetic Association Complete Food and Nutrition Guide*, 2nd ed. New York: Wiley, 2002.
An excellent resource for basic nutritional information.

Kedesdy, Jurgen H. and Budd, Karen S. *Childhood Feeding Disorders: Biobehavioral Assessment and Intervention*. Baltimore: Paul H. Brookes, 1998.
Although written for professionals, this book has good chapters on a number of feeding problems including over- and under-eating, pica, and rumination.

Legge, Brenda. *Can't Eat, Won't Eat: Dietary Difficulties and Autistic Spectrum Disorders*. London: Jessica Kingsley, 2002. (www.jkp.com)
A highly readable discussion of dietary issues in autism and related conditions.

Medlen, Joan E. Guthrie. *The Down Syndrome Nutrition Handbook: A Guide to Promoting Healthy Lifestyles*. Bethesda,MD: Woodbine House, 2002.

Although written for parents of children with Down syndrome, this is an excellent book for parents of children with any developmental disability, covering common problems such as picky eating, texture aversion, and obesity. Also a good resource for helping you plan daily diets.

Tamborlane, William V., M.D., Ed. *The Yale Guide to Children's Nutrition*. New Haven, CT: Yale University Press, 1997.

An excellent resource on nutrition. This book includes chapters on nutrition at different ages, common concerns, special problems in nutrition, growth charts, and recipes.

Chapter 7: Safety and Your Child

American Red Cross and Kathleen A. Handal. *The American Red Cross First Aid and Safety Handbook*. Boston: Little, Brown, 1992.

Step-by-step instructions, with illustrations, for administering emergency first aid.

Chavelle, R.M., Strauss, D.J., and Picket, J. (2001). Causes of Death in Autism. *Journal of Autism and Developmental Disorders*, 31, 569-76.

Jagoda, Andy. *Good Housekeeping Family First Aid Book*. New York: Hearst Books, 2000.

Step-by-step instructions and good illustrations make this a handy introduction to first aid.

Johns Hopkins Children's Center. *First Aid for Children Fast*. Dorling Kindersley, 2002.

A helpful guide for handling minor childhood injuries as well as life-threatening emergencies.

Rodgers, George C., Jr. and Matyunas, Nancy J. *Handbook of Common Poisonings in Children*, 3rd ed. Elk Grove Village, IL: American Academy of Pediatrics, 1994.

Shaw, Ellen. *Keep Kids Safe: A Parent's Guide to Child Safety*. Appleton, WI: Quality Life Resources, 2001.

A short guide to child safety with many illustrations.

Shore, Kenneth. *Keeping Kids Safe*. New York: Prentice Hall, 2001.

A book written for parents of all children but many parts are applicable to children with autism spectrum disorders.

Unintentional Injuries in Children. The Future of Children (a publication of the Packard Foundation), Vol. 10, 2000. www.futureofchildren.org.

Chapter 8: Sleep and Sleep Problems

Durand, V. Mark. *Sleep Better! A Guide to Improving Sleep for Children with Special Needs.* Baltimore: Paul H. Brookes, 1998.
   This book provides practical strategies for encouraging children with special needs to sleep predictably.

Ferber, Richard. *Solve Your Child's Sleep Problems.* New York: Simon and Schuster, 1985.
   Although a bit dated, this book still has much valuable information.

Weissbluth, M. *Healthy Sleep Habits, Happy Child.* New York: Ballantine Books, 1999.
   This helpful introduction to sleep problems in children provides useful information on sleep and sleeping problems.

Chapter 9: Seizure Disorders

*Freeman, John, Vining, Eileen P.J., and Pillas, Diana J. *Seizures and Epilepsy in Childhood: A Guide.* Baltimore: Johns Hopkins University Press, 2002.
   A parent-oriented book discussing seizure disorders.

Hollins, Sheila, Bernal, Jane, and Thacker, Alice. *Getting on with Epilepsy.* London: St. George's Hospital Medical School and Gaskell, 1999.
   A picture book for children with epilepsy.

MD Volkmar, F. R. and Nelson, D. S. (1990). Seizure Disorders in Autism. *Journal of the American Academy of Child & Adolescent Psychiatry*, 29(1),127-29.
   One of only a handful of studies on seizures in autism.

Chapter 10: Dental Care

*Acs, George, and Ng Man Wai. "Dental Care for Your Child with Special Needs." In *When Your Child Has a Disability: The Complete Sourcebook for Daily and Medical Care.* Mark L. Batshaw, M.D., Ed. Baltimore: Paul H. Brookes, 2001.
   An excellent chapter on issues in dental care for children with special needs.

Civardi, Anne and Bates, M. *Going to the Dentist (First Experiences).* Tulsa: EDC Publishing, 2001.
   A children's book with well-done illustrations.

Mayer, Mercer. *Just Going to the Dentist.* New York, NY: Golden Books, 1990.
   A child's book, featuring "Little Critter," about visiting the dentist.

Murkoff, Heidi. *What to Expect When You Go to the Dentist*. New York, NY: Harper Festival, 2002.

An illustrated children's book on visiting the dentist (there is a similar book by the same author on going to the doctor).

Chapter 11: Sensory Issues

Kranowitz, Carol S., Sava, Deane I., Haber, Elizabeth, Balzer-Martin, Lynn, and Szklut, Stacey. *Answers to Questions Teachers Ask about Sensory Integration*, 2nd ed. Las Vegas, NV: Sensory Resources, 2001.

This book is designed for teachers but also will address many questions that parents have about sensory integration.

Kranowitz, Carol S. *101 Activities for Kids in Tight Spaces: At the Doctor's Office, on Car, Train, and Plane Trips, Home Sick in Bed*. New York, NY: St. Martin's Press, 1995.

Activities for restless children, many of which would be applicable for children with autism spectrum disorders.

Smith Myles, B. et al. *Asperger Syndrome and Sensory Issues: Practical Solutions for Making Sense of the World*. Shawnee Mission, KS: Autism Asperger Publishing Co., 2001. (www.asperger.net).

This book covers the impact of the sensory system on behavior, reviews relevant assessment tools, and discusses practical interventions for parents and educators.

Chapter 12: Common Challenging Behaviors

Clements, John and Zarkowska, Ewa. *Behavioural Concerns and Autism Spectrum Disorders: Explanations and Strategies for Change*. London: Jessica Kingsley, 2000. (www.jkp.com)

A concise and very readable introduction to dealing with behavior problems in autism.

Hodgdon, Linda. *Solving Behavior Problems in Autism: Improving Communication with Visual Strategies*. Troy, MI: QuirkRoberts, 1999.

Explains how to use visual strategies to diffuse difficult behavior and self-management challenges in children with autism. Includes information for parents.

Hodgdon, Linda. *Visual Strategies for Improving Communication. Volume 1: Practical Supports for School and Home*. Troy, MI: QuirkRoberts, 1995.

Explains how to use visual methods to structure and organize classroom routines to enable children with autism to succeed. Includes information for parents.

Schopler, Eric, Ed. *Parent Survival Manual: A Guide to Crisis Resolution in Autism and Related Developmental Disorders*. New York: Plenum Press, 1995.

This is a well-done, quite practical book concerned with common problems; the many wonderful examples add to the book.

Schopler, Eric and Mesibov, Gary. *Behavioral Issues in Autism*. New York, NY: Plenum Press, 1994.

Part of a very worthwhile series of books. This book provides perspectives on different approaches to behavior problems in autism.

Chapter 13: Medications for Challenging Behaviors

^MDKeltner, N.L. and Folks, D.G. *Psychotropic Drugs*, 3rd ed. St. Louis: Mosby,1993.

This book, of greatest value to physicians and healthcare providers, provides both short discussions of specific medications as well as more detailed information. It covers drugs used for seizures as well as drugs intended primarily for behavioral problems.

Kutcher, Stan, Ed. *Practical Child and Adolescent Psychopharmacology*. Cambridge: Cambridge University Press, 2002.

As the name implies, a very straightforward book of special interest to physicians. There is a very good chapter on autism and related disorders.

McCracken, J.T., McGough, J., Shah, B., Cronin, P., Hong, D., Aman, M.G., et al. (2002). Risperidone in Children with Autism and Serious Behavioral Problems. *New England Journal of Medicine*, 347(5), 314-21.

[MD] Martin, Andres, Scahill, Lawrence, Charney, Denis S., and Leckman, James F. *Pediatric Psychopharmacology*. Oxford: Oxford University Press, 2003.

The most current and comprehensive summary of drugs used in the treatment of children with behavioral, developmental, and emotional disorders.

Tsai, Luke K. *Taking the Mystery Out of Medication in Autism/Asperger Syndrome: A Guide for Parents and Non-Medical Professionals*. Arlington, TX: Future Horizons, 2001.

Based on more than 20 years of clinical experience working with more than 1,000 individuals with autism spectrum disorders (ASDs) and their caregivers, Dr. Tsai's book explores the role of medication in ASDs; good coverage of many medications.

[MD] Werry, John S. and Aman, Michael G. *Practioner's Guide to Psychoactive Drugs for Children and Adolescents*, 2nd ed. New York: Plenum Press, 1999.

An excellent resource on psychoactive drugs for physicians.

Wilens, T.E. *Straight Talk about Psychiatric Medications for Kids*. New York: Guilford Press, 2001.

Written specifically for parents, this is a high readable summary of information on medications prescribed for various psychiatric problems. It includes an excellent discussion of potential benefits and side effects of medications.

Chapter 14: Adolescence and Sexuality

Crary, Elizabeth and Casebolt, Pati. *Pick Up Your Socks... and Other Skills Growing Children Need*. Seattle, WA: Parenting Press, 1990.

A very helpful guide to teaching responsibility, this book is particularly relevant to parents of more able children on the autism spectrum.

Fegan, Lydia, Rauch, Anne, and McCarthy, Wendy. *Sexuality and People with Intellectual Disability*. 2nd ed. Baltimore: Paul H. Brookes, 1993.

An excellent resource for parents of children with intellectual disabilities. There is a short chapter on autism; the chapters on sex education are particularly helpful.

Hingsburger, Dave. *Just Say Know!: Understanding and Reducing the Risk of Sexual Victimization of People with Developmental Disabilities*. Quebec, Canada: Diverse City Press, 1995.

A short book that discusses various aspects of the potential for sexual abuse.

Hollins, Sheila and Downer, Jackie. *Keeping Healthy "Down Below."* London: Gaskell and St. George's Hospital Medical School, 2000.

A picture book for girls/women.

Hollins, Sheila and Perez, Wendy. *Looking After My Breasts*. London: Gaskell and St. George's Hospital Medical School, 2000.

A picture book for girls/women.

Hollins, Sheila and Roth, Terry. *Hug Me, Touch Me*. London: St. George's Mental Health Library, 1994.

A picture book on appropriate touching and intimacy.

Schopler, Eric and Mesibov, Gary. *Autism in Adolescents and Adults*. New York: Plenum Press, 1983.

Part of the TEACCH series, this book includes chapters on sexuality and behavior and development in adolescents.

Schwier, Karin Melberg and Hingsburger, David. *Sexuality: Your Sons and Daughters with Intellectual Disabilities*. Baltimore: Paul H. Brookes, 2000.

Advice and strategies for teaching young people with intellectual disabilities (especially Down syndrome) about sex and relationships.

Smith Myles, B. and Adreon, D. *Asperger Syndrome and Adolescence: Practical Solutions for School Success.* Shawnee Mission, KS: Autism Asperger Publishing Company, 2001. (www.asperger.net).

The focus of this book is on strategies and supports necessary to ensure a successful school experience for students with Asperger's disorder at the middle and secondary levels.

Taymans, Juliana M and West, Lynda L. *Unlocking Potential: College and Other Choices for People with LD and AD/HD.* Bethesda, MD: Woodbine House, 2000.

Although not written for parents of children with autism spectrum disorders, this book has much practical advice for parents of higher functioning individuals for whom college and employment are strong possibilities.

Wrobel, Mary J. *Taking Care of Myself.* Arlington, TX: Future Horizons, 2003.

This book provides some guidance on encouraging independence and self-care skills.

Videos available from James Stanfield Company (P.O. Box 41058, Santa Barbara, CA 93140; 800-421-6534/www.stansfield.com):

Circles 1: Intimacy & Relationships (social boundaries)
Circles 2: Stop Abuse (recognize and avoid sexual abuse)
Circles 3: Safer Ways (avoiding sexually transmitted diseases)
The Gyn Exam
Janet's Got Her Period
No-Go-Tell

Chapter 15: Dealing with Developmental Deterioration

Catalano, Robert A. *When Autism Strikes: Families Cope with Childhood Disintegrative Disorder.* New York: Perseus Publishing, 1998.

Eight parents describe their experiences raising children diagnosed with CDD.

Lewis, Jackie and Wilson, Debbie. *Pathways to Learning in Rett Syndrome.* London: David Fulton, 1998.

Provides good advice on the special needs of children with Rett's.

Parker, James and Parker, Philip, Eds. *The Official Parent's Sourcebook on Rett's Syndrome.* San Diego: Icon Health Publications, 2002.

A well-researched guide to Rett's disorder including summaries of recent research and Internet resources.

Schulze, Craig. *When Snow Turns to Rain: One Family's Struggle to Solve the Riddle of Autism*. Bethesda, MD: Woodbine House, 1996.
   Although the parents were not aware of it when writing this book, this is a story of a child who has childhood disintegrative disorder. The book is out of print, but available second hand and in libraries.

Van Acker, Richard. "Rett's Syndrome." In *Handbook of Autism and Pervasive Developmental Disorders*, 2nd ed., D.J. Cohen and F.R. Volkmar, M.D., Eds. New York: John Wiley & Sons, 1997, pp. 60-93.
   Summary of work on Rett's disorder.

Volkmar, Fred R., Klin, Ami, Marans, Wendy, and Cohen, Donald J. "Childhood Disintegrative Disorder." In *Handbook of Autism and Pervasive Developmental Disorders*, 2nd ed., D.J. Cohen and F.R. Volkmar, M.D., Eds. New York: John Wiley & Sons, 1997, pp. 47-59.
   Summary of research on childhood disintegrative disorder.

Chapter 16: Complementary and Alternative Treatments

[MD] Chez, M.G., Buchanan, C.P., Bagan, B.T., Hammer, M.S., McCarthy, K.S., Ovrutskaya, I., Nowinski, C.V. et al.(2000). Secretin and Autism: A Two-Part Clinical Investigation. *Journal of Autism and Developmental Disorders, 30,* 87-94.
   A study of secretin in autism.

[MD] Coniglio, S.J., Lewis, J.D., Lang, C., Burns, T.G., Subhani-Siddique, R., Weintraub, A., Schub, H., et al. (2001). A Randomized, Double-blind, Placebo-controlled Trial of Single-dose Intravenous Secretin as Treatment for Children with Autism. *Journal of Pediatrics, 138,* 649-55.
   Another study of secretin in autism.

[MD] Dunn-Geier, J., Ho, H.H., Auersperg, E., Doyle, D., Eaves, L., Matsuba, C., Orrbine, E. et al. (2000). Effect of Secretin on Children with Autism: A Randomized Controlled Trial. *Developmental Medicine and Child Neurology, 42,* 796-802.
   More work on Secretin.

Escalona, A., Field, T., Singer-Strunch, R., Cullen, C., and Hartshorn, K. Brief Report: Improvements in Behavior of Children with Autism Following Massage Therapy. *Journal of Autism and Developmental Disorder, 31,* 513-516.
   Paper presenting data on improvement with massage therapy.

Gerlach, Elizabeth. *Autism Treatment Guide*, rev. ed. Eugene, OR: Four Leaf Press, 1998.
   Review of many of the treatments—traditional and alternative—for children with autism.

Hansen, R. L. and S. Ozonoff. "Alternative Theories: Assessment and Therapy Options." In *Autism Spectrum Disorders: A Research Review for Practitioners.* S. Ozonoff, S. J. Rogers, and R. L. Hendren, Eds. Washington, D.C.: American Psychiatry Association Press, 2003.
An excellent review of a variety of alternative treatments proposed for autism.

[MD]Horvath, K., Stefanatos, G., Sokolski, K.N., Wachtel, R., Nabors, L., and Tildon, J.T. (1998). Improved Social and Language Skills after Secretin Administration in Patients with Autistic Spectrum Disorders. *Journal of the Association for Academic Minority Physicians, 9,* 9-15.
The original secretin paper.

Hyman, S. L. and S. E. Levy. (2000). Autistic Spectrum Disorders: When Traditional Medicine Is Not Enough. *Contemporary Pediatrics 17,* 101-116.
A very helpful summary of some of the issues involved in alternative therapies in autism.

[MD]Owley, T., McMahon, W., Cook ,E.H., Laulhere, T.M., South, M., Mays, L.Z., and Shernoff, E.S., et al. (2001). Multi-site, Double-blind, Placebo-controlled Trial of Porcine Secretin in Autism. *Journal of the American Academy of Child and Adolescent Psychiatry, 40,*1293-1299.
Another study of secretin.

Park, R., *Voodoo Science: The Road from Foolishness to Fraud.* Oxford, England: Oxford University Press, 2000.
A very readable discussion of some of the problems raised in evaluating unusual treatments.

[MD] Roberts, W., Weaver, L., Brian, J., Bryson, S., Emelianova, S., Griffiths, A.M., MacKinnon, B., et al. (2001). Repeated Doses of Porcine Secretin in the Treatment of Autism: A Randomized, Placebo-Controlled Trial. *Pediatrics,107,* E71.
Another study of secretin.

[MD]Sandler, A.D. and Bodfish, J.W. (2000). Placebo Effects in Autism: Lessons from Secretin. *Journal of Developmental & Behavioral Pediatrics, 21,* 347-50.
A discussion of what we can learn from the many studies of secretin.

[MD] Sandler, A.D., Sutton, K.A., DeWeese, J., Girardi, M.A., Sheppard, V., and Bodfish, J.W. (1999). Lack of Benefit of a Single Dose of Synthetic Human Secretin in the Treatment of Autism and Pervasive Developmental Disorder. *New England Journal of Medicine, 341,*1801-6.
Another study of secretin.

Shapiro, Arthur K. and Shapiro, Elaine. *The Powerful Placebo*. Baltimore: Johns Hopkins University Press, 1997.
  A detailed and scholarly discussion of the placebo effect and all the various factors that contribute to it.

MD Volkmar, F. R. (1999). Editorial - Lessons from Secretin. *New England Journal of Medicine*, 341, 1842-44.
  Discussion of one of the first secretin papers.

Afterword

Harris, Sandra L. *Siblings of Children with Autism: A Guide for Families*. Bethesda, MD: Woodbine House, 1994.
  A useful guide to understanding sibling relationships, how autism affects them and how parents can support their children in living and growing with a sibling with autism.

Meyer, Donald, Vadasy, Patricia, and Fewell, Rebecca. *Living with a Brother or Sister with Special Needs: A Book for Sibs,* 2nd ed. Seattle, WA: University of Washington Press, 1996.
  An excellent introduction to the subject of disabilities for siblings. Reviews specific disabilities and discusses what it is like to be a sibling of a child with a disability.

Miller, Nancy and Sammons, Catherine. *Everybody's Different: Understanding and Changing Our Reactions to Disabilities*. Baltimore: Paul H. Brookes, 1999.
  This book explores the reactions of people to those who have disabilities, and provides advice on how to change attitudes.

*Siegel, Byrna and Silverstein, Stuart. *What About Me? Growing Up with a Developmentally Disabled Sibling*. New York: Insight Books, 1994.
  Written by a sibling of a person with a disability, this book discusses the emotions of siblings of children with disabilities.

Sullivan, Ruth C. "Diagnosis Autism: You Can Handle It." In *Handbook of Autism and Pervasive Developmental Disorders*, 2nd ed., D.J. Cohen and F.R. Volkmar, M.D., Eds. New York: John Wiley & Sons, 1997.
  A parent reviews her experience in coping with the diagnosis of autism in her child.

Sperry, Virginia W. *Fragile Success: Ten Autistic Children, Childhood to Adulthood*. Baltimore: Paul H. Brookes, 2000.
  An account (from a teacher) of the life course of children with autism from childhood to adulthood.

INDEX

Paradoxical reaction, 99, 103, 151-52, 175
Parenting issues, 297-300
Paroxetine, 234
Partial seizures. *See* Seizures, partial
Patching, 195
Paxil®, 234
PDD. *See also* Autism spectrum disorders
  compared to autism spectrum disorder, 2
  compared to PDD-NOS, 1-2
  types of, 1-2
PDD-NOS. *See also* Autism spectrum disorders
  and nonverbal learning disability, 8
  attention and, 232
  cause of, 23
  compared to PDD, 1-2
  depression and, 214
  diagnosis of, 51, 306
  early signs of, 29
  incidence of, 12
  overview of, 10-11
  prognosis, 10
  seizures and, 170
Peabody Picture Vocabulary Test, 41
PECS, 77, 217
Pediasure®, 115
Pediatricians
  ages seen by, 258
  and referrals to specialists, 67
  preparing child to see, 61-62
  selecting, 59-60, 295-96
  switching, 74
  working with on medication treatment
    plan, 223-24
Peer-reviewed journals. *See* Journals, peer-
    reviewed
Pelvic exams, 254, 259
Perphenazine, 229
Perseveration. *See* Behavior, perseverative
Pervasive developmental disorder. *See* PDD
Pharmacists, 69, 71
Phenobarbital, 165
Phenytoin, 166
Photographs, as teaching aids, 100, 250, 252
Photoscreening, 194
Physical activity. *See* Exercise
Physical exams, 62, 97-98
Physical therapist
  as part of assessment team, 33, 43
  sensory issues and, 196
Physician's statement of need, 123
Physicians. *See* Doctors; Pediatricians
Pica, 63, 119-20
Picture Exchange Communication System.
  See PECS
Pimples. *See* Acne
Pineal gland, 151

Pink eye, 84
Pinworms, 81
PKU, 19-20
Placebo, 222
Placebo effect, 223, 276
Plants, 131-32
Plaque, 179
Plasmapharesis, 287
Playgrounds, 130
Play skills, 217
PMS, 253-54
Pneumococcal disease, 64
Point-of-service insurance plans, 309
Poison Control Center, 136
Poisoning, 132, 135,-37. *See also* Lead poisoning
Polio, 63, 64
Polypharmacy, 239
Pools, 130
Postictal period, 155
Posture, 15
PPOs, 310-11
Preexisting disorder, condition, 313
Pregnancy
  and onset of autism, 16
  in individuals with ASDs, 257
Premenstrual syndrome, 253
Prenatal tests, 18
Preschool Language Scale, 41
Pressure equalizing tubes, 83, 92
Preventive care, 60-61, 65
Primary care physician
  involving in medication issues, 224
  referrals from, 308
Primidone, 165
Prisms, 292
Privacy, 249-50, 256
Pronoun reversal, 40
Propranolol, 237
Proprioception, 195
Prosody, 40
Prozac®, 234
Psychiatrists, 216, 223
Psychological testing, 33, 36-40. *See also* IQ tests
Psychologists, 119, 152
  behavioral, 74, 177, 204, 216
  developmental, 216
  school, 217
Psychosis, 263
Psychotherapy, 8, 274
Puberty, 204, 245-47, 257
Publications, evaluating, 279
Quetiapine, 227
Rabies, 134
Rashes, 131, 165
Rating scales, autism, 43-44
Reactive attachment disorder, 48

Tourette syndrome, 205
Toxicology screens, 98
Tranquilizers, major. *See* Neuroleptics
Tranquilizers, minor, 237
Transitional objects, 29
Transitions, 210. *See also* Behavior, rigidity;
    Change, resistance to
Tranxene®, 167
Trazodone, 234
Treatments. *See* Alternative and controversial
    treatments; Behavioral interventions;
    Medications; Therapies
Trexan®, 239
Trifluoperazine, 229
Trilafon®, 229
Trileptal®, 167, 236
Tuberous sclerosis
    and autism, 19, 72
    incidence of, 18
    inheritance of, 19
    symptoms of, 18-19, 72-73
Tubes, ear, 83, 84, 92
Twain, Mark, 276
Twins, 21
Tylenol®. *See* acetaminophen
United States Dept. of Agriculture, 108, 123
Urinary tract infections, 80-81, 148
Urine
    reflux of, 80-81
    taking specimens of, 80
    tests, 266
Vaccinations
    anesthetic cream for, 65
    as cause of autism, 66, 287
    MMR, 65, 66
    required in the U.S., 64-65
    side effects of, 65
Vagus nerve stimulation, 168
Validity, 44-45
Valium®, 151, 167
Valproic acid, 166, 235, 236
Varicella, 65
Venlafaxine, 234
Vestibular stimulation, 270
Vest, weighted, 197
Victor the Wild Boy, 24
Vineland Adaptive Behavior Scales, 39, 42
Vision. *See also* Eye contact
    exams, 193-94
    stereotyped behavior and, 193
    therapies for, 291-92
    treating problems, 194-95
Visual aids, for teaching, 77, 100, 250, 252, 254
Visual-spatial skills, 26, 193
Vitamins
    A, 112

B₆, 286
B₁₂, 112
    deficiencies of, 113
    folic acid, 286
    "mega" doses of, 286
    recommended amounts of, 112
    supplements, 112, 225
Vocabulary, 41
Vodka, 93
Voiding cystourethrogram, 80
Volkmar, Fred R., 378
Vomiting, 79, 80, 88, 122, 136. *See also* Rumination
Walking, 15, 195, 205, 269-70
Wandering, 127, 128, 147
Water
    drinking, 112, 113, 179
    temperature of, 132
Water Pik®, 178
Wax, ear, 82, 83, 191
Wechsler Intelligence Scales, 39. *See also* IQ tests
Weight
    excessive, 117-18
    inadequate, 115, 118-19
    sudden changes in, 118
Wellbutrin®, 233, 234
Well child visits, 66-67, 68
Wet dreams, 254
Wetting, 80
Wheat, 122
Wheezing, 122. *See also* Asthma
White noise, 144
Wiesner, Lisa A., 378
Windows, 102, 126, 127
Wing, Lorna, 7
Wisdom teeth. *See* Teeth, wisdom
X-rays, 161, 266
Yeast, 285, 289
Zarontin®, 167
Ziprasidone, 227
Zoloft®, 208, 234
Zonegran®, 167
Zyprexa®. *See* Olanzepine
Zyrtec®, 86

ABOUT THE AUTHORS

Fred R. Volkmar, M.D., is the Irving B. Harris Professor of Child Psychiatry, Pediatrics, and Psychology at the Yale University Child Study Center. He is the primary author of the American Psychiatric Association's DSM-IV section on autism and pervasive developmental disorders. Dr. Volkmar is the director of autism research at Yale, and the coauthor of a number of books, including *ASPERGER SYNDROME* and *THE HANDBOOK OF AUTISM AND PERVASIVE DEVELOPMENTAL DISORDERS*. Dr. Volkmar has served as an associate editor of the *Journal of Child Psychology and Psychiatry*, the *Journal of Autism*, and the *American Journal of Psychiatry*. He is the author of several hundred research papers and book chapters on autism and related disorders.

Lisa A. Wiesner, M.D., is a pediatrician in private practice in Orange, Connecticut. She is a graduate of Harvard College and Case Western Reserve School of Medicine. She completed her pediatric training at Yale New Haven Hospital and a fellowship in Adolescent Medicine at Yale and is an Assistant Clinical Professor of Pediatrics at Yale.